o that the gift may

wish to found and
l Gloucester a free
e of furnishing gratu
abitants of that city
treatment therein and
to George J. Marsh,
n E. Somes John K.
ester Cunningham all
hereby named and

...as they may need

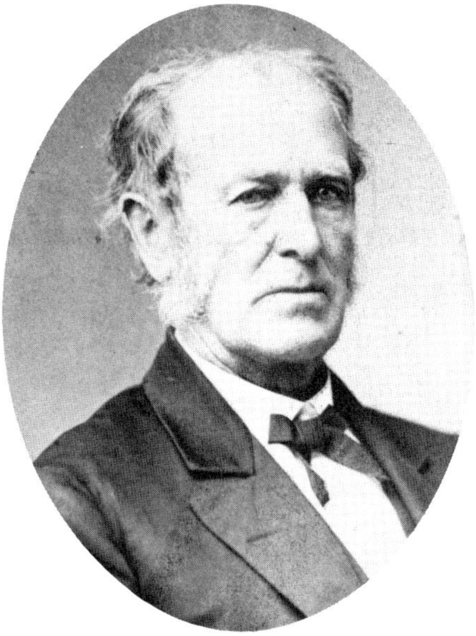

Addison Gilbert 1808-1888

"It is my wish to found and establish in the City of Gloucester a hospital . . . to admit as patients therein such citizens and such inhabitants of the city . . . as may need medical or surgical aid and treatment . . . "

From clause 35 of the last will and testament of Addison Gilbert.

...as they may need

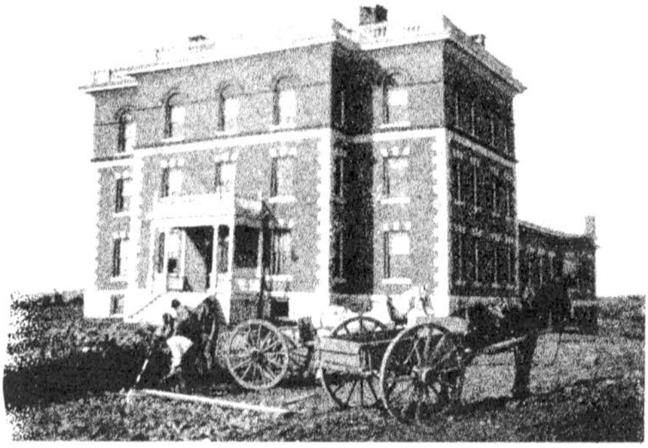

a history of the Addison Gilbert Hospital

By

Laurence F. Brooks

and

W. Warren Babson, MD

Published for the

Addison Gilbert Hospital

by

Phoenix Publishing

West Kennebunk, Maine

Library of Congress Cataloging-in-Publication Data

Brooks, Laurence F., 1915-
As they may need: a history of the Addison Gilbert Hospital, 1889-1989 / by Laurence F. Brooks and W. Warren Babson.
p. cm.
ISBN 0-914659-43-X
1. Addison Gilbert Hospital — History. 2. Medicine — Massachusetts — Gloucester — History. I. Babson, W. Warren. 1905-1987. II. Addison Gilbert Foundation. III. Title.
RA982.G52A343 1989
362.1'1'097445 — dc20 89-16395
CIP

Printed in the United States of America

To the many people,
past and present,
who for one hundred years
have labored at all levels
to make this hospital
what it is today.

Contents

Foreword

When it was again suggested, prior proposals having been made in 1950 and 1970, that a history of the Addison Gilbert Hospital be written, it was perhaps visualized as simply the story of the institution itself, using as its basis the records from its founding to its present. As the prospective authors thought about the matter, however, this approach began to seem somewhat pedestrian. Instead we planned a story that would explore behind the somewhat spare minutes of Trustee and Medical Staff meetings, medical and other statistics, and other source material available.

Such records would be necessary, of course, but we wanted to get behind the scenes if we could, discovering *why* things happened, *who* caused them to happen and *how* they were carried to conclusion. To do this we needed insofar as it was possible to talk to those who were there when the events took place. We were fortunate in that people still among us could take us back to explore more than half the almost one hundred years of our hospital's existence. In talking to them we taped hours of conversation, all to be deciphered and typed by a corps of patient and often frustrated hospital transcriptionists, chief among them Betty Doyle, at that time the hospital's medical librarian.

We are grateful to those interviewees: Administrator Tucker Vye and longtime President Bill Webber; Drs. Earle Andrews, Ronald Hallett, Larry Ross, George Taylor and Ed Wells; nurses Marjory Howlett,

Madge Noble, Dotty Oleson and Muriel Walker; Leona Mitchell and others who patiently answered our questions as they helped to fill the gaps in the records while bringing to life the times and the people involved. We appreciate also those who, like Dr. Abbott Hooper in connection with the Manning family, offered memorabilia and documents from the early days.

In going further back and to enlarge on those other sources, we turned to the staffs at the Sawyer Free Library, the Gloucester City Clerk's office and the Cape Ann Historical Society, who guided us in searching through old newspaper files and other records. For the story of the Women's Auxiliary we are grateful to Kay Steele, who took on the task of delving into voluminous handwritten records.

It was soon obvious that the hospital did not simply rise from nowhere. We felt background was needed to explore how it related to the times at its founding and before. This raised questions of what medicine was like here on Cape Ann and elsewhere before Addison Gilbert's dream became reality. From such questions came the idea of going all the way back to *Mayflower* days and the first settlement on Cape Ann to trace the area's medical history. The several prior histories of Gloucester and Rockport all had referred to it, but none addressed it specifically. Only our prestigious local historian, Joe Garland, seems to have considered the idea and indeed had already done some preliminary research on the subject.

A prologue therefore attempts to provide this background, with primary emphasis on Cape Ann and its immediate vicinity. Such other information as seemed necessary — developments outside the area, for example — has also been included, but only as it appeared essential to the local story. Those who wish to explore general medical history will find ample material with which to work. In preparing the pre-hospital segment we were given significant assistance by Joe Garland, who generously shared his research and expertise with us. We are grateful also to the Essex Institute in Salem and to the Harvard Medical School Library, both of which are repositories of original records and prior work.

When the medical history of Cape Ann extends into the story of the hospital we have incorporated those elements into the major subject since, after all, they are part of an interwoven whole.

Some will criticize the lack of many accouterments of proper history – bibliography, sources, copious footnotes, etc. – but we are not proper historians and chose to omit such details. The hospital material comes from records of the Board of Trustees and Medical Staff, annual reports, old newspaper files and from the taped recollections of individuals. Where it seemed appropriate we have documented the source of quotations or other information as part of the text. For all this we ask forgiveness of the purists and hope they understand.

In closing we must also acknowledge the valuable assistance given us by our "board of advisors," those who read the rough first draft segments and critiqued the work, its content and its method. Our thanks for this go to Joseph E. Garland, whose enthusiasm for the project was further encouraged by the fact that his grandfather and great-grandfather were both members of the hospital's first Medical Staff. We are grateful also to Helen E. Rees, Ed.D., and Elizabeth D. Robinton, Ph.D., both Smith College professors emeritus now living in Rockport, and to their friend Genevieve Miller, Ph.D., whose knowledge as medical historian and curator helped in our research of the early days of medicine. Others – Ted Scharfenstein, Kay Steele and our wives – also read the first draft to be sure we were making things clear. Our warm thanks go to that long-suffering group.

Laurence F. Brooks
W. Warren Babson, MD

Gloucester, Massachusetts
May, 1987

Postscript

Dr. Babson became ill shortly after this foreword was prepared and died on September 26, 1987. I am most grateful for the long hours of work he did in connection with the medical aspects of our joint project, which had been almost completely drafted prior to his death. His place as medical advisor was taken by his friend and colleague, Robert N. Lundberg, MD, who as a participant in the events from 1974 through 1983 helped interpret the medical side of those years.

L.F.B.

March, 1988

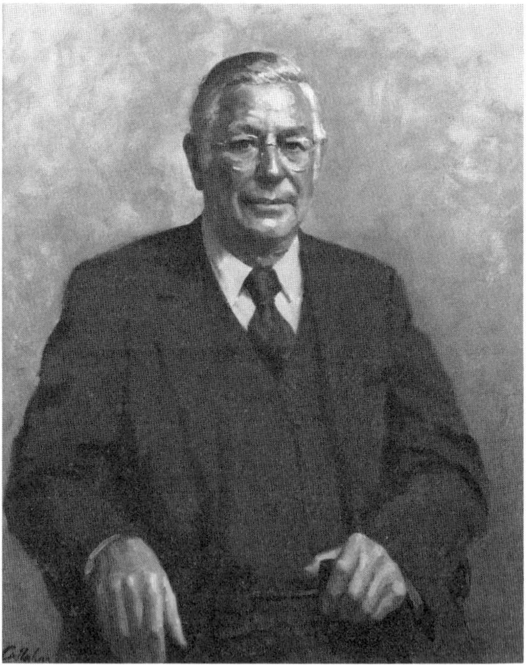

Dr. W. Warren Babson from a portrait by Jack Callahan of Rockport, commissioned by the Trustees in 1974.

...as they may need

PROLOGUE

TRADITION places the earliest English arrivals at Gloucester in 1623, when Roger Conant led a band of men there to establish a fishing stage, a project they abandoned two years later when they left to join the newly founded settlement at Salem. Cape Ann awaited further habitation until 1630, when a larger group of men and women of the Winthrop company, having arrived at Massachusetts Bay a short time earlier, came to establish the first permanent settlement and take advantage of the opportunities offered by a large harbor.

In order to further promote and encourage fishing, in 1639 the General Court of the Massachusetts Bay Colony ordered the allotment of sites for the structures necessary to fishing operations. At the same time it ordered assignment of land "both for their fishing and for keeping of cattle and for corn, &c; and that such other fishermen as will join in the way of fishing, and inhabit there, shall have such lands and other liberties as shall be needful and fit for their occasions." By 1641 Cape Ann and similar nearby settlements had reached a point where the General Court appointed a commission to establish boundaries for Ipswich, Cape Ann, and Manchester (then known as Jeffries Creek). The records of a few years later, in 1650, list eighty-one male settlers which, adding wives and children, suggests a population of perhaps two hundred.

The Early Settlement

The first recorded physician in the Bay Colony was Samuel Fuller, known as "Deacon," a member of the Mayflower company. Although not an ordained minister, he preached regularly at Plymouth and on his travels. He had studied medicine in England and Holland and this training served well, as illness often struck hard during those first years. In addition to serving as physician and spiritual leader at Plymouth he traveled throughout the infant colony, and in 1628 he visited Boston and Salem at the request of Governor Endicott to treat settlers ill with "ye scurvy, and others of other diseases by letting blood and other means."

Deacon Fuller died of smallpox in 1633, leaving a widow who was a midwife. The colony was to wait several years longer before it had the services of another trained doctor, English physicians often being satisfied to remain at home with more lucrative and sometimes prestigious practices. Colonial medicine was left to develop on its own, and, for better or worse, practice was left to those without specific training for it. Governor Winthrop, for example, was well read in science and, judging by his letters to those seeking his advice, was reasonably well versed in the medicine of the time.

Many ministers, although without formal training, developed a skill in medicine through experience and self-teaching. Among these was Reverend Thomas Thatcher, pastor of Old South Church in Boston, an authority on smallpox and regarded by his fellow colonists as a competent physician. Others engaged in medical practice were barbers who did minor surgery and schoolmasters who, like the ministers, were usually among the better educated. Most people spent a great deal of time outdoors, and fresh air probably was as effective a treatment as anything except for those times when epidemic disease or accidents occurred, and the simple home remedies of the day sufficed for most problems.

The mainstay of medical treatment was the family medicine chest. This was found in nearly every home and contained mostly "simples" and herbal medicines, along with concoctions containing what today seem absurd and even abhorrent ingredients. Cow-bugs, found under damp wood, were used along with natural excretions and other secretions — vegetable, animal, and human. Some of those early remedies may not have been too far off the mark; after all, today's penicillin is based on a refined but natural mold. Bleeding was also a common treatment into the nineteenth century and was used in a wide variety of illnesses.

Along with the medicine chest most families had one or more medical books or pamphlets which described various illnesses and offered prescriptions for their treatment. One of the more bizarre remedies, grandly named "The Quintessence of Snakes, Adders, or Vipers," appeared in a 1661 publication entitled *A Treatise of the Choicest Spagyricall Preparations*. Prescribed for "purifying the blood, flesh and skin, and consequently all diseases therein, it cures also the falling sickness & strengthens the Brain, Sight and Hearing, and preserveth from gray hairs, reneweth Youth, cureth the Gout and Consumption, causeth Sweat, is very good in and against Pestilential infections." Another, a compound of ants, ants' eggs, woodlice, bees, and soot mixed together with "Spirit of Wine," would appear, based on the last ingredient, to be designed to make the patient forget his problem.

It is obvious that the medical knowledge of the time was largely conjectural and primitive, with even the best-trained physicians knowing little about the cause and treatment of illness and disease. The colonists, most of whom subscribed to the theories of Cotton Mather, were convinced that such things were the work of the devil and accepted as gospel Mather's pronouncement as to "how easily can he shoot the deleterious Miasms into the Juices and Bowels of Men's Bodies."

There is no indication in the scanty records available from the settlement period of any resident practitioner on Cape Ann until 1637, when one Isabel Babson, a midwife, came from Salem to Gloucester. The widowed Mrs. Babson and her son James had emigrated from England a few years earlier, and, finding a community in need of her specialty and her knowledge of simple medicine, she remained until her death in 1661 at eighty-four.

Isabel Babson was a useful and respected member of the community for almost twenty-five years. Even after the Cape Ann settlement had been recognized by the General Court as a formal "township," with its boundary extending to the Essex line, she seems to have remained the sole practitioner until her death. The people relied on her advice, their own ingenuity, and the simple remedies available to them from the land and from apothecaries in the larger towns of Boston, Ipswich, and Salem. She also seems to have done well materially since, in addition to her homestead located on two acres in what is now Main Street's West End, she owned several acres of moor and marshland in today's East Gloucester, near Good Harbor Beach. These holdings were further increased in 1657 when, probably as an expression of appreciation for her services, the town fathers granted her a plot near what was then called Fishermen's Field, not far from the present Stage Fort Park.

Through James Babson a family dynasty was begun, and there are descendants of Isabel Babson throughout the United States today. She is, in fact, the many times removed ancestress of the coauthors of this history, one being a namesake descendant and the other related through James's daughter Abigail. A direct tie to Addison Gilbert Hospital is found more than three centuries after she came to Gloucester in the naming of a new wing in her honor. The name she bore would also be that of many of the hospital's protagonists, and therefore will appear again as the story develops.

The nearest physician with some training was John Winthrop, Jr., the Governor's son, who had a practice in Ipswich, then a larger community than Gloucester. Reverend John Emerson, a 1656 Harvard graduate, came to Gloucester in 1663 and carried on a medical practice. Mr. Emerson may even have been "recruited" to take up residence here, since records show him granted a sum of money by the town with which to establish his home. His grant brought him property located on thirty acres from the Meeting House Green along what is now Washington Street toward Riverdale Mills where, as one of the principal mill owners in town, he may also have operated the old gristmill at the head of Mill River.

History also records the name of Ann Millet, who was paid two pounds, six shillings by the town "for curing Elinor Gooding" in 1700. Also recorded are instances when the Selectmen paid to send cases to practitioners in other communities — John Winthrop, Jr., in Ipswich and Dr. James Kibber in Lynn after 1690.

Meanwhile, here and elsewhere, for lack of preventive and curative medicine, illness and epidemic diseases had to be coped with as they arose. Smallpox was perhaps the earliest and worst. It had occurred among the coastal and Merrimack Valley Indian tribes shortly before the first settlers arrived, probably introduced by early traders, and decimated the previously unexposed natives. With no means of treatment, once smallpox invaded a community there was little to be done but to let it run its course. The sick could be segregated, but poor sanitation and the violently contagious nature of the scourge thwarted all efforts to contain it. The seacoast towns seem to have suffered especially badly, as it spread from passengers and crews of visiting vessels. Marblehead, Newburyport, and Salem were all hard hit before 1700.

As the eighteenth century approached shipbuilding had been added to fishing and farming. This required utilization of Cape Ann's relatively sparse timber, and lumbering became a further occupation. At least three "meetinghouses" attested to the growth and permanency of the community, the population of which then stood at seven hundred. The Harbor Village, as the waterfront part of Gloucester was called, was well established with permanent homes and small shops, while to the north the Annisquam Parish had also attracted settlers as a microcosm of the larger village and, like it, was given over to sea-related pursuits.

A quarter of the people in the Cape Ann settlement were by then located in the West Parish, where the land was better suited for agriculture. It was accessible by land over what was then as now called "the Cut," first opened through the beach and marshes at the harbor and bridged by Reverend Richard Blynman in 1643. The West Parish could also be reached by a rowboat ferry established in 1694 from Trynell Cove at the foot of what is now Ferry Street and running to Stony Cove in Little River. By 1725 its largest farm was one developed by William Coffin on five hundred acres of timberland and open pasture located between the Annisquam and Essex rivers.

Out on the northeast tip of the Cape another settlement, politically a part of Gloucester, was developing individuality and independence. Sandy Bay, as it was called until it finally broke away from Gloucester more than a hundred years later, was geographically isolated, accessible only by sea or across a stony moor. It had a life of its own with fishing, farming, and, later, quarrying of its ubiquitous granite ledges as its natural occupations.

Medicine in the now-maturing colonies was profiting to some degree from more advanced work being done in England and France, although the best European physicians still preferred to stay at home with secure practices. English medicine found its way to America chiefly through the printed word, and such books and pamphlets as crossed the sea were eagerly sought and studied. Some were copied, such as *The English Physician,* which first appeared in England in 1643. When first printed in Boston in 1708 it became popular among laymen as well as practitioners.

Most illnesses of the period were vaguely characterized as "agues and fevers." When the family medicine chest did not suffice and the doctor was called in, bleeding and purging were still standard practice. Surgery was making small advances in going beyond the amputation of injured limbs to the setting of fractures, treatment of wounds, and the excision of benign tumors.

Early Epidemics

By 1700 smallpox was being attacked as experiments began in inoculation as a preventive measure. The method had its start in the folk medicine of Turkey and China and some parts of Africa. A slave of Cotton Mather described the treatment to his master as practiced in his tribe and convinced him that he was immune because of it. Crude by modern standards, the procedure consisted simply of using matter from the sores of one already ill to infect another who, developing a mild case, was thereafter immune. Mather, who had read about similar practices by Greek and Italian physicians, urged the use of it in this country in his 1721 "Address to the Physicians of Boston."

The method was extremely controversial. Few practitioners had the courage to try it, and some town governments strictly banned the practice. Dr. Zabdiel Boylston of Boston was among the more venturesome who heeded

Mather's exhortations, inoculating first his six-year-old son and, a month later, his older son John, age thirteen. By the end of 1721 Boylston had inoculated 242 patients, and other Boston physicians, encouraged by his apparent success, had treated another 40. Of the 282 only 6 died; the rest thenceforth enjoyed immunity. The epidemic raging in Boston that year came to an end, but outside the city, where the procedure was either unknown or forbidden, the death toll ranged as high as 15 percent of the population. Even in Boston, the disease was far from eliminated, and despite all measures it was to remain a major problem everywhere into the next century.

Cape Ann suffered equally with the rest of the world from this disease, which was without question the most serious health problem of the day. But despite Dr. Boylston's success with inoculation the people here, like so many elsewhere, feared the method and preferred taking their chances. According to Marshall Swan's delightful history, *Town on Sandy Bay,* Sandy Bay was the first to accept the procedure, in February 1752, when the Parish voted "to have the Enoculation [*sic*] in Mr. Baker's and Mr. Witham's houses." From the same source we learn that inoculation was again tried in 1779, using five houses, again including Baker's.

Gloucester remained adamant until a severe outbreak in 1778. John Babson's *History of Gloucester* tells the story, which also offers insight to feelings in many small communities regarding it:

During the first four months of 1778, great excitement prevailed in the town, on account of the smallpox. The people had taken a firm stand against inoculation, having voted 'to have no inoculation in town on any terms,' but in October they were obliged to recede and provide hospitals [pest-houses] in different parts of town to accommodate the inoculated. The disease seems to have spread all over town at this time, but we have no knowledge [as to numbers].

Control was difficult. Gloucester put guards along the waterfront during outbreaks in an attempt to keep out seafaring strangers who might carry the contagion. In 1730 a barricade was mounted at the Cut in a similar attempt to screen strangers arriving by land. This watch station, manned by burly citizens, was to be set up whenever an epidemic threatened, with all outsiders held there until they could be fumigated.

In *Guns Off Gloucester* Joseph E. Garland tells of one such barricade. Describing an outbreak in nearby Marblehead in June 1773, he says:

The nearby coast, of course, shrank from Marblehead in horror. Gloucester rushed Adam Hufflin and John Avery over to Watch House Point to ward off contaminated strangers by sea and hied husky John McKean off to the Cut to watch the gate and hustle all out-of-towners and suspects into his smoke house for a fumigation, which was thought to be the most effective preventative. . . .

It was undoubtedly during this scare that the services of John McKean at the Cut were enlisted by Captain Foster against a two-legged plague far more detested than the pox by the patriotic freetraders of Gloucester. A schooner of Foster's had come in during the night, no doubt from the West Indies.

According to custom, the hatches were immediately opened, and the landing of the cargo was commenced, the owner himself assisting. A considerable part was landed and stored before daybreak, but more than half was still on board, and, early in the morning, a tidewaiter [customs officer] was expected from Salem. The fertile mind of Foster hit at once upon an expedient. On the Cut was a watchhouse, where John McKean, a stout Irishman, had been employed, in a time of alarm about the smallpox, to stop all strangers entering the Town and subject them to a fumigating process. It is sufficient to say that his Majesty's officer of the customs was on that morning ushered into the watchhouse by John McKean; that he was kept there all day and released after dark, purified from all infectious diseases, so far as a thorough smoking could do it.

The Captain Foster of Garland's story, obviously not one to bow to British taxes and rules, resided on Middle Street in what is now the Trust Department of the Bank of New England, Cape Ann branch. He naturally joined the Revolution and came out of that war a Colonel of Militia.

There were at least four severe epidemics of smallpox in Gloucester between 1764 and 1779. Essex County had been swept in 1773 and 1774, possibly due to troop movements through the towns along the highways, and Sandy Bay, frequently visited by the disease through the years, suffered especially heavily in 1752 and 1760 and with Gloucester during the 1770s.

Other than inoculation and screening, the primary control method was isolation, whereby the victims were segregated in "pesthouses," sometimes spoken of as hospitals but basically little more than collection stations. As far as can be determined there were none of these on Cape Ann until 1777, when one was built just west of Bond's Hill on the mainland. Prior to that time the nearest seems to have been the Essex Hospital on Cat Island, off Marblehead, established in 1773. Privately owned, with eighty beds, it was burned the next year by neighbors who feared its proximity. Others were located in Newburyport, Salem, and Boston, with at least two in the latter city staffed by physicians and set aside for a relatively wealthy clientele.

The pesthouse in Salem seems to have been used off and on for several years. Reverend William Bentley, a Salem diarist and raconteur, speaks of it as "the Hospital of the Natural Small Pox" and describes how, after permitting some inoculation in 1792, opinion changed the following year, as "the Selectmen of Salem have informed the public that all the hospitals are cleansed & that no further inoculation will be permitted." He also tells of its later reopening during another epidemic in 1798.

Diphtheria, or "throat distemper," and its companion, scarlet fever, were other killing epidemic diseases of the time. It seems to have hit Sandy Bay with special virulence, with at least two major outbreaks recorded. One in 1738 took thirty-one children — a heavy toll indeed, since there were only twenty-seven families residing there at the time. All of John Gott's children died, and the John Pools lost most of their grandchildren. Typical of the attitude of that era, the village took the long view: "We have reason to bless God for sparing so many [for] there is still living in our neighborhood more than 140 persons."

An epidemic again struck the village in 1793, killing sixty-two more children. Dr. James Goss, Sandy Bay's only trained physician, did his best with the primitive treatment available, but was unable to control the spread of the disease. It was shortly after this outbreak that Salem's Dr. Edward Holyoke successfully developed an effective treatment, using antimony, mercury, opium, and quinine in a prescription that became widely accepted during the next century.

Scarlet fever was another of the ravaging diseases that periodically struck the area, occurring first in Kingston, N.H. in 1735 and spreading the next year to Boston, where four thousand were stricken. Cape Ann had its share of this disease, not only during colonial times but into the twentieth century. Dr. William Douglas of Boston was perhaps the first to diagnose, treat, and cure scarlet fever. His carefully documented clinical observations during the Boston epidemic were important in distinguishing scarlet fever from diphtheria, with which it was often confused, and preceded John Fothergill's so-called classical description of that disease by a dozen years.

Typhoid fever was another epidemic disease that raged through the colonies. In 1797 it struck one hundred people in Sandy Bay. Although that seems to have been the worst outbreak recorded on isolated Cape Ann, it swept through nearby Manchester in 1794, visiting every home but two and killing sixty-four people.

Tuberculosis (or consumption, to use its then common name), was another frequent cause of death. It seems to have become more prevalent after the Revolution, when it began to afflict the young in great numbers. This debilitating illness would remain a problem and cause of death until the present century, although it does not seem to have been as serious a problem on Cape Ann as some other diseases of the day. A study by the Massachusetts Board of Health in 1871 found it here among those of "sedentary habits [with] neglected or mismanaged skin diseases . . . [or] an innutritious diet," so perhaps the largely outdoor life and "the influence of the sea-winds" kept the area relatively free of it.

The control of illness and disease from the seventeenth century through the nineteenth was further complicated by a lack of all but the most elementary sanitary measures. Open privies, no refrigeration, poor garbage disposal, and a general laxity in personal hygiene all contributed to the problem. Illness hit hardest among the poor, those least able to establish such controls, whose plight was simply accepted as part of the natural human condition.

Care of the poor, and especially the aged poor without families, was at first considered a function of the church, but by 1700 this responsibility was shifting to tax-supported town governments. Free care of the poor was also accepted as a necessary part of the physician's service, and this, along with generally low fees of often doubtful collectibility or with payment in goods instead of money, was certainly a factor in forcing many of those early practitioners to engage in other lines of work.

Pioneer Doctors

In addition to being ministers or teachers, doctors engaged in commercial enterprises or took paid government positions until well into the nineteenth century. Dr. Harold Bowditch describes this diversity in his introduction to Russell Leigh Jackson's 1948 *The Physicians of Essex County,* published by Essex Institute and containing brief biographies of many area physicians of the seventeenth and eighteenth centuries:

> *A striking feature is the record of employments other than professional in which our early Essex County physicians have engaged before, during or after their medical careers. Here we find the ferryman, the farmer, the shipmaster and trader, the town officer, politician, statesman and one college president, the cordwainer, tailor, weaver and scrivener, the preacher, judge, lawyer and school teacher, the mill owner, manufacturer, inventor and astronomer, the tavern keeper and of course the apothecary.*

Those on Cape Ann were no different. The first to call himself "doctor" here was Thomas Bray, born in Gloucester in 1687 and a shoemaker by trade.

Self-taught, he practiced until his death in 1743. John Newman, a schoolteacher, came in 1712, and six years later we find Edward Thompson, also a teacher, who served as town Selectman in 1725–26 before moving on to Haverhill the next year. Reverend Nicholas Webster came to Gloucester from Manchester in 1717 to teach and practice medicine, both of which he seems to have preferred to pastoral duties, which he abandoned after leaving Manchester. Another early female practitioner was Mrs. Enys Herrick, who, by order of the Selectmen in 1712, was to be paid for the treatment of Elizabeth Hoping "five pounds if she did cure the woman's brist [*sic*] and if she could not cure it, she should have three pounds."

Cape Ann was doubtless not unique in having a number of families in which the practice of medicine was passed from father to son. Dr. David Plummer began the tradition when he came from Ipswich in 1723 to marry Ann Newman (believed to be the daughter of John Newman). Plummer practiced in Gloucester until his death in 1748, when his place was taken by his son Samuel, a very highly regarded man who was also the owner of Thatcher's Island. Samuel Plummer was in turn joined by his own son, Joshua, a Harvard graduate of 1773, who gained recognition as a well-regarded physician and surgeon. Joshua's practice here was short, however, and he moved to Salem following his father's death in 1778; his own death followed soon thereafter in 1791, at age thirty-five — young even for that time. His daughter made sure that he would be remembered, however, in her endowment in his name of the Plummer Professorship of Morals at Harvard.

Not so honorable was his brother, Dr. Samuel Plummer, Jr. Also a Harvard graduate, he joined his father and brother in practice here, but a short time later, accused of murdering one of his father's slaves, who was pregnant by him, he fled "by way of the Squam Ferry and the Ipswich Road." Never caught, he returned home just once, slipping back for a short, surreptitious visit some thirty years later.

Daniel Witham, Isabel Babson's great-grandson, carried that family's medical tradition forward when he began a practice here in 1730. A civic-minded man, also a schoolteacher, he served as Town Clerk for forty-two years and as Selectman during most of them, dying as a respected physician and citizen in 1776.

The Mannings of Sandy Bay formed another of these family dynasties. Dr. John Manning, Jr., son of Dr. John Manning of Ipswich, established his first practice in Gloucester in 1786 and moved to Sandy Bay twelve years later. Described as "a man of considerable eccentricity of character," he was like many others of his time in keeping a detailed journal of each day's events that proves him to have had a keen eye for the world around him. His second son, Charles, joined him in practice in 1822 but died, at age forty-three, only two years after his father's own death in 1841.

An older Manning son, a third John, had just joined his brother in 1842, having left a flourishing practice in Waldoboro, Maine after their father's death. John Manning, 3rd carried on the family practice until his death in 1852, at age fifty-three, and was succeeded by his son Joseph, whom he had called from their practice in Waldoboro that year. Joseph Manning, who also practiced dentistry, maintained the family practice in Rockport until 1890, thus rounding out a span of more than one hundred years on Cape Ann.[1]

Sandy Bay got its first resident physician in 1748, when Caleb Rea came at the age of twenty-one from Danvers. He remained only eight years before returning whence he had come, leaving the village without a physician until Dr. Goss arrived in 1792. James Goss was another multifaceted doctor, a State Representative in 1832 and a schoolteacher. He is described by Jackson as "often employed in writing deeds and other instruments . . . [who] by his various services, secured the respect of society and the reputation of usefulness." His practice coincided with those of the first Mannings, and he remained active until his death in 1842.[2]

It is impossible not to include also Dr. Edward Augustus Holyoke in any discussion of the physicians of the prerevolutionary period and beyond. Although he was not in practice on Cape Ann, his influence on medicine as practiced in New England and elsewhere at the time makes him a factor. The son of one of Harvard's early presidents, Reverend Edward Holyoke, he was born in 1728 as the first of eight children. Entering Harvard at fourteen, he graduated second in his class in 1746 and, after a brief stint as a teacher, apprenticed himself for two years of medical training under Thomas Berry of Ipswich. This "training," typical of the day, consisted of following his mentor on his daily rounds, compounding his prescriptions, and learning what he could by precept and observation.

He began his own practice in Salem in 1749 and was soon known throughout the area as a highly regarded physician, gentle and considerate. He was not only a studious researcher of disease but was also well versed in meteorology and astronomy. A meticulous record keeper, Dr. Holyoke left copious notes along with his daily journal detailing his cases with descriptions of symptoms, his diagnoses, and careful observations as to the effectiveness of treatment. Many of these are preserved at Salem's Essex Institute and offer valuable insight into the medicine and the mores of the time. Among them are exchanges of letters with patients and physicians seeking his advice from all parts of the North Shore.

In recognition of his many accomplishments Harvard Medical School awarded him its first Doctor of Medicine degree in 1782, long after his graduation. Some years later his alma mater also gave him an honorary LL.D. Dr. Holyoke practiced in Salem for seventy-nine years to within five months of his death, at 101, on March 31, 1829.

A New Nation and a New Century

With the American colonies' freedom from British rule and domination would come change — political, commercial, social — to a nation now in control of its own destiny. Eminence would come and leadership would emerge, but it would be a long process, full of trial and error.

This was true also in medicine, where adequate training and effective regulation were both conspicuous by their absence. Although training was becoming more formalized, with the College of Philadelphia (now University of Pennsylvania) having organized a medical school before the Revolution and that at Harvard established in 1782, it was in many ways only an improvement over the older apprenticeships. In the rush to establish training too many schools were being formed and taught by unqualified people, and even the best of them, those affiliated with universities and hospitals, were able to do little more than expose their students to lectures and demonstrations.

In the early years of the new century some thirty-five to forty of these schools, good, bad, or indifferent, were established. Their students could leave after one or two years, often with little real training but calling themselves "doctor." The better trained, more qualified among them soon recognized that higher standards and some regulation would be needed, but with a government still preoccupied with more urgent problems this was slow to come.

The profession was therefore largely left to set its own standards, and this it did by grouping itself into "societies." Among the first of these was the Massachusetts Medical Society, chartered in 1781 in a spin-off from the only slightly older Boston Medical Society. Among the founders of the new group was its first President, Dr. Holyoke. It and similar bodies attempted to establish ethical codes and some degree of standards for practice and, through control of membership, to separate the qualified, trained physicians from those they regarded as quacks.

Their regular meetings also offered opportunities for further learning through discussion, the reading of papers by leading physicians and surgeons, and general exchange of information. The Massachusetts society also established the state's first medical library in 1782, drawing on the meager literature then available. But as voluntary groups with no authority, the societies were all largely ineffective in any regulatory sense.

A lack of easy communication further hampered control and learning. While doctors in the larger urban centers could exchange ideas and experience, those in outlying areas were forced to rely on what they had learned in medical school, supplemented by such reading material as became available to them. Many of the leading physicians and surgeons regularly published papers on their work privately, and such sharing of ideas was enhanced in 1812 when Dr. John Warren of Boston established the *New England Journal of Medicine*. But while Warren and his colleagues could meet monthly to discuss their work, outside the cities keeping informed about medical progress depended on individual ambition and diligence, and was doubtless all too often neglected. The country doctor and those in smaller communities were thus limited in their access to knowledge. Most did their best, but their best was sometimes not good enough.

To some degree the layman was still about as capable as the doctors of the period in treating ordinary sickness. Home care handbooks were numerous and made it possible for the country householder to diagnose and treat many problems. One such was *Domestic Medicine*, originally published in Scotland by William Buchan, which went through some thirty editions in the United States between 1790 and 1850. It put in simple terms a general exposition of the causes and prevention of disease and offered detailed descriptions of symptoms and treatment of specific disorders. Buchan emphasized diet, exercise, fresh air, and simple preventive measures rather than drugs and medicine, but he and others in similar works continued to advocate bloodletting, purging, and blistering. For the most part such books were eminently practical, however, and their authors were sufficiently advanced to have abandoned earlier beliefs and superstitions concerning evil spirits as a cause of disease.

Hospitals, except for the pestilence isolation units and almshouses, were nonexistent until after the Revolution, with a single exception: Philadelphia, the seat of medical knowledge in the colonies, did have its Pennsylvania Hospital, founded in 1752. It was only after the war, during which assembly and treatment centers for the wounded of both sides had been established, that impetus was given to the formation of hospitals, some of which were located on the same sites as the wartime centers and even then only in the larger cities.

The New York General Hospital was founded in 1791, followed by the Boston Dispensary in 1796. The latter, an ambulatory treatment clinic for the poor, was not a true hospital; the Massachusetts General Hospital, chartered in 1811, was the first in-patient treatment center in New England. By 1850 the larger centers – Philadelphia, New York, Baltimore, and Boston – all had one or more functioning hospitals, but smaller communities had few until after the Civil War. Before that there was little demand for hospitals – they were regarded with fear, and no one chose to go there. The few who did went because of special circumstances – the homeless poor, the aged without family or servants to care for them at home, seamen or other travelers unlucky enough to fall ill in a strange city.

Even so, the "state of the art" was advancing. Discoveries made in Europe during the last days of the previous century were beginning to make their way to the United States. Jenner's development of an efficient, safe vaccine against smallpox in 1798, for example, was introduced in Boston by Dr. Benjamin Waterhouse, who had considerable success with it.

France, after its own revolution, became a leading center for medical research and discovery. Its physicians utilized hospitalized patients for clinical observations which, covering many cases, could be correlated with subsequent postmortem studies. From these came new theories as to the nature and treatment of illness, an important one of which held that previously accepted heroic techniques such as bleeding and purging had no therapeutic value.

This particular school of thought held that nature itself was "the great agent of cure," so described by Dr. Jacob Bigelow of Harvard. As the use of heroic medicine declined, a new school of homeopathy, although far from universally accepted, was growing, and by 1850 it had led to a theory of practice that recalled the earliest days of herbal medicine and the more recent work of Buchan. Its credo was the "law of similars" or "like cures like," which taught that illness could be cured by drugs or other materials that produced the symptoms of that illness in a healthy person. Onion, to suggest one example, makes the eyes water and the nose run; therefore, an extract of onion was advocated to cure the cold, which produces those symptoms. The effects of the remedy could further be heightened by administering it in diluted doses, the homeopathic rationale being that the disease would then be displaced by a weaker but similar artificial illness that the body could more easily overcome.

Like all new theories, it had strong opposition. Although many of his colleagues joined Bigelow in his enthusiasm, others followed Oliver Wendell Holmes in opposing it as "the nature trusting heresy." It had its greatest credibility on this side of the Atlantic after 1850, with most of its followers graduates of specialized medical schools and entitled to carry the MD after their names.

Oliver Wendell Holmes, MD, famous as poet-philosopher-jurist, was also one of the outstanding physicians of his time. An 1836 graduate of Harvard Medical School, he was among many young doctors who studied under Pierre Louis in Paris. Holmes is considered by many authorities one of the more important figures in the development of medicine in this country. His work with childbed fever, in which he demonstrated that contagion frequently was conveyed by the physician himself from one patient to another, was an early step in proving the importance of asepsis and absolute cleanliness on the part of those treating patients. A member of the Medical Staff at Massachusetts General Hospital, he taught anatomy at Harvard Medical School, and remained in practice until his death in 1894.

But despite Holmes, Warren, Jenner, Waterhouse, Bigelow, and others at the top of their profession, medicine in outlying areas did not share in their advances before 1850. Although there were conscientious physicians in the smaller communities, they were not the professional equals of their urban colleagues, with their medical societies, their hospitals, and their generally easier access to consultation and the exchange of ideas. The country doctors continued to face competition, although on a diminishing scale as time passed, from the lay practitioners who still used the old folk methods, free of any regulation and regarding medical practice as their right regardless of training and heedless of new theories and beliefs.

Meanwhile the post-Revolution Cape Ann community was moving forward with the nation. Its population by 1800 stood at 5,000, with almost 400 living at Sandy Bay. Thirty years later there were 7,500 on the Cape, and Sandy Bay had grown sufficiently to make its residents begin to yearn for their own independence. This came on February 27, 1840 with the signing of a bill combining Sandy Bay, Pigeon Cove, and the eastern portion of the old Squam Parish into the Town of Rockport, a community of 2,650 with the right to govern its own affairs.

The old Harbor Village was now Gloucester's center of population, as the residents built new homes nearer the burgeoning waterfront. Although the area extending from Meeting House Green to Annisquam remained a popular residential choice, it ceased to attract many new homes until later in the century. Dogtown Common had a brief spell of life during this time, its poor and rocky soil being all that many returning soldiers or soldiers' widows, often poverty-stricken, could afford. After 1830 it was again largely abandoned to the open moorland that we know today.

The West Parish seems to have remained much as it had been for the preceding hundred years. Coffin's farm had, however, deteriorated from well-tended timberland and open tilled fields to what John Babson describes as "a collection of barren sand-hills," perhaps an early example of too ambitious clear-cutting and sodbreaking. Today Coffin's Beach, its dunes, and the sandy expanse behind them are all that remain of that five hundred-acre empire.

Foreign trade was becoming of considerable importance to Gloucester and would be the source of several fortunes, some of which were destined to generate significant philanthropic benefactions in the years ahead. Historian John Babson estimated that at the peak of this trade some forty to fifty vessels called Gloucester their home port, from which they carried on a lively two-way commerce with Europe and other parts of the world. Perhaps the most romantic, and profitable, was the Surinam trade. Surinam, or Dutch Guiana, through its chief port at Paramaribo, received fish, beef, pork, flour, and other goods that had passed through Gloucester for shipment; in return from Paramaribo back through Gloucester came molasses, sugar, cocoa, and coffee. By 1850 this trade accounted for an important share of the town's economy.

Fishing and the coastal trade were also major factors in the life of Cape Ann. The latter included supplying lumber to Boston, until the timberlands were exhausted, after which Gloucester served for a brief period as a transshipment port for Nova Scotia lumber. Fishing was then, as now, a leading occupation, although its greatest years were not to come until after 1850. Stonecutting on a commercial scale also had its beginnings during this period, with the first quarry opened in Sandy Bay during 1824.

Early Cape Ann Physicians

As the Cape Ann community grew, so did the number of its medical practitioners. Dr. Goss and the Mannings were joined about 1790 in Sandy Bay by Dr. Ephraim Davis, who like them was to live out his days there. We find Reverend Eli Forbes arriving during the war at Gloucester, where he came in 1775 to preach and practice medicine until his decease in 1804. Forbes is described by William Bentley as "most known by his experiments of the Dockroot in Cancer."

Dr. William Coffin, son of farmer Peter Coffin, began practice in 1779 with an office at Front (now Main) and Short streets in Gloucester, serving here until his death in 1827. Trained in Boston, he returned home to open his practice after wartime service as surgeon aboard the armed ship *Tyrannicide*. Another who became part of Gloucester's history during the early postwar period is John Kittredge, son of the then well-known Dr. Thomas Kittredge of Andover. Young Dr. Kittredge came here from Harvard in 1795, practiced for ten years, then abandoned medicine when he was appointed the port's Collector of Customs and named President of the town's bank.

It is interesting to note that he replaced Dr. William Tuck, a physician from Manchester, as customs officer.[3]

Physicians of varying interests seem to have continued to be the case among those arriving after 1800. Many came for short stays, leaving for greener pastures elsewhere. Others adopted more or less permanent residence here, remaining in practice for periods of ten years or more. The total number suggests that the Cape Ann population was reasonably well served.

The first to come after the turn of the century was Ebenezar Dale, for whom Gloucester's Dale Avenue was later named. Trained under Dr. Thomas Kittredge, he opened his practice here in 1810 because, according to John Babson, "the Republicans wanted a doctor of that belief in town, the others being Federalists." He practiced until his death in 1834. Henry Prentiss, a Harvard Medical School gradute of 1817, came in 1820 and then succeeded to Dr. Coffin's practice in 1827, holding it until his own death in 1839.

Dr. Samuel Gott was a native of Sandy Bay who trained at Harvard and Massachusetts General Hospital before returning home to practice in 1836. He was deeply interested in education and was Chairman of the Gloucester School Board until Rockport separated and he took the same post there. In 1854, not long before he left Rockport for Berlin, Massachusetts, he prepared and delivered a four-hour lecture on the Sandy Bay saga, a discourse that some thirty-five years later was assembled and published as the first *History of Rockport.*

Joseph Reynolds, MD, also trained at Harvard, practiced not only in Sandy Bay (1833—40) but also in Gloucester from 1840 to 1853, when he moved to Concord. He was an apothecary on the side and was apparently not held in esteem by his colleagues, one of whom, Dr. Joseph Garland, much later said of him: "He had the theory thoroughly but failed in diagnosis and therefore failed in treatment."

Dr. Benjamin Haskell, a homeopathic practitioner and thus a bridge from the old to a newer school of thought, came to Sandy Bay in 1839. He was well thought of by his fellow citizens as well as by his peers, who knew him as a frequent contributor to the medical journals of the day. He died after a short illness in 1878, having given forty years of distinguished service to the people of Rockport.[4]

Two others with long service records who arrived in Gloucester after 1840 are worthy of special note. One, Dr. Joseph Garland, was another who sired a medical family. He was also the only physician from this era to survive to join the first medical staff of the Addison Gilbert Hospital when it opened late in the century. A native of Hampton, New Hampshire, he received his medical degree at Jefferson Medical College in 1840 and came to Gloucester in 1849. His namesake grandson, Joseph Garland, MD, a noted Boston pediatrician and later editor of the *New England Journal of Medicine*, described him almost a century later as among the last of the allopathic school of "bleeders, purgers and pukers," techniques he later abandoned.

The tribute to him in the hospital's *Annual Report* following his death in 1902 describes his fifty years in Gloucester as a continuous learning period during a time of great change in medicine and himself as endeavoring "by reading and observation, to keep pace with the advance of medical knowledge, especially when corroborated by the results of his long experience." Dr. Garland's medical peers elected him President of the Essex South Medical Society in 1870, and his fellow citizens further recognized him by electing him Mayor of Gloucester for two terms, in 1880 and 1881.

Dr. Herman E. Davidson came to Cape Ann to establish a Gloucester practice in 1842. Holder of a Harvard medical degree, he was described in 1901 by his former colleague, Dr. Garland, as "thoroughly educated [and a] skilled physician of the modern school of his day, willing to wait on nature and ever ready to assist her efforts."[5] In this he would seem to have leaned toward the homeopathic school rather than the heroic or allopathic school of Dr. Garland and others. Dr. Davidson gave thirty-five years of service to his fellow citizens.

The Post-1850 Period

As the nation entered the second half of the nineteenth century, the medical state of the art was moving ahead. An event of vast importance to surgery had had its first public demonstration at Massachusetts General Hospital in 1846 when, in a surgical amphitheatre still in existence today known as the Ether Dome, practical anesthesia was proven viable. The use of ether meant the end of the crude and hurried surgery prevalent until that time and, by making surgical exploration possible, opened new avenues for treatment and care. The surgical possibilities were carried even further by the work of Lord Joseph Lister in England, who by 1867 was demonstrating his findings in antiseptic techniques from which came new concepts of aseptic surgery and the diminution of surgical infection.

New instruments available — the stethoscope and microscope from 1819 and 1832 respectively, the spirometer of 1844, the ophthalmoscope in 1851, and the laryngoscope after 1855 — meant also that diagnosis was no longer solely dependent on the patient's description of symptoms interpreted by the physician's use of his five senses and sometimes superficial observation.

Chemical and bacteriological testing followed Louis Pasteur's research in Europe and, together with new instruments, produced information independent of the doctor's judgment, or the patient's. These tools and others were soon to be widely found in doctors' offices and emerging hospitals.

The origins of disease became clearer with Louis Pasteur's research, through which he identified bacteria. His discovery of the anthrax bacillus in 1877 led to the further work of Robert Koch, who isolated *Bacillus tuberculosis* and linked it to the widespread "consumption." Other researchers, most of them in Europe, carried their work forward. The era of discovery was flourishing.

The most visible, and therefore the most dramatic, advances, however, were being made in surgery. By the 1850s Dr. Jacob Bigelow was doing orthopedic and genitourinary work in Boston, and would shortly develop a means of crushing bladder stones. Chest surgery was introduced in Boston by Dr. Henry I. Bowditch in 1850. But until Joseph Lister's use of antiseptics in surgery became generally accepted, after 1880, surgery was still a risky business of limited range and volume. Infection took a heavy toll; the mortality rate for amputations was about 40 percent, and penetration of the major body cavities was rare, even by men like Bowditch. Lister's method relied on antisepsis, usually by carbolic acid spray, during the operation to kill microorganisms in the air.

Others, carrying on Lister's study, improved his somewhat crude method of hygienic control with the introduction of asepsis, which relied on sterile conditions – the surgeons' and nurses' hands and arms, towels, sheets, sponges, instruments, and sutures – and the use of gowns, gloves, caps and masks. With control over infection possible, the surgeon could more safely explore the abdomen, chest and skull.

As diagnosis and treatment improved with the advent of more and better equipment and technique, so too did the need for greater capital investment. The surgeon wanted a more suitable place to work than in his office or, as was often the case, at a household kitchen table. The physician's office itself required the purchase of many of the new tools if he expected to keep up with developments. By the end of the Civil War, therefore, the United States was ready for the hospital concept to flower. By 1865, there were about 200 across the nation.

Quackery and Nostrums

In spite of the relatively far-reaching advances in the state of the art, however, practices still remained that seem strange today. Quackery was rampant in those almost unregulated times, and medical practitioners of whatever degree of skill were supplemented by other sources of treatment available to the lay householder.

The patent medicine manufacturers, advertising liberally in newspapers and magazines, offered therapy and advice along with their potions. A mutual antipathy between them and the physicians ran high. The nostrum peddlers derided the professionals, whom they depicted as eager to cut people up or to give prolonged and expensive treatment. The medicine makers, for their part, touted "sure cures" that would provide "instant relief" for any ache and at low cost.

It would be almost impossible to detail the hundreds of medicines and cures offered. Many were utter fakes, such as the Radam Microbe Killer, a concoction sold during the eighties of water with minute traces of red wine and hydrochloric and sulphuric acids. Lydia Pinkham's Vegetable Compound and others created a doubt as to the physician's ability to cure and urged use of their mixtures to avoid undergoing surgery or having a stranger touch one's body. Many of them relied on what are today called "controlled substances." Opium (or laudanum, as it was then called), was widely prescribed by doctors and found its way into many of the patent medicines for treating insomnia, nervousness, coughing, diarrhea and all manner of aches and pains.

The *Gloucester Telegraph*, the *Cape Ann Advertiser* and their successor, the *Gloucester Daily Times*, all carried their share of this type of advertising and medical advice. Through them we learn of such things as Dr. McLane's Celebrated Vermifuge Liver Pills — "for expelling Worms, the cure of Liver Complaints, all Bilious Derangements, Sick Head Ache, &c." Winter's Balsam of Wild Cherry, "for all who suffer with any disease of the Throat, Lungs or Chest," offered signed testimonials. Or perhaps one preferred Dr. Langley's Root and Herb Compound, "for the cure of Liver Complaints, Jaundice in its worst forms, Hot Blood or Skin, all Bilious Diseases, Dyspepsia, every disease arising from Indigestion, Bad Habits of Life, Headache, Dizziness, Heartburn, Pains in the Side or Bowels, Loss of Appetite and every problem arising from Impurities of the Blood." Dr. P. Humphrey & Co. of New York City affered "Specific Homeopathic Remedies for the People," complete with testimonials, symptoms and remedy, all neatly tied in with a price list and instructions for receiving their cures by mail.

The editorial pages were equally full of good advice. One could learn "How to Cure a Cold," "How to Discover Small Pox in its Early Stage," and how to make a "Cure for a Rattlesnake Bite," a "Simple Cure for the Dysentary," a "Cure for Nervous Headache," and a treatment for "Diphtheria or Putrid Sore Throat." One writer inserted "A Note for the Doctors — A Remedy for Diphtheria," by Dr. A. DeGrande of "Boulogne and Vice Consul at Havana."

Attempts at Regulation

Meanwhile, on the more legitimate side of medicine, the broadening responsibilities of practice also meant better training and more effective regulation. The fly-by-night schools of earlier years were giving way to medical schools almost exclusively affiliated with universities and hospitals. By 1880 there were almost twelve thousand students attending some eighty recognized schools, which in 1890 formed the Association of American Medical Colleges.

The medical associations had become factors as self-governing guardians of the profession. The American Medical Association, founded in 1847 and opposed by what it called "irregular" practitioners who accused it of monopolistic practices, established ethical codes governing physician-physician and physician-patient relationships, handling of fees, and other issues. It was active in opposing what it saw as unconventional schools of medical theory – Thompsonianism and eclecticism, whose followers held to botanic remedies, the Christian Scientists, homeopaths and, later, osteopaths. The AMA was, like any other political body, divided by internal jealousies, but it did at least begin to bring order to the system and raise its standards.

The desire for similar control expressed itself also in the smaller cities and towns. In 1850 four of the town's leading physicians formed what they grandly called the Gloucester Medical Association. Its founders, Dr. Davidson, Dr. Joseph Garland, Dr. Reynolds, and Dr. Isaac Smith, were soon joined by doctors Bacon and Barber and others. Some of the association's records are among Dr. Garland's effects and provide an interesting insight into what control meant.

The constitution of the GMA mandated quarterly meetings to set fees and exchange information regarding delinquent payers. It provided for new members drawn from those it considered "regular" physicians, declaring that "any such Physician who refuses to conform to our fee Bill shall be deemed by us, irregular." Its members further agreed to be governed "in our intercourse with each other" by the Code of Ethics of the American Medical Association.

Fees were a major concern to these pragmatic men, and most of the constitution was devoted to covering all conceivable situations. Some degree of professional self-interest and perhaps earlier jealousies can be detected in the section on medical charges: "For the purpose of promoting mutual good understanding, and of advancing our own interests and the responsibility of the profession in town, we agree to . . . the following rules in our charges." Those rules contain some interesting judgments:

1. The charge for medical visits to strangers at Hotels, boarding houses, & private houses, shall be one dollar for each visit, in the village. Out of the village, 50 cents shall be added to the usual fee in the neighborhood where the patient is.

2. For visits on board vessels, inside the Fort, one dollar & fifty cents, outside of do. from two to three dollars according to weather and distance.

3. The charge for visits in the night shall be double the usual charge in the day.

4. Visits made between 9 oclk and sunrise shall be considered night visits.

5. In consultations one doll. and fifty cents shall be added to the usual charge for visit.

6. Where more than one patient is sick in a family at the same time, twenty five cents shall be added to the usual fee, for each patient.

7. In addition to the ordinary fee for visit and medicine, fifty cents shall be charged for Venesections and the same sum for the minor operations of surgery in general.

8. The obstetric fee shall be $5.00 and this shall cover ordinary attendance for one week. Extraordinary attendance shall be charged in addition. The charge for twins shall be ten dollars.

9. In the operations of Surgery, and in other things not specified above, we will adopt the Salem fee bills.

10. Our charges shall be as follows, within the geographical bounds specified.

Between the Cut and the top of Union Hill, fifty cents a visit. From the top of Union Hill to Lufkins, 62½ cents. From Lufkins to Abraham Williams (Gardner's Brook), 75 cents. From thence to Rockport line, $1.00.

From Lufkins Hill, south to the foot of Saywards Hill, 75 cents. From thence to the gate (H. Robinson) opening onto the Beach, $1.00. To Niles' $1.25. To Lighthouse on the Point, $1.50. To the Island and to Rocky Neck, $1.50.

To the houses on the hill to the eastward of the Methodist Meetinghouse, 62½¢. From the Cut to Cressy's Hill, 75 cents. Beyond and to the neighborhood of Freshwater Cove, $1.00. To Kettle Cove $1.50, for single visit. For continued visits, $1.25. To the further end of the new road, 75 cents. To Freeman's $1.00. To Essex line $1.50 to 2.00.

On the north, to Flat Rock, 50 cents, thence to Burying Ground lane, 62½¢, thence to Isaac Hodgkins 75 cents, thence to the meeting house beyond the mill, $1.00.

11. For consultation visits on the Cape, beyond the limits specified above, five dollars.

12. Medical service shall be rendered to clergymen whose meetings we attend, gratuitously. To other clergymen the usual charge shall be made.

When payment was not forthcoming, the good doctors acted decisively. At their first meeting, on January 17, 1850, they "completed the list of names and engage that we will not render them medical service, except in cases of emergency, until they have made some satisfactory settlement."

An attempt to have themselves recognized by the Massachusetts Medical Society as a District Society with "the usual privileges" thereof was apparently unsuccessful; the state group seems to have considered the Essex South Medical Society, founded some fifty years earlier, sufficient to cover the area. The Gloucester association does not appear to have survived more than a few years, and the last act shown on the records left by Dr. Garland was a fee revision dated September 1, 1864. Today we might question its motives and its apparent machinations, but that's the way it was in those days, at least in Gloucester.

Medical Practice in the Nineteenth Century

As medical practitioners the doctors of Cape Ann at that time were no better or worse than their colleagues elsewhere. They were small-town and country doctors, public servants ready at all hours to attend the needs of their patients. They were for the most part beloved by those patients and held the respect of their communities, which were beginning to judge them for their knowledge and skill. They made daily rounds from house to house or saw their patients in offices, which were almost invariably a part of their own residences.

A good description of the country doctor's rounds can be found in the tribute to the deceased Dr. Garland in the hospital's *Annual Report* of 1902:

Dr. Garland could be seen driving his little white mare, by night and by day, from Eastern Point to West Gloucester, and Annisquam to Kettle Cove, until it seemed a marvel how horse or man could stand such continuous work; nor could they, had not each been given a wonderful endurance. As Dr. Garland's practice grew, he became especially successful and popular as an obstetrician, attending at times more than 200 cases in a year. When one thinks of the miles that were travelled, the sleepless nights, the care and anxi-

ety that are always present when human life is at stake, one begins to realize what a busy man he was, and how little time he had for anything but professional duties.

Small-town surgery, before the day of the hospital, was also an adventure. That undertaking was well described by Dr. Garland's namesake grandson in an address to the hospital's nursing school graduates in 1933:

It was not long [after 1879 that] my father (Dr. Joseph Everett Garland) began to perform abdominal surgery on Cape Ann. . . . Of these early ventures into surgery Mr. Fred Barker could tell you much more than I, for he was the anesthetist. The time was usually on a Sunday morning when other matters did not press and pious people were at church. . . . The operating room was usually the kitchen of the house, the table a sturdy kitchen table or two. The instruments were boiled on the convenient stove from which, however, we trust the ether can was kept at a safe distance.

The Gloucester doctors had one class of patient peculiar to the seagoing community. The fishermen, basically healthy in their outdoor life, suffered illness and accidents relating to their work. Erysipelas, a severe rash caused by chafing and salt-infected wounds, was common, as were colds and other respiratory problems. Gurry poisoning, caused when fish bones or fins pierced the skin, and fishhooks themselves, which often caught fingers, were other sources of trouble. Rheumatism and dyspepsia were fairly common, as was frostbite, especially on the winter banks. Cooks were sometimes scalded. And delirium tremens was not unknown.

The skipper or the cook was the doctor when at sea. Like the housewife ashore, he relied on books and experience to handle most cases, hoping that serious illness or accident would stay away but willing to do his best when they occurred. Druggist Fred Barker supplied one of the most popular instruction books, and his *Handbook for Fishermen* was found aboard almost every Gloucester vessel. Another staple aboard was the vessel's medicine chest, supplied and replenished as needed from Barker's Drug Store on Main Street.[6]

After another war had been fought, this one the fratricidal Civil War between North and South, Cape Ann's communities continued to grow and prosper. During this period Gloucester's fishing industry reached its time of greatest prosperity, with its large schooner fleet. The best years of the Grand Banks fishery came between 1870 and 1900. With a population then approaching fifteen thousand, Gloucester became a city in May 1873 and elected its first Mayor after a contest in which Robert R. Fears defeated a wealthy merchant-banker named Addison Gilbert by four hundred votes.

Rockport during those years had a population of about 3500. The inshore fishery was a large employer of the town's men, with quarrying next. Rockport's granite was used for city streets and buildings wherever water could take it. Attempts at unrelated industry were largely unsuccessful, and enterprises such as the Manning Organ Company, organized by Dr. Joseph Manning's son William, and the Rockport Steam Cotton Mill were short-lived. Except for the Cape Ann Tool Company, which was incorporated from a small quarry tool shop in 1891, Rockport was, then as now, essentially given over to the sea, tourism and local trade.

Some Prominent Physicians

There seems to have been an ample supply of physicians to serve the growing community, most (but surely not all) considered "regular" by the Gloucester Medical Association. Some had held over from before 1850; of those coming later, we can do little more than list most of them.[7]

Dr. J. Franklin Dyer opened an Annisquam practice in 1851 and remained there until his death in 1879. Plagued by frail health stemming from his Civil War service as Division Surgeon, Dr. Dyer was nonetheless able to serve as one of Gloucester's earliest mayors. His colleague Joseph Garland described him as "of genial manner [and giving] prompt and efficient service."

Charles H. Hildreth, MD, a graduate of Harvard Medical School with further training at Massachusetts General Hospital, began his practice in 1852. Described by Dr. Garland as "a gifted writer [with] much skill and broad ideas of progress," his name lived on in the Hildreth School, itself now only a memory to old-timers. Dr. Hildreth died in 1884, "and in that death," wrote Dr. Garland, "Gloucester lost one of its brightest intellects."

It is a possibility that Addison Gilbert's personal physician was Dr. George B. Stevens who, although not mentioned in Garland's 1901 lecture,[5] practiced at 62 Middle Street and was a witness to the Gilbert will. Dr. Stevens came to Gloucester about 1875 and was last listed as a physician in an 1888 city directory. Another whom Dr. Garland fails to mention was Dr. Charles B. Hall, who practiced in Rockport from 1880 to 1923. Surprisingly little is recalled of him except that he had a home at Land's End and, according to Swan's history, treated James Davis's fractured shoulder.

Not so neglected was Augustus M. Tupper, MD. Dr. Tupper arrived in Rockport in 1870 after completing his study at Harvard Medical School. He soon joined Dr. Haskell in practice and succeeded to his residence at his death in 1878. More than simply a well-loved and respected physician, Dr. Tupper was one of the town's leading citizens, among the founders of St. Mary's Episcopal Church and Carnegie Library. He was also active in establishing

Rockport's short-lived Haskins Hospital, in 1906. The popular Dr. Tupper served his fellow townsmen with devoted skill for more than fifty years.

Completing the roll of Cape Ann physicians of this period are the fourteen men and one woman who were to comprise the original medical staff at Addison Gilbert Hospital. The first of these was Albert S. Garland, MD, nephew of Dr. Joseph Garland, who opened his practice in 1866 after Harvard Medical School and remained until his death in 1921. He was followed the next year by Edward S. Eveleth, MD, a graduate of the College of Physicians and Surgeons in 1867, who was a member of the hospital's Medical Staff until 1919.

Dr. Thomas Conant, also from Harvard Medical School and one of the series of homeopathic practitioners here, succeeded to the practice of Dr. Samuel Worcester in 1868. Dr. Conant was well thought of by his peers, who selected him as a member of the hospital's first Medical Board; his service also lasted until 1919. George and Abbie Morse were, like Dr. Conant, homeopathic believers; both graduated from Boston University School of Medicine in 1875 and came to Gloucester the same year. He practiced until his death in 1904 and she until hers in 1914.

Another Garland joined the family in practice here when Joseph Everett Garland, MD returned to his hometown in 1879, following his 1877 degree from Harvard and a period of study in Europe. J. Everett Garland had planned to practice in the midwest after honing his skills in Europe, but came home at his father's urging to assist him in practice after he became Gloucester's Mayor.

Next came Sumner F. Quimby, MD, direct from New York University Medical School in 1882 to minister to the people of Gloucester until his death in 1914. Philip Mooney, class of 1882 at Vermont Union Medical School, arrived in 1884 and remained for thirty years of practice. He was closely followed by Charles H. Morrow with his 1885 MD from the University of Pennsylvania Medical School; Dr. Morrow was a Medical Staff member until 1919.

Long service was also given by Dr. Snow P. F. Cook, who came in 1886 from the University of Pennsylvania and remained until his death in 1934, serving as Staff Oculist. Another Pennsylvania graduate was Dr. James H. Knowles, class of 1886, who served from 1890 to 1919. Also coming in 1890 was Edward B. Hallett, MD, an 1887 graduate of Dartmouth Medical School. Dr. Hallett, whose son Ronald was also to become a Medical Staff member some years later, was a revered figure in the community until his death in 1939.

Dr. William Rowley, Harvard Medical School 1893, practiced in Gloucester from 1894 until his death in 1924. Percy C. Rowley by a year at Harvard and opened his practice ing until 1919. The junior man on that first staff was other whose son would follow him in a Gloucester rived fresh from medical school in late 1896 and mai in his residence on Dale Avenue until his death in 19 original staff still in active practice, he was the senior cal Staff at the time of his death.[8]

Genesis of the Addison Gilbert Hospital

The time had come when kitchen table surgery, the doctor's office and his daily wearying rounds of his patients' homes were not enough. Doctors were beginning to turn to the hospitals as a place for treatment and care, and by 1880 there were almost a thousand such institutions nationwide. The first in the vicinity of Cape Ann was Salem Hospital, which had been established during 1874 in a converted residence. Anna Jaques (often incorrectly spelled "Jacques") Hospital for the people of Newburyport followed ten years later. Next came Beverly Hospital, chartered in 1893; it emerged from what had been called Dr. Torrey's Hospital, which had opened in 1889. Beverly and Salem hospitals both operated for several years in converted private residences, a common practice in those days.

Undoubtedly there had been discussion among the local medical community concerning the subject, but the first public expression of the need for a hospital here seems to have been an editorial in the *Cape Ann Advertiser* of October 31, 1884. Couched in the style of the day, it rather skillfully stated the case and requested funds as would any fund raiser today.

One of the city's activists of the time was Addison Gilbert, a businessman whose ancestor John Gilbert had come to Gloucester in 1704. Addison Gilbert was born November 23, 1808 to Samuel and Sally (Woodbury) Gilbert. His birthplace on what is now Main Street's West End was destroyed in the Great Fire of 1830.

Samuel Gilbert was a prosperous ship's chandler whose wealth was based on the midcentury Surinam trade. His son carried on the family business, adding other ventures as the fisheries also prospered, and by age forty he was already one of the town's wealthiest citizens. Active in town affairs as Moderator and Selectman while Gloucester was still a town, he had also served as Representative to the General Court of Massachusetts. He was a Trustee of the Cape Ann Savings Bank from its founding in 1846 (three others among the charter corporators were Dr. Joseph Reynolds, doctor-businessman William Ferson, and historian John J. Babson) and became its president in 1880. Conflict of interest being more easily tolerated then, it

ossible for Mr. Gilbert also to be an incorporator and the first Presi-
nt of the City National (later Gloucester National) Bank when it was established in 1876.

Young Addison's mother died shortly after his birth and four years later his father remarried. The boy was brought up by his stepmother, Mary Hayes, herself a lifelong Gloucesterite, descended on her mother's side from the Warner, Sargent, and Prince families, all early Cape Ann settlers. She and Addison, a lifelong bachelor, resided together at the family home on Western Avenue at Angle Street from the time of his father's death in 1860 until her own, at age 102, only a few months prior to Addison's. They would appear to have been alike in many ways despite the lack of blood ties; she has been described as autocratic and overbearing, as was he, and they also shared a reputation for penuriousness.

What sort of man was this community leader? Little is known of his personality except as it was remembered years later by Alfred Mansfield Brooks, a next-door neighbor as a boy of ten or twelve, whose book *Gloucester Recollected* draws something of a portrait.

Addison Gilbert impressed me as an old man [who always] looked dissatisfied. Even as a little boy I knew he was rich, better off than anybody in the neighborhood. I also knew that he and his step-mother (with whom he lived) quarrelled without cease. He had the reputation of being niggardly about small things and generous with the large [and had] a depth of sympathy which is far rarer than generosity with money.

Addison never got over an affront. He did not speak to Eliza Haskell from the day she refused to marry him when she was 18 to the day of her death at 75. Their paths crossed frequently in the houses of friends, at church and on the street, and as Eliza said, "He looks stony at me still."

He loved to rule - anything, anybody, anywhere and at any time [and] had little praise from any side until he was an old man and known to be rich.

Brooks recalls a conversation his mother had with a neighbor at the time of Mary Gilbert's death "I wonder what Addison will put on her stone," the neighbor remarked. To which his mother replied, "Nothing, Abby, because though he's honest as the day is long, he's narrow as a crack." It is curious, perhaps indicative of their personalities, that Addison's name was not mentioned in his stepmother's obituary nor hers in his, although it can be assumed that he must have had considerable say in preparing hers.

But all of that may have been the older, somehow soured Addison Gilbert. Another side is revealed in his obituary: "As a young man, Mr. Gilbert was popular among his associates in social life and took a leading part in the festivities of the day, being active in amateur theatricals and other forms of social enjoyment." His sociability is further evidenced by his description in that same source as "a prominent Odd Fellow having been admitted to Ocean Lodge Jan. 10, 1846, four months after the lodge was instituted."

This many-faceted man's life was spent in close proximity to the waterfront, and he could not help but be aware that the nature of the industry there, along with Cape Ann's other occupation in the quarries, created many hazards. He knew that there were frequent accidents and that often the victims were forced to endure a torturous journey by land or sea to Boston or Salem for treatment. Even before the *Advertiser* editorial he could be expected to have discussed the subject with his friends and almost certainly with J. Everett Garland, George Stevens and others among Gloucester's physicians.

However he was viewed by his contemporaries, the sympathetic nature of which Alfred Brooks was aware combined in the end with the side of him that prompted generosity in big things. At his death on July 2, 1888, he left a will bequeathing his wealth to benefit the people of his native city. In his obituary the *Times* estimated his financial worth at "three hundred thousand to nearly half a million dollars," a very large estate in that day, when $25 per week was a high salary indeed and there was no income tax.

The will, drawn February 13, 1888, made specific bequests totaling $234,700, of which $31,000 went to twenty-two relatives, servants, and friends. Perhaps typical of the man were the wishes and sentiments expressed: the bequest of $4,000 "to Addison Gilbert Procter, my namesake, now at the West . . . hoping he will invest it safely and use only the income thereof"; "to Miss Mary Williams . . . my late mother's maidservant, who was faithful to the end, $4,000"; "to Mrs. Ann M. Williams . . . mother of Mary Williams, $3,000, hoping she will deposit it in some safe institution, drawing only the income thereof."

Six bequests were made to his associates at the two banks, some of whom were also left specific items from his home. His "portrait, painted in oil" went to City National Bank, and "my large portrait, in crayon, executed by Adams, now in my parlor" was designated for the Cape Ann Savings Bank. The Sawyer Library was given oil portraits of his parents and of himself plus "all my other pictures, albums and books." It appears possible that the portraits of his father and himself now hanging at the hospital were those left the library. George J. Marsh and Henry A. Parmenter, his executors, were given $4,000 and $1,000 respectively.

Nine organizations received a total of $28,700, and again perhaps the bequests help portray their maker. To the Female Charitable Association of Gloucester he left $2,000; the Massachusetts Society for the Prevention of Cruelty to Animals received $4,000. To the Gloucester Fishermen's and Seamen's Widows' and Orphans' Society went $10,000 in trust; $5,000 in trust to the Fireman's Relief Association; $4,000 in trust to the Cape Ann Scientific and Literary (now Cape Ann Historical) Association; $2,000 in trust to the Independent Christian Society of Gloucester; and $1,000 to the Odd Fellows. There was also $500 to the city provided that "income thereof only shall be used annually to improve and beautify the old burial ground in Bridge Street, report thereof to be made annually, so that the gift may not be lost sight of." The sum of $200 was given to Oak Grove Cemetery for care of his lot and monument there.

His residence and $75,000 in trust were designated "to found and establish in the City of Gloucester a home for Aged and Indigent Persons, not under sixty years of age. . . . I wish it to be an institution to keep those who have yet held their heads up in the world from sinking; to keep alive the spirit of a decent household when poverty is in danger of crushing it; to assist those who are the most willing, but not always the most able to assist themselves." This became the Gilbert Home, which survived until 1982, when it was sold and the trust dissolved.

His largest bequest was for $100,000, to gratify his wish "to found and establish . . . a free hospital." After naming five trustees, he made further stipulations:

I wish the building to be of brick, with the name 'The Gilbert Hospital' in marble or granite, in front . . . the grounds to be of ample extent and properly embellished . . . to admit as patients therein such citizens and such inhabitants of the city, and in cases of emergency such others as [the trustees] may see fit, as may need medical or surgical aid and treatment, and to provide, gratuitously, such aid and treatment to the indigent . . . to receive in aid of maintaining [it] such compensation as may be paid by patients . . . who shall be able to make such compensation.

The residue of the estate, amounting to about $50,000, was left to his named trustees to establish a permanent fund for "the relief and benefit of the deserving poor of the city . . . as have seen better days and have, without fault, fallen into distress."

And that is how it all began!

NOTES

[1]Other father-son practices – Egan, Garland, and Hallett – would follow that same tradition. We will hear their stories later.

[2]Other mid-eighteenth-century practitioners were Mary Ellery and Elizabeth Gardner, both recorded as having been voted payment by town officials for successful treatment of men and women; Nathan Lakeman, 1725–30; Samuel Holten, 1758–60; Samuel Rogers, commander of a militia company during the Revolution and in Gloucester from 1767 to 1777; and Israel Woodbury, c. 1767–97.

[3]Also included on the immediate postwar list of practitioners: Thomas Babbit from 1787 to 1789; Ebenezar Davis from Essex in 1780 to practice in Annisquam; John Herrick at Lanesville for a few years from 1785; Henry Phelps, trained under Dr. Joshua Plummer in Salem as physician and apothecary from 1790, who shortly thereafter left medicine to become a magistrate and Gloucester's postmaster; and in Sandy Bay two women, "Nursewoman" Ruth Dorcas Dresser and Mrs. Mary Gammage.

[4]Others of shorter stays or lesser importance on Cape Ann during this period are: Amasa D. Bacon, in Annisquam from 1837 to 1857, when he moved to Sharon, Massachusetts; Joseph S. Barber, Annisquam, 1832 to c. 1850; William Ferson, Sandy Bay from 1802 to 1805, when he moved to Gloucester to take a town office and become treasurer of Cape Ann Savings Bank and a member of the State Senate; Edwin P. Grosvenor, in Gloucester for a short time during the 1840s; John P. Moriarty, Gloucester from c. 1835 to 1840, when he was forced to leave because of his unpopular views regarding the fishing industry; Adam Nichols and David Preston at Sandy Bay and Gloucester respectively during the 1830s; Rev. Daniel D. Smith, probably the last minister-physician on Cape Ann, who held a pastorate in the Harbor Village during the 1840s; and Isaac Smith, also in Harbor Village from 1831 to his retirement about 1851.

[5]This was a New Year's Day lecture titled "Physicians and Progress of Medicine of the Nineteenth Century in Gloucester" and reprinted in full by the *Times*. It contained candid descriptions of Garland's predecessors and colleagues.

[6]Another well-thumbed book was *The Mariner's Medical Guide*, edited and published in Boston by James Folsom, who described it as "designed for the use of Ships, Families and Plantations" and called himself "Ship Druggist."

[7]Less well-known physicians of the post-1850 period in Gloucester were: W. Bergengren (1869–71); H. K. Bryant (1875); Sarah Coly (c. 1860); George C. Estabrook (c. 1869); Walter F. Fuller (1886–93); D. B. Gifford (1870–73); Daniel Goodenow (1896–97); William Hale (1885–1900); A. B. Hoyt (c. 1858); H. P. Huntoon (1879); J. J. Johnson (1879); Gilbert V. Jones (1890–97); A. C. McLellan (1894–95); Dana P. Richardson (1888); Levi Saunders, in practice in Lanesville from 1857 to about 1900; George W. Smith (c. 1854); J. Ranlet Smith (c. 1873–1905); Lawrence S. Smith (1888); P. S. Stearns (1880); Charles W. Stockman (1880–93); James A. Thompson (1892–93); and Cape Ann's first homeopaths, Dr. Walters (1855–60) and his successor, Samuel Worcester (1860–67); and Samuel L. Young, a Lanesville native and physician-businessman (1852–79).
In Rockport: Oscar D. Abbott (1852–60); Edward E. Barden (1873–75); E. M. Dolloff (1894–95); A. K. Gould (1875); T. R. Grow (1888–91); F. Haigh (1892–93); O. St. Clair O'Brien (1886–1913); and John E. Sanborn (1870–85).

[8]These and all who have followed them as members of the Addison Gilbert Hospital Medical Staff are listed in Appendix H. Cape Ann physicians who came after those listed previously and who were not hospital Medical Staff members are to be found in various city directories which, after 1900, are quite comprehensive and reliable.

ENTERED AT POST OFFICE, GLOUCESTER,
AS SECOND-CLASS MATTER.

Cape Ann Advertiser,

PUBLISHED EVERY FRIDAY MORNING,

—BY—

PROCTER BROTHERS,

EDITORS AND PROPRIETORS.

OFFICE, 108 AND 110 MAIN STREET, PROCTER BUILDING.

I. N. STORY, PRINTER.

TERMS:—Subscribers out of Essex County, $2.65 per year, which includes postage; within Essex Co., $2.50 per year strictly in advance, $2.75 within six months, or $3.00 at the end of the year.

All advertisements, to insure insertion, must be handed in by Thursday noon.

Obituary notices inserted for 12 1-2 cents per line.

FRIDAY, Oct. 31, 1884.

A City Hospital.

Among the actual requirements of Gloucester, which shall place her on an equality with her sister sisters of the Commonwealth, is a hospital where those of the sick who wish can have the best of attendance, and where those who are injured, as is frequently the case, especially among our sea-faring population, can be taken in and properly cared for.

A correspondent in another column calls attention to the Anna Jacques Hospital at Newburyport, which he has recently visited, and the query again presents itself, why cannot Gloucester be similarly blessed? A donation from some public-spirited individual who has the good of our city at heart, and who has the wherewith to carry out his good intentions, would be warmly welcomed and properly applied, and there is not the least doubt but that others would follow suit and a sufficient sum be realized to provide for its needs.

Then again, as is the case with this hospital at Newburyport, and others, various societies and corporations contribute sums which provide a bed for any one or more of their members who may need to avail themselves of the privileges offered, and philanthropic people remember such institutions in their wills.

We learn that there is one gentleman who stands ready to give substantial assistance to a hospital in this city. So far as we can understand, he wishes the city to make the first effort in obtaining the building, and then he will be ...dy with his offering. This is indeed praise- ... city was in condi- ... thus start

PART I
THE EARLY YEARS
1889 - 1908

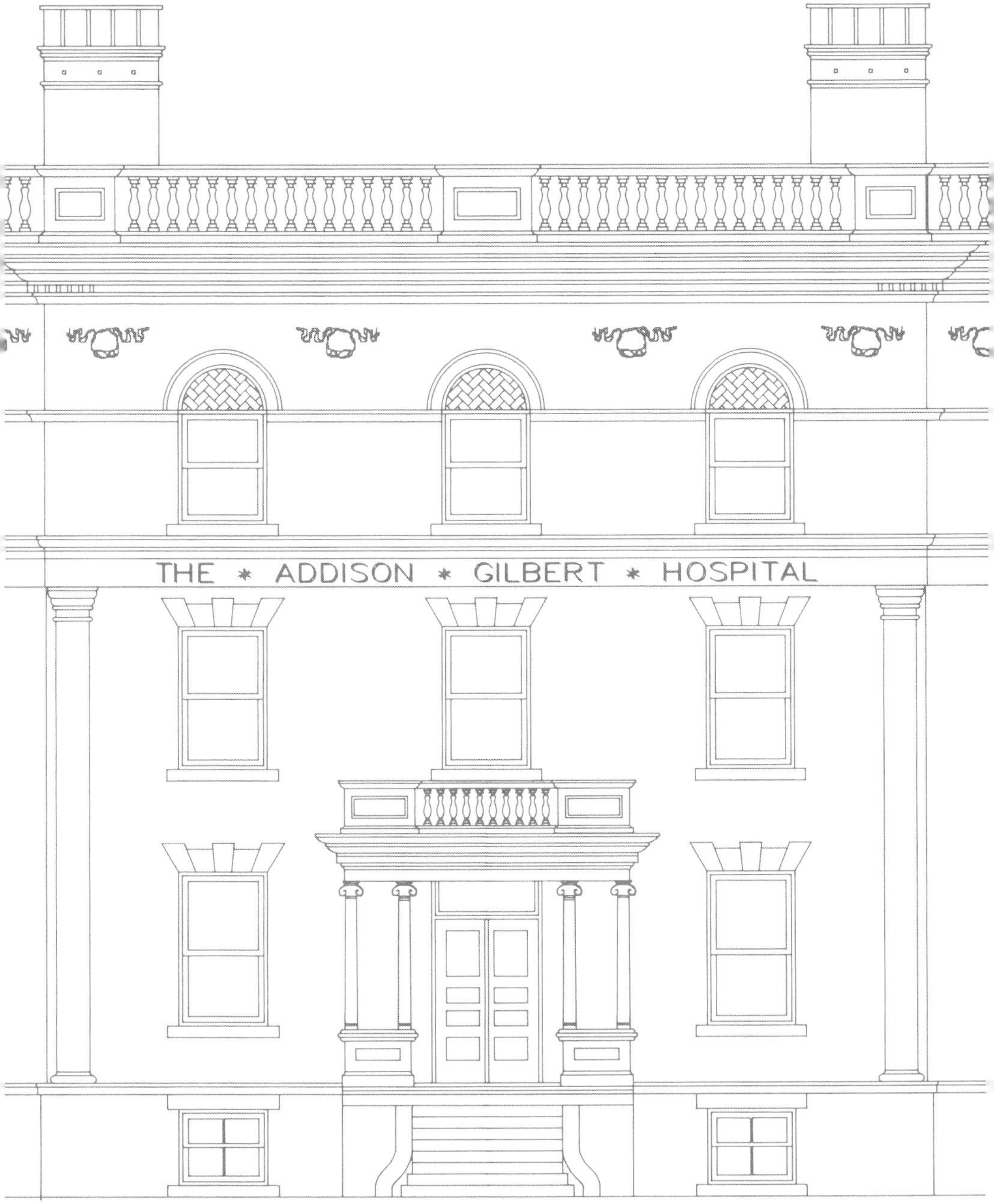

Architects' design of front elevation of the original Addison Gilbert Hospital.

1

Planning and Construction

ADDISON GILBERT'S WILL was quickly probated, and on February 18, 1889 the five Trustees held their first official meeting. The designees, Sylvester Cunningham, John K. Dustin, Jr., George J. Marsh, Henry A. Parmenter and John E. Somes, were all connected in one way or other to the fisheries, and all but one were also bankers. The five invited two others, John Corliss and Allan Rogers, to join them as Corporators and Trustees of the proposed hospital, and all were present at the initial session at Cape Ann Savings Bank.

Sylvester Cunningham was born in Gloucester in 1850. He had spent his adult life as partner in Cunningham & Thompson, Commercial Street fish brokers, a firm which, somewhat incongruously, also had large Western real estate holdings among which was the Knutsford House, at that time the largest hotel in Salt Lake City. Mr. Cunningham was President of both City National Bank and Cape Ann Savings Bank. His obituary of January 23, 1909 described him as "reserved in his manner, but at all times courteous and genial in his quiet way."

John Dustin, born in 1843 at Topsham, Vermont, came to Lanesville in early adulthood to help out in his father's grocery store, a veteran of the Civil War and the only one of the seven Trustees to have served in that conflict. He went on to become a partner in John Pew & Son and was with that firm when it and others merged to become Gorton-Pew Fisheries Company, of which he became part of the management group. He was also Vice President of Gloucester Safe Deposit & Trust Company. His 1909 obituary de-

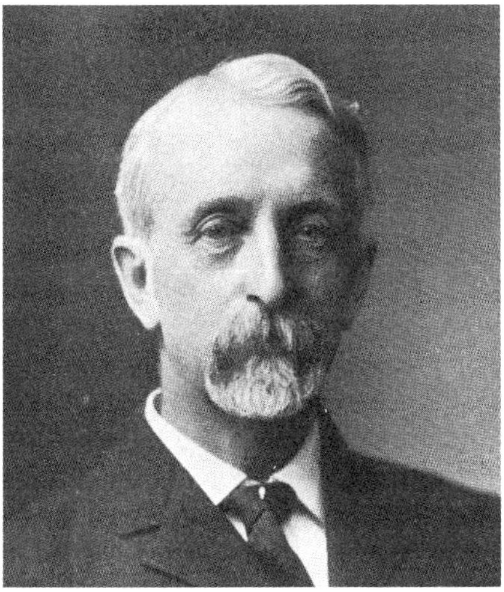

John K. Dustin was the first president and a member of the original building committee.

scribed him as "never . . . unduly hurried or excited [and of a] nature which, under the stress of greatest activity, maintained a coolness and deliberate quality which could always be relied upon."

The third Gilbert Trustee, George J. Marsh, was perhaps closest to him and was coexecutor of his estate. His parents were Eben and Nancy (Rogers) Marsh of Boston, where he had been born in 1835. His father was a Boston merchant, and his mother, a Gloucester native, was the sister of George H. Rogers, a Gloucester merchant and shipowner with whom George Marsh was at one time associated. By 1889, however, he had become full-time Treasurer of Cape Ann Savings Bank.

Henry Parmenter, coexecutor with Marsh of the Gilbert estate, was President of City National Bank, succeeding Addison Gilbert in that post. A native of Marlboro, Massachusetts, born in 1832, he began a career as a teacher and had come to Gloucester in 1857 as principal of the old Collins School, which stood where McPherson Park now looms. He resigned that position to form a fisheries partnership, Parmenter, Rice & Garland, which became one of the important local firms of the late 1800s. His 1891 obituary pictures him "a man of strong convictions, shrewd business habits and unquestioned integrity."

John E. Somes, born in 1840 in Gloucester, was President of Cape Ann National Bank and Vice-President of Cape Ann Savings Bank. He was a partner in Clark & Somes, a fish broker on Rogers Street. Having married into the longtime resident Presson family, he had a summer home on Presson's Point, overlooking Little River.

John Corliss was Vice-President of City National Bank at the time and later became its President. He moved to Boston in 1900, severing his Gloucester connections. Allan Rogers was a partner in John C. Calef & Company, a dry-goods retail firm. A civic-minded man, he served two terms as Mayor of Gloucester, in 1876 and 1877, a term in the State Senate, in 1879, and on the Gloucester School Committee from 1880 until 1904.[1]

The seven had, on February 5, 1889, incorporated as The Addison Gilbert Hospital choosing to honor the full name of its benefactor instead of simply calling it by his surname, as suggested in his will. George Marsh, who seems to have been the leader of the group and who signed the call to the organizational meeting of February 18, took the chair to open it and requested nominations. John Corliss was chosen as Chairman and John Dustin was sworn in as temporary clerk.

A set of bylaws, obviously worked up ahead of time, was presented by Mr. Cunningham and adopted unanimously. These contained no radical departures from normal bylaw provisions in establishing the corporation, its meetings, and for the addition to it of "any citizen or inhabitant of the Commonwealth." It provided for a seven-member Board of Trustees who "may fill vacancies in their own body" with the usual officers to "be elected by written ballot." Its bonded Treasurer could "when duly authorized by the Board of Trustees, sell and convey, transfer or release, any real or personal property or any interest therein held in trust or owned by the corporation."

Bylaws in hand, the Corporators then elected the Board, and, no surprise, the seven were named thereto. Mr. Marsh was elected Clerk-Treasurer with an Auditing Committee of Corliss, Cunningham, and Somes. On adjournment to a meeting of the Board, John Dustin was elected President and John Corliss Vice-President, and Cunningham, Rogers, and Somes became the Finance Committee.

The Charter was issued on March 13, 1889 by Henry B. Pierce, Secretary of the Commonwealth, and with that the hospital became officially recognized, with its purpose stated in terms compliant with the Gilbert will. The organization was then in place and ready to proceed with its business, the most immediate of which was the investment of its funds and planning for a hospital building.

The Gilbert Fund of $100,000 in cash, a single bond series, and mortgages was turned over to the Trustees on April 27 following the issuance of the Charter. The mortgages represented seventeen holdings in the West totaling $20,345.60, reflecting Mr. Gilbert's interest in that region, as did $11,343.33 in Oregon Short Line Railroad 6 percent bonds. The Finance

Committee kept the mortgages and the bonds and, except for $10,000 deposited at Cape Ann Savings Bank and $2,500 held as cash on hand, followed the then-favored investment preference for railroad bonds for the balance. This "rails only" policy was followed for several years thereafter, except for a later investment of $17,500 in New Hampshire Trust Company and Oregon Improvement bonds, both of which showed losses at sale, when much of the portfolio was converted to meet construction and other expenses.

Most of the mortgages were eventually paid off without problem, but Mr. Gilbert's judgment of them was not infallible. One piece, described as the Krueger property in Newton, Kansas, was foreclosed in 1893, but title problems prevented sale until late 1898. Bennett's Information Agency, advertising "Inquiries of Any Nature Answered for $2 Each," described the holding to the Trustees as "not desirable [since] the town of Newton overgrew several years ago, and there is any amount of vacant and valueless property there. The house is a one story four room with well and cistern on back porch and cost perhaps $600 to build it ten years ago, now unoccupied, and it is doubtful if you could find anyone who would give $200 for it with complete title." By June 1899, however, someone was found to buy it for $550, the Trustees having made the best of a bad bargain while proving that Cape Ann Yankee bankers weren't too bad with a dollar.

Their primary concern, however, was getting a hospital built. They first had to find a suitable location to meet the mandate of the will that "the grounds be of ample extent and properly embellished, [large enough for] a building to be of brick . . . attractive in appearance." At a meeting on April 5, 1889 the President and Treasurer "were chosen a committee to see what the Eben Brown estate could be bought for." The Brown farm was reasonably close to the old Harbor Village and, located as it was on the main road around the Cape, it was also handy to the outlying areas.

The only other site recorded as having been considered was a three-acre plot belonging to Gorham P. Low between the old Meeting House Green and the river, near where Ashland Place is today. At a price of $7,000 this was a possible location, but the lot was far smaller, and the committee decided in December "that no action be taken until it is decided whether or not the Brown lot can be purchased."

The committee apparently did not meet formally again until June 1890, and the cause of the delay is not clear. It may be that Eben Brown was reluctant to sell, but whatever the reason the committee recorded its opinion at that meeting that "no suitable site could be obtained at present." Another year was to pass before the owner was persuaded to sell the property for

$10,000 subject to "a good and clear title thereto, free of all encumbrances."

An encumbrance soon appeared. It lay in the will of Jonathan Brown, Eben's grandfather (which by coincidence had Addison Gilbert as one of its three witnesses). The restricting clause—"I give and devise to my grandson Eben Brown, the son of my son, Jonathan, the farm as hereinbefore described subject to the life estate therein given to my son Jonathan, and subject also to the limitation that if said Eben die without issue, then this devise is to go to other son or sons of my son Jonathan if any there should be and if not to the heirs of my son Jonathan forever"—was taken to flaw the title pending determination of the existence of other heirs.

And there the matter rested while the parties pursued the problem through the legalities[2] until finally, on January 1, 1896, the purchase price was paid and the deed registered. Cash for the payment was raised through sale of bonds, and $11,887.98 including interest and court costs was paid Mr. Brown. The long period of waiting had not been wasted, however, as the Trustees, confident of eventual acquisition, had proceeded with site survey and planning for the building.

Much of this activity and any other business during the waiting period was done on an informal basis, as between January 1890 and June 1895 only ten Board meetings recorded any business. Other meetings, duly entered at regular intervals, were all adjourned for lack of a quorum or the minutes simply stated "Nothing done." Although a Building Committee (President, Treasurer, and a new Trustee, Dr. Isaac Adams) was appointed at the Corporation's Annual Meeting in June 1892, the only record of its work appears undated between the minutes of that meeting and the Annual Meeting of June 1893. That record advises that "sundry irregular meetings were held during the year and plans of Gardner, Pyne & Gardner of Springfield [Massachusetts] considered."

Isaac Adams, elected a Trustee at the same meeting at which he was named to the Building Committee, seems a peculiar choice to replace Henry Parmenter, who had died the previous December. He was a summer resident of Annisquam and owned much of what is known today as Adams Hill in that village. His winter home was in Cambridge, although after his election to the hospital Board he registered to vote in Gloucester. A graduate of Harvard Medical School, he maintained a small private practice in Boston, but his larger interests lay in the business world. An inventor, he developed a workable incandescent lamp almost simultaneously with Thomas Edison, to whom he lost in the patent procedure. His later invention of a new nickel plating process was more successful, and he accumulated a fortune through his United Nickel Plating Company. His commitment to the hospital would seem to have been minimal; he is recorded as attending only one Board meeting during his incumbency, and since the Building Committee records, if they kept any, have not survived, we cannot testify as to his contribution thereto.

Addison Gilbert's hospital was unusual in that it was to be built as such in a time when many, possible most, small community hospitals were initially opened in converted private residences with obvious deficiencies of design and operation. Although they were expanded or totally replaced as soon as feasible, the Gilbert bequest made it possible to plan his hospital to its purpose from the start.

By April 1895 Gardner, Pyne and the committee, assisted by a consulting committee of Drs. J. Everett Garland, Thomas Conant and Gilbert Jones[3], had assembled plans for submission to the full Board. These called for a main building of four floors, with twelve rooms of two or three beds each on the two upper levels and offices and ancillary facilities on the first and ground floors in what today is called North Wing. Connected to it was a single-story ell containing the surgical suite, with further ancillary space below it on the ground floor. The architects' original plan also included a one-story ward of ten beds extending southward from the west end of the ell.

It was soon apparent that $100,000 would not build and equip the plant envisioned in those first plans, and the committee was requested to investigate eventual disposition of the Brown house and barn to raise funds and also to cut back on the building and landscaping to spend less on them. On June 28, 1895 the committee reported that grading would only be done to bring the foundation to street level and that the ten-bed ward would be eliminated. They insisted, surely supported by Dr. Garland, that all else remain as planned.

The summer passed while specifications were put out for contractor consideration, and when next the Board met in September four bids were submitted. Two Gloucester firms, Maddix Brothers and the Jackman Company, were high, Blanchard of Lynn at $40,971 was also high, and the contract was awarded to the low bidder, H. P. Cummings of Ware, Massachusetts at $34,850 with a bond of $5,000. The architects were asked to remain as construction supervisors, the committee was "authorized to make such changes in plans as they may deem expedient," and finally, with the passing of the deed, the work got under way early in 1896.

Things seem to have gone smoothly and on schedule and by October the Board was beginning to plan for opening sometime during the ensuing year. Then came what can only be described as a terrifying event, although no indication of its trauma or even its occurence is evident in the records. It became public knowledge in the *Gloucester Times* of October 6, 1896 under the headline "APPALLING TRAGEDY," and the story that followed broke the news that George Marsh had shot and killed himself the previous day.

The story detailed the events leading up to the tragedy, which began when the Directors of Cape Ann Savings Bank, of which he was Treasurer and where he kept bachelor quarters upstairs, had become uneasy during a routine bank examination. They had called a special meeting for October 5 to go into Mr. Marsh's books and inventory the bank's securities, but when they assembled, instead of Mr. Marsh himself, they found a note revealing his plan to kill himself. A delegation was immediately sent to his summer home overlooking Cambridge Beach and the river in Annisquam, where it found a scene which the newspaper described in graphic detail. Dr. J. E. Garland was summoned, but there was nothing he could do.

There was a small run of worried depositors at the bank the next business day, but it soon appeared that its funds were not in any difficulty. Such was not the case for the hospital, the Gilbert Home, and the residuary trust, however. Securities totaling over $40,000 were missing, $18,300 of them the property of the hospital which, despite the fact that its Treasurer was bonded for $10,000, stood to lose a large portion of its equity. Further investigation revealed that Mr. Marsh had invested heavily in Diamond Match Company on margin and had been caught up in the stock market panic of 1896, and his Boston brokers were demanding settlement. Doubtless with every intention of soon replacing what he regarded as borrowed funds, he covered his immediate cash requirements with bearer bonds entrusted to his custody.

It was learned later that several estates for which he was trustee or executor also suffered losses. A remarkable statement in the *Times* reported that "the representatives of the estates held Mr. Marsh in such esteem that they decline to further smirch his memory by divulging anything regarding any shortages which may have resulted from his acts." It did disclose, however, that "the Dr. Charles H. Hildreth estate was entirely wiped out [and] there is no doubt that there is a large shortage." In closing its coverage of the affair the newspaper editorialized in the style of the day over "the sad termination of what promised to be an unusually successful career [which] carries with it a warning to every man, young or old, who holds a position of trust, to beware of the first step in a career which, if persisted in, will, sooner or later, blast their prospects and bring ruin in their path."

A terse note in the hospital cash journal closed the matter. On a page headed "George J. Marsh (Loss by his defalcation)" entries from October 1896 to February 1897 showed $10,000 received from the bondsman and the loss of $11,600 from three separate railroad bonds, written off as "taken for his own use." Other than that, except for later replacing him on the Board and

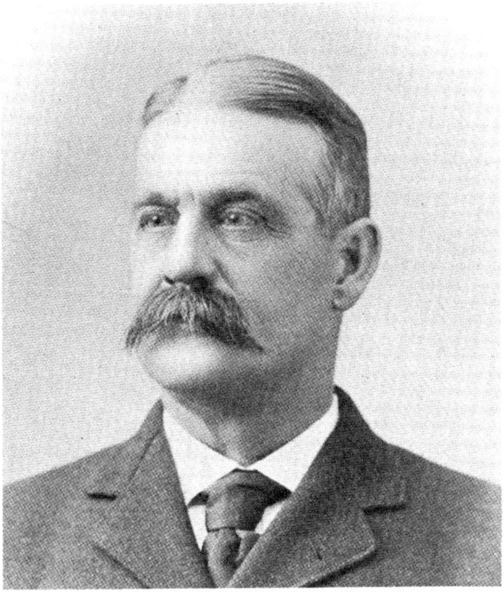

Charles H. Pew was elected to the presidency in 1897 shortly before the new hospital was to open.

as Treasurer, the matter was relegated to history, and only a 1901 entry for $1,000 received "on account" from the Marsh estate mentions the episode further.

The general desire to forgive and forget notwithstanding, the hospital had been severely damaged. It had lost over 10 percent of its total funds when well into a costly construction program, and its Trustees also faced opening in a few months with what were, at best, already limited operating funds.

President Dustin was authorized to act as Treasurer pro tem, and John Corliss was appointed Clerk. With only five active Trustees at a time when so much had to be done, "it seemed absolutely necessary to elect some person to the vacancy in the Board of Trustees who could become an active officer in the development of the work, also to elect a Treasurer . . . .and Secretary." At a special meeting of the Corporation on April 5, 1897, with only three members present, Charles H. Pew was elected Corporator, and, since he was present, he took his seat, giving the meeting its quorum. The four then elected Sylvanus Smith to the Corporation and Mr. Pew to the Board.

Mr. Dustin had earlier expressed his wish to be relieved of the presidency before the hospital opened for business. John Corliss declared himself unable to devote the time required and did in fact shortly thereafter resign from the Board, and apparently the others were unwilling to take on the responsibility. So it was that, after adjourning to a Board of Trustees meeting that April day, Charles H. Pew, the new member, was elected President.

He was almost a preordained choice, born in Gloucester in 1835 and having spent his adult life with John Pew & Son, the family fisheries firm, of which John Dustin was also a part.

Dustin was elected Clerk and the new Corporator, Sylvanus Smith, became the Treasurer, although not voted a Trustee until the next Annual Meeting. Captain Smith was described in the *Times* obituary of him in November 1916 as "the last survivor of the old-time native fish skippers." Of old Cape Ann stock, after giving up active fishing, he became one of Gloucester's business and civic leaders and was elected to two terms each in the Massachusetts General Court and State Senate, from 1892 through 1895. He was a charter incorporator of the old Gloucester Safe Deposit & Trust Company and served as its President for many years. In addition to the vessel outfitting business, Sylvanus Smith & Co., Inc., which he founded, he was President of Gloucester Net & Twine Company and Treasurer of Cape Ann Anchor Works.

By April 1897, with the new building practically complete except for furnishing, it was time to find someone to manage and staff it. The administrative head of most small hospitals at that time was the Matron, usually a nurse, responsible only to the Trustees and with complete power within the hospital, a situation often frustrating to medical staffs. Hers was an autocratic rule – hiring and firing, directing the nurses in their work and in many aspects of their personal lives, overseeing the kitchen and, at least at the Addison Gilbert Hospital, even keeping the account books.

To fill that position the Trustees hired Emma J. Gordon, then Matron at Somerville Hospital, under a two-year contract at $1,000 annually. She took charge May 1 to work under President Pew who, with Dr. Adams, was authorized as a "committee with full powers." Her first task was to hire a staff of nurses and prepare the hospital for its expected opening in August.

The Trustees also had to provide a suitable residence for the nurses, appoint and organize the Medical Staff and draw up rules and regulations. They also, with a prescience that began a tradition to continue through the years, voted on April 29 "that Mr. Rogers be authorized to prepare a circular letter soliciting contributions for support which shall be sent to former residents and natives of Gloucester who may feel a desire to assist the hospital in any way."

The regulations prepared by the Trustees, with counsel from Dr. Garland, were approved in June. They governed the in-hospital activities of the Medical Staff, which was to be overseen by a Medical Board of three physicians appointed by the Trustees and working under their governance. The Staff was classified as consulting physicians, visiting staff and assistant physicians with rotating assignment to the Ward Service. They also detailed the responsibilities of the Matron and the terms under which patients were to be admitted.[4]

Essential to any hospital is the presence in the community of a solid corps of good physicians who have the confidence and respect of its citizens. Gloucester had such a corps. Its dean was the venerable Joseph Garland, and its accepted leader was his son Everett. Dr. Everett Garland, long a proponent of a hospital for Gloucester and surely influential in Addison Gilbert's decision, had worked with the Trustees in planning it. Like the rest of the community, they respected his influence and experience, and he was their obvious and logical choice as Chairman of the Medical Board.[5] Dr. Thomas Conant, the only other appointee to that original Board, was joined a year later by Dr. Edward S. Eveleth as the required third member. They were joined by the eleven men and one woman described in the prologue, all of whom became the active Medical Staff. The senior Dr. Garland, then approaching eighty, was appointed consulting physician as the Staff's sixteenth member.

It was Miss Gordon's assignment to enlist the nursing staff. For this she had no choice but to go off-Cape, since there were few if any "trained" nurses here. Any such would have been employed in physician's offices or doing private duty for them and could be assumed to have been unwilling to join the hospital's closely supervised and hard-worked staff. She, therefore, turned to her former hospital in Somerville where, using the attractions of Cape Ann and the opportunity offered by a new hospital as bait, she was able to assemble the nucleus of her staff. Among them was a young Swede named Martin Lofquist, a male nurse and therefore a rare prize. Martin became a popular and valuable member of the team and stayed for about twenty years before leaving to become nurse-valet for John Hays Hammond, Sr.

The nursing staff was reasonably complete in June and its eight members — a head, one each for the operating and accident rooms, four female floor nurses and Martin — were ready for whatever came their way. All but Martin moved into the somewhat renovated Brown residence, located about fifty yards south from the circular drive at the front of the hospital and midway between the street and what today is called Webber House.

A nurse's life was strictly supervised in 1897. These daughters of Florence Nightingale were expected to be examples of propriety and hew to a very fine line. Few if any married, since they were expected to live in quarters provided by the hospital, taking all their meals there, and, on the rare day off, to report in to the Matron personally on their return from a day in town or, on Sunday, from their few hours off to attend church. They were

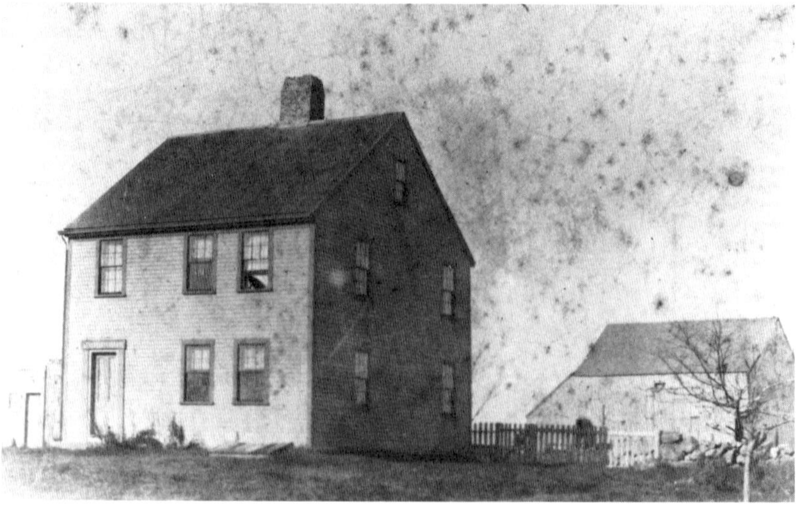

The old Brown farmhouse housed the first nursing staff until a new nurses' residence was built in 1903.

expected to wear starched and pristine white on duty, but they were also the housekeeping crew, sweeping the floors, making the beds, cleaning up the operating rooms, serving the meals and, with all that, caring for the patients. For all this they were paid $10 per month plus room and board to start and $12 to $15 after a year of experience. The head nurse was paid $30 per month.

By late spring of 1897 the bricks-and-mortar phase of the work was complete and Washington Street above Meeting House Green had a new appearance, dominated by the three-story hospital building. It was the brick structure specified by Mr. Gilbert with accent trim of Cape Ann granite, which except for the entrance has remained unchanged to this day. Its upper windows looked out on a broad vista with the town to the south, the entire Cape across Dogtown Common to the east, Ipswich Bay to the north and to the west the river and the West Gloucester hills.

A *Times* reporter had a guided tour of the facility in early June. He probably arrived via the new electric car line, which passed the hospital along unpaved Washington Street en route to Lanesville, and entered over eight granite steps and under the white pillared porch to the front door.

We were welcomed by the Matron, Miss Emma J. Gordon, who escorted the party over the building. It shows on every hand the most complete, up-

to-date arrangements and has an air of comfort, bright and homelike, every room having a delightful outlook, as the situation is such that look which way you may, the prospect is charming.

The arrangements for heating and ventilation are perfect, so that a standard of heat can always be maintained. The new hospital starts out with the most favorable prospects and will fill a long-felt want and bids fair to be well-endowed as the years go by.

Our city is fortunate in having so well arranged a hospital, and the plans of the far-sighted donor have been in excellent hands, and from the fact that so many have already endowed beds and shown a personal interest in the future welfare will no doubt attract other persons of means and generous impulse.

At the right of the entrance was a reception room, which doubled as an office; connected to this, about where the Gift Shop was until 1986, was the Trustees' Room. The Doctors' Room, entered from either the hall or the operating room area, adjoined that of the Trustees. Of this area the fireplace in the front lobby is all that survives. Across the hall, where the Coffee Shop was later located, was the two-room apartment where the Matron, by custom unmarried, lived. A dining room for use by the nurse was located just behind these rooms.

Off the hall a single wooden stairway connected all floors. Over this the nurses (probably relying heavily on Martin Lofquist) had to carry nonambulatory patients; there would be no elevator until many years later. The two patient floors each had five quite spacious rooms plus a smaller one with a single bed for paying patients or isolation. Painted wooden nameplates identified the $300 benefactor of each room. These floors also had two bathrooms with tub; there were no private baths, and even the newfangled flush toilets may have been strange to some of the patients. The second floor, primarily for paying patients, also had a sun porch looking westward. The five larger rooms on each floor had marble-mantled fireplaces, of which seven have survived intact in rooms that would be readily recognized as John Dustin, Dr. Garland, and others among their planners. A linen room completed the layout.

The other important element of the hospital was its surgical area on the first floor. En route the corridor passed the ambulance entrance, about where the elevator now hums. Down the corridor and on the right, where today we find computer territory, was the surgery with its waiting room and dispensary. An etherizing room, the main operating room and an isolation room occupied the rest of the single-story ell in space now used by the hospi-

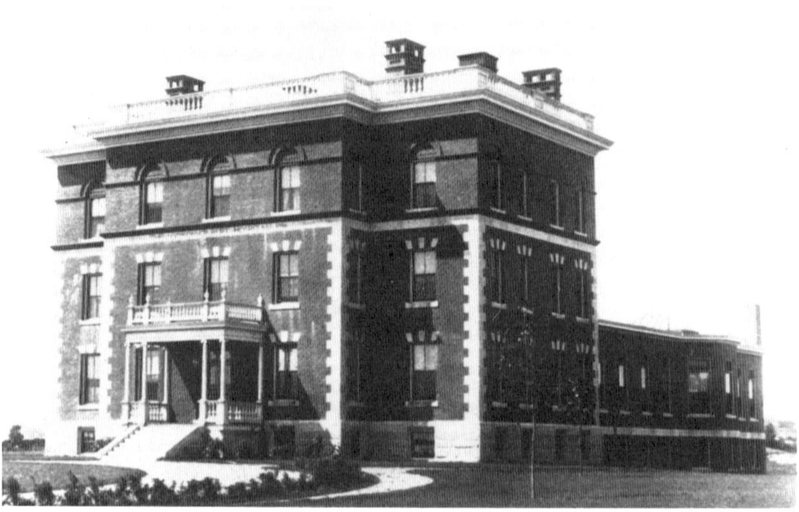

The Addison Gilbert Hospital shortly after completion of the original landscaping.

tal's financial department. Like the rest of the building, it relied on gas lighting until 1901, when the electric power line was extended from downtown. Across the corridor, now replaced by the President's office, was an open porch over which the doctors could arrive privately, leaving their teams at convenient hitching posts.

The basement contained a small kitchen, the Servants' Dining Room and an iced storeroom beneath the Matron's apartment and the Nurses' Room. Under the Trustees Room were a dry storeroom and two coal bins for the hospital's fuel supply. The ground floor of the ell, today's kitchen, housed the boiler room and laundry.

The new hospital had cost $51,061.38 including land, architectural plans for $2,067, the building with heat and plumbing at $35,953.81 and the balance for such miscellaneous items as a domed cesspool, walls, fences and minimal landscaping. For equipment, furnishings and supplies, renovations in the old farmhouse to make it usable as nurses' quarters, and operating expenses, the Trustees found themselves with about $37,000 left of Addison Gilbert's bequest.

Gifts were the factor that could make the difference. An accounting and receipt dated February 14, 1898 to Female Charitable Association lists the furnishings for the Abbie I. Sawyer Room at a total of $71.98, for which the room was supplied with bed, mattress, two pillows, two straight chairs and a rocker, wardrobe, screen, bureau, washstand and hospital stand. The dollar bought a lot in those days, but with funds getting tight regardless, it would have been forbearance indeed if the conversation in the Trustees' Room didn't occasionally include some mention of the suddenly departed George Marsh and the funds that departed with him.

NOTES

[1]These men and all who followed them as Trustees of Addison Gilbert Hospital are listed in Appendix E.

[2]See Appendix A for further details of the legal problems.

[3]Dr. Jones was in Gloucester from 1890 to 1897, when his practice ceased.

[4]See Appendix B for the complete Regulations of the Staff.

[5]See Appendix I for a list of Dr. Garland's successors through the years.

2

Open and Functioning

WITH THE HOSPITAL ready to open the Trustees and Medical Staff faced for the first time the matter of its effective operation. It is important to understand these two groups in order to appreciate some of the problems that lay ahead.

As governing body, the Trustees were the final authority. They were sincere, earnest men, but they lacked hospital experience and had no form of guidance in their task of managing such an institution. Obviously intelligent as successful businessmen, they could only rely on that intelligence and their common sense in doing their best to cope with a new public responsibility. They were on their own and would make mistakes, but gradually they would gain experience and, some years in the future, would eventually have outside guidance.

The Medical Staff, on the other hand, consisted of men trained to the work they had to do. Equally sincere, they too had a public responsibility, coupled with strong convictions as to what they required to meet that responsibility. They could not be blamed for sometimes becoming frustrated at the problems of the Trustees, but through sharing experiences with their peers at medical society meetings they knew they were not alone in this frustration. Other outside guidance was available to them through the American Medical Association and, later, the American College of Surgeons.

Between these two groups stood the Matron, legally responsible to the Trustees, but also needing to work with the Staff. Hers was the task of supervising the hospital's day-to-day operation while trying to please two very diverse bodies. Torn between the governing board on one side and the working doctors on the other , she must have felt at times that she could please neither. Only rarely did the two groups to whom she answered communicate directly, always going through her or communicating in writing — a fact that made the Matron's work even harder.

This early period was one of learning and development for the inexperienced Trustees. It was not an easy time, and it is apparent that too few of the seven were anxious to bear a hand in the work. During those early years the Board often held meetings with only two or three present. Although guidance and supervision of the Matron was a major responsibility and one or two Trustees visited the hospital to consult with her almost daily, it was usually the same ones who attended the meetings. They attempted to improve that situation in 1903, when these daily visits were allocated among the whole Board by a vote to appoint a Visiting Trustee after each monthly meeting to serve until the next session. One-man committees "with full power" were also appointed frequently, and many decisions seem to have been made on that basis.

The Board was greatly fortified in 1900 by the election of Nathaniel Babson, who soon became a leader in hospital affairs. Retired since age forty, he was a well-to-do retail merchant with energy and time plus a keen financial acumen. He was elected to the seat vacated by John Somes' resignation, and by 1904 he was so deep in the work that he was "appointed to act as managing Trustee for the remainder of the year . . . to have charge of all detail matters connected with the management of the hospital and to take the place of the visiting Trustees." He remained a leading figure in the work of the hospital until his death in 1927, one of the outstanding people who have served it.

But by the Annual Meeting of June 1906 it was apparent that even with a Nat Babson, seven Trustees were not enough. The bylaws were amended to permit an increase, and six new members were added to supplement the six then serving, President Pew having died that spring.

The First Patients

The hospital was scheduled to open in July 1897, but it was ready in June when a young fishermen named Dennis McNeary was brought in with fractures of the arm and pelvis, major injury to the brachial plexis, his left arm paralyzed, severe facial lacerations and heavy bruises. Rumor had it that Dennis had been imbibing at Howard Blackburn's saloon, a rumor vigorously denied by Mr. Blackburn, who was already in some difficulty with the city's licensing authorities. In any case, considerably influenced by John

Barleycorn, Dennis was en route to his Manchester boardinghouse walking the railroad track when he was struck by the engine of a train coming down from Boston, about midafternoon.

Ready or not, the hospital had its first case, and Dr. J. E. Garland his first hospitalized patient. Nursing records of the case have survived through the years on plain ruled notebook paper with penciled columns. The medical record of the case, kept in accordance with the rules, was only slightly more formal and filled the first three pages of Volume I of the handwritten record book. Dr. Garland's record of the case was brief by today's standard, but each detail of treatment is carefully entered. After a month, on July 9, he wrote: "Electrical exam. of muscles give partial reaction of degeneration of muscles of arm, those muscles supplied by the inner and posterior cord, i.e. the extensor of the arm and hand, reacting only feebly to strong stimuli." A few days later he noted, "Muscles react better, especially the flexor muscles." By July 19, five weeks after his accident, Dennis was deemed "well except for paralysis of arm [and] recommended for transfer to [the state operated poorhouse at] Tewksbury. [Patient] refuses transfer and is discharged on own responsibility."

The second patient, a forty-five year-old housewife, came in on June 15 with what was diagnosed as an inflammatory breast cancer, on which Dr. Garland performed the indicated surgery. Dr. Percy Procter is recorded as making a "microscopic examination of tumor." By the end of the month three more patients had been admitted; if a formal opening had ever been considered, all thought of it was abandoned. In a way it seems unfortunate that, after ten years of labor and considerable trauma, there wasn't some form of celebration with perhaps speeches and a ribbon cutting. If there was it was never mentioned, but perhaps just being ready at last to serve the people of Gloucester was enough.

Financial Problems and Support

The Trustees faced problems from the start of operations. The most serious were financial and rested on their literal interpretation of a sentence in the Gilbert will: "It is my wish to found . . . . a free hospital, for the purpose of furnishing gratuitously to citizens and inhabitants of that city medical and surgical treatment therein." He modified the words "free" and "gratuitously" a few paragraphs later by specifying that compensation should be made by those "who shall be able to make such compensation."

Already short of operating funds, the Trustees only exacerbated the problem as they leaned toward free care plus a general lack of decisiveness in collecting from those who could be expected to pay. They also perhaps did not set fees high enough, at $10 a week for ward patients able to pay and ranging from $15 to $25 weekly for others. Costs per average patient were calculated at "about $14 per week – a fair average for a cottage hospital."

During the first two years there was a cushion in the remaining Gilbert funds along with early gift support, but in May 1899 the Treasurer told the Board that "about $450 of the March accounts are still unpaid for want of funds. The amount due . . . over and above cash on hand will be about $700 [and it is] estimated that there is due for board and attendance from public and private sources about $800." By the end of June, when the fiscal year closed, he showed a balance of cash on hand of $188. It could and did get worse; the monthly reports of the Board occasionally showed a negative balance, and by the close of 1903, with the national economy suffering a recession, the *Annual Report* indicated a cash balance of $43.03.

Such results were probably to be expected when income from fees and charges rarely exceeded the total from all other sources. But although they were separate from operations, some remedies were available. Financial support was stimulated from whatever sources were at hand.

Almost every annual report carried a sentence or two on the subject of gifts. The end page of each issue was devoted to a listing of "How to Help the Hospital," together with a reminder of the importance of bequests and offering the proper form for making them. The modern "wish list" had its precursor in 1900 when the Trustees "expressed their wish that plans for the future extensions of the wards and buildings should be determined upon that could be examined by any person desiring to donate money for a building."

In December 1900 Nathaniel Babson reported on his "examination of bills and accounts due from patients," with the result that starting "Jan. 1, 1901, bills [shall] be rendered as due and collected weekly." Mr. Babson was put in charge of collections. The Board even "sold the standing grass to Osman Babson for twenty dollars" that summer.[1] In 1903 President Charles Pew offered "to make up the increase personally if necessary" so Miss Carrie Davis, the Head Nurse, could have a raise in pay. The next year, with uncollected accounts standing at $1000, the Trustees voted to cancel the hospital's subscription to *The Medical and Surgical Journal* as "an unnecessary expense."

Much of the early giving to the hospital was designated for the support of free care. The Trustees had decided before it opened that a gift of $5000 would be required to endow a free bed permanently, and that one of $300 would cover such a bed for a year. This was the standard used by Allan Rogers in his gift solicitation letter of April 1897 and in subsequent requests made via the newspaper and in the hospital's annual report. The endowment of a free-care bed also carried with it the right to designate admission to it, a provision then common among hospitals that was discarded a few years later.

Public support was more generous during the first three or four years of operation than it was after the opening enthusiasm waned. Free-bed gifts totaled $25,400 between 1897 and 1907, with half being received during the first two years. Other gifts totaled just over $16,000, and eight bequests added $60,000 as endowment. One of them, by Benjamin Corliss of $5000 for a free bed, had been received in 1895 and thus has the honor of being the first recorded after that of Addison Gilbert.

Individuals and groups sponsored events of all types. One children's group that called itself "The Little Helpers" raised more than $500 over a three-year period. Summer residents, particularly in the popular Magnolia resort and at Eastern Point, were also active in sponsoring annual fairs. The Magnolia regulars at the Oceanside Hotel endowed one of the permanent free beds in this way and later supported the Ambulance Fund.

There were spasmodic attempts by individuals to enlist support among the fishermen, but they were largely fruitless. Some of the vessels and their crews made gifts for special events, and the larger processors, especially those whose owners were involved at the hospital, were generous. One lady, wishing to remain anonymous, contributed annually "in memory of poor fishermen" and gave $50 to $100 for years even after she moved away from Gloucester, a loyal record that continued until her death in 1925.

The Volunteers

Another source of assistance lay in volunteers. The first such group to come forward was the Addison Gilbert Hospital Aid Association, with twenty-six men comprising its membership. Established "to assist the Addison Gilbert Hospital by raising a fund to further its charitable purposes," its first meeting was held October 20, 1897, when the members elected its organizers, Freeman D. Hodson and Thomas J. Carroll, as President and Vice-President. Hodson was an East Gloucester grocer then serving the last of three terms as city Alderman, and Carroll, then cutting shed foreman for Slade Gorton, was also an Alderman. Tom Carroll, who later was made a partner in Slade Gorton Company, went on to become President and Chairman of Gorton-Pew Fisheries Company as well as President of Cape Ann Fisheries, Producers Fish Company and Gloucester National Bank. He was a hospital Trustee from 1930 until his death in 1947.

Their plan was to reach out to the community through the various fraternal organizations for cooperation in organizing events, the chief of which was to be an annual Thanksgiving Night Ball. The first of these, held in 1897, was given a rave review by the *Times*, which described it as "the largest indoor gathering of Gloucester citizens of which there is any record." With attendance estimated at 1,750 it taxed the capacity of the City Hall Auditorium, then the city's home for social, athletic and political affairs. Two policemen at each door were kept busy with a roisterous but apparently orderly crowd. It would seem that, although no problems were reported and everyone was said to have enjoyed the affair, the crowd that year discouraged future attendance, as the next two balls were about half that size. All were gala dance parties, however, and combined raised $2403 for the benefit of the hospital.

Despite its ambitions and its party-organizing abilities, the Aid Association had a very short life. Its twelfth and final meeting was held March 14, 1900, when it turned $600 over to the hospital, leaving $3.46 in its treasury. The *Annual Report* of 1901 described its demise: "The Aid Association has not been active for the past year, doubtless feeling that . . . the Ladies would afford . . . all the opportunity of contributing to the work that was judicious or necessary."

The ladies responded enthusiastically. First proposed by the men's group as "The Ladies Gilbert Hospital Association," which would work under it, the women decided that they could do better on their own. And so it was that on October 13, 1898 eighty-four ladies met at the Butler's Point (Bay View) home of Mrs. Jonas French to form "a permanent organization." The Ladies Aid Society, as it was called that day, met again two weeks later when its members adopted a constitution and bylaws and renamed themselves the Women's Auxiliary to the Addison Gilbert Hospital. A year later its membership stood at 462 dedicated women working together to assist their hospital by raising money and promoting goodwill on its behalf.

Miscellaneous fund-raising activities enabled them to make their first contribution in May 1899, with the Trustees extending thanks "to the Ladies Auxiliary Association for the timely contribution of $500 toward expenses." This sum came from a variety of sources, not least among them being gifts left with calling cards on January 1, 1899, at which time "nine ladies opened their houses for New Year's Receptions." Annual Donation Days also brought in collections of home preserves, linens and other items deemed useful at the hospital.

The infant Auxiliary, however, faced a crisis before it was six months old. At issue was a further literal interpretation of the Gilbert will by the Trustees, namely: "to admit as patients therein such citizens and inhabitants of the city, and . . . such others as [the Trustees] may see fit." They took this

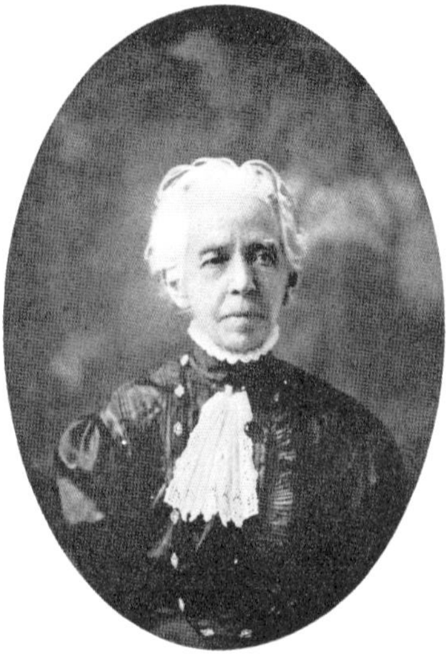

Maria Bray was the second president of the Women's Auxiliary and served it well for fifteen years. Strong-willed and articulate during a time when women hesitated to speak out, she was a powerful representative for the Auxiliary at trustees' meetings.

as limiting its use to Gloucester residents, an interpretation meaning that Rockporters must either be cared for at their homes or make the trip to Beverly or Salem.

Mrs. French, elected as the Auxiliary's first President, was well aware of the issue, since some of her husband's Cape Ann Granite Company quarries were located at Rockport. She had also recruited several Rockport women to membership, and with their backing she raised the question of Rockport's exclusion from what she and they saw as Cape Ann's hospital.

A conference with the Trustees brought the matter into the open in April 1899, when "the Secretary was instructed to write Mrs. Jonas H. French . . . that according to the terms of the founder's will we cannot admit cases outside of Gloucester except in emergency and by special arrangement with the Trustees." Mrs. French, refusing to accept this situation, resigned as President and took the Rockport members with her. The Board maintained its position in spite of the Auxiliary's continuing pleas for a policy change, and Gloucester and Rockport continued to go their separate ways on the matter. The impasse forced the Auxiliary to reorganize; Mrs. Maria H. Bray was persuaded to take the presidency six months later and occupied that office with distinction for the next fifteen years.

The revived Auxiliary made its first report of activities in the *Annual Report* of 1900. Each monthly meeting at the Washington Street Grand Army Hall featured a program to educate and entertain the membership. Through these they learned about "Wives, Widows and Wills"; "Parliamentary Law";

"Day Nurseries"; "Charity, Club, Hospital"; "Woman to Woman"; "Hypnotism"; "Tuberculosis"; "The Scenery of New England and Why It Is So"; "Celia Thaxter and Her Writings"; "One Year Upon the Mediterranean"; "Travels Through Spain" and, appropriately, "Philanthropy, Its Pain and Pleasure." The report added that "meetings are well attended."

It also recognized the work of the Entertainment Committee for the 1899 "Colonial Entertainment" at City Hall, which made $116.25, and the 1900 "New Year's Reception netting $220 in spite of a severe snowstorm which made traveling almost impossible." Also among its first year's support were "articles and money furnished the Hospital: bottle of brandy, 8 face cloths; 12 night shirts; 8 screen covers; 6 pieces [bolts?] of cheese cloth; 4 woolen sheets; 12 surgeon's gowns; 12 bottles of preserves; porter; palm leaf fans; 4 dozen fringed napkins; one gallon each of brandy, whisky and sherry; $15 and bills sent from the hospital to the amount of $113.74 have been paid."

Although they may not have done so at first, the Trustees soon came to appreciate the importance of an ambitious Women's Auxiliary (even though they at first weren't sure of its name) and didn't hesitate to call on it for help. In July 1899 they received "$1,000 from the Ladies Auxiliary Society, a sum just needed to pay the outstanding bills of the past financial year."

Nor were the ladies hesitant about conferring with the Trustees. In the spring of 1900 President Bray led a delegation to the Board with a proposal "for use of the grounds for an elaborate social festivity sometime in July." This became the fabulously successful *Fête Champetre* which took place on July 10, 1900. The committee arranged twenty-two booths and exhibits representing and selling the goods of many nations, staffing them throughout a perfect Cape Ann summer day with 245 women workers and twelve "boys attired in white suits," who ran the peanut booth.

Admiral William T. Sampson and Lieutenant Governor John L. Bates were escorted to the grounds by a parade from City Hall that featured Clark's Military Band and Company G, Eighth Regiment, under command of Captain Edward J. Horton. Mayor George E. Merchant surely summed up the feelings of all as he officially opened the Fête: "The ladies, God bless 'em, have labored as in no other cause, and they richly deserve the success which I feel assured will come to them."

How right he was! The affair raised $4,950.63, which can be extrapolated into something well over $50,000 in today's dollars. The Fête Champêtre was followed by other such events: a Japanese Tombola at City Hall in April 1902 netted $3394.63; a Swastika Carnival was followed in 1906 by a controversial Pop Concert planned for New Year's Eve at City Hall. This was a joint effort by the Auxiliary and various church women's groups, but the latter felt "Pop" music too indecorous and withdrew. The Auxiliary's Ways and Means Committee resigned with angry tears, and New Year's Eve 1906 began to look like Custer's Last Stand. Calmer heads prevailed, however, and a Colonial Reception, presumably more suitable, was hosted instead.

Historian Joseph Garland describes another source of funds in his biography of Howard Blackburn, *Lone Voyager*. As told by Mr. Garland's grandmother, Mrs. J. Everett Garland," [Mr. Blackburn] also presented the Women's Auxiliary . . . with a large jar full of pennies that had been accumulating on the bar all year. The ladies, wearing white gloves lest they be contaminated by germs, counted the Blackburn coppers one by one; there were 7,181 of them."

All these efforts helped make it possible for the Yankee banker Trustees to avoid the dread necessity of dipping into endowment principal during those first difficult years. And the Auxiliary had begun a tradition of support that would seldom flag as they carried forward Mrs. Bray's exhortation to her fellow members — "Let us not be weary in well-doing."

Public Relations

A further function of the Trustees involved communication with the public. The people of Gloucester obviously looked on their hospital as above reproach, and there was no unfavorable publicity involving it; in fact there was little in the newspaper about it at all. In 1906 the Board appointed one of its members, Fred A. Shackelford, "to interview the newspapers in regard to news items," and he was able to generate some interest in that way. But for the most part the hospital was left to go its own way, uncriticized and unpublicized.

The issuance of printed annual reports was seen as another way to share news of what the hospital was doing. The first was released in June 1898 and established a format that endured for many years. It listed the Members of the Corporation, the Board of Trustees and the Medical Staff and included reports by the Board, the Treasurer, the Matron, the Nursing School, and, starting in 1899, the Auxiliary. Also included were detailed statistics covering "The Work of the Hospital." These tabulated the medical and surgical cases treated, listing utilization figures and demographic details of those admitted, giving age, sex, occupation and birthplace. Early issues also contained lists of donors along with the items contributed, and later a listing of Training School graduates was maintained. However, the reports only said what the public was supposed to hear, and with 500 maximum printed each year they didn't receive wide circulation. Nevertheless, they are revealing of the past and are especially helpful in their tables of financial and patient statistics.

The School of Nursing

A problem facing all hospitals at the time was an inability to find enough trained nurses. Trained nurses were virtually nonexistent prior to 1870, and until the first training schools were established in 1873 hospital nursing was considered a menial, unskilled occupation. Although at first resisted by the medical profession out of an unjustified, perhaps jealous, fear that educated nurses would not do as they were told, the training concept spread rapidly. By 1900 there were more than four hundred such schools in the United States, the majority of them hospital based.

Since having its own school was about the only way a community hospital could obtain nurses, most found it expedient to establish one. The Addison Gilbert was no exception, and at a Trustee meeting in October 1897 the "matter of opening a training school for nurses was brought up and thought to be necessary in the near future." The near future came quickly and, since her duties included the superintendency of the training-school-to-be, Miss Gordon began to recruit students.

The young women of the area were apparently eager to join the profession. She had thirty applicants, of whom she could accept seven for the scheduled two-year program and twelve more for a probationary period, following which they could be reexamined for enrollment. Under the rules of the Training School "candidates will be received as accommodations in the Home permit. They must be between the ages of 21 and 35 years; must have received at least a good common school education and must present certificates of good character and health."

The Medical Staff appears to have cooperated generously in the teaching, its members regularly presenting lectures and demonstrations. Textbooks and manuals of nursing, plus hands-on work under the Matron and Head Nurse, bolstered the curriculum, which covered anatomy, physiology, hygiene, disease, surgery and obstetrics along with such essentials as dressings, use of catheter and enema, working with helpless patients, cooking and record keeping. Inevitably the "pupil nurses" were also called upon to perform the housekeeping chores and other unwelcome duties of the regular staff nurses. They were paid $9 per month during their first year of study and $12 thereafter.

Of the seven students accepted for study when the school opened early in 1898, Mary M. Brown and Laura M. Hubley completed the course in May

1899 and were awarded their diplomas at the first graduation ceremony, held November 22, 1899. Dr. J. E. Garland and Vice-President Sylvester Cunningham addressed the small assembly, the Matron passed out the pins, and the school was embarked on a path that it would follow for the next half-century. Over the years it would grow in size and in depth of curriculum, changing to a three-year program in 1903 but remaining, as it began, an adjunct of the hospital that converted young women into trained, and later registered, nurses — twenty-nine of them by 1907.

Nurses' Residence

It soon became obvious that the relatively small rehabilitated farmhouse, which a few years later would be sold and removed, would not allow the nursing staff and school to expand as they should. Grace E. Pillsbury, by then the Matron, wrote in her first annual report in June 1900: "We could do much toward reducing the expenses of the Hospital if we had more room for nurses and thus be able to have more nurses in the Training School. [Also] as we are now situated, we are often unable to provide nurses in private families when called upon to do so."

In a coincidence of good timing the Trustees were told in November 1900 that "a gift of $5,000 was in prospect [and it is] the wish of the donor that the money be used for the construction of a building of just that cost." Dr. Garland, who was instrumental in obtaining the gift, wanted a contagious ward but was persuaded by the Trustees that a nurses' residence was of first priority. A month later architect Ezra Phillips had completed plans for a residence to be erected "on the Ferry Lane side of the Main Hospital building." The donor, by then revealed as Mrs. Fred A. (Mabel) Barker, the wife of Dr. Garland's kitchen table anesthetist, agreed, and construction of the home was scheduled for spring.

Mrs. Barker, who came to the rescue so fortuitously, is described by her cousin, Alfred Mansfield Brooks, in *Gloucester Recollected* as "frail in health and protected on every hand by her devoted husband. . . . Her attitude toward life was unbelievably Victorian, and every propriety had to be observed in her presence. At the same time she was plagued by a sense of humor which found amusing things which should have shocked her. She was the descendant of an old Gloucester family."

The plans called for a clapboarded frame building of four floors, including the basement. A covered porch was to span the entire front, and a balustraded widow's walk on the main roof would match that on the hospital. The first floor had six rooms, designated as parlor, reception room, library,

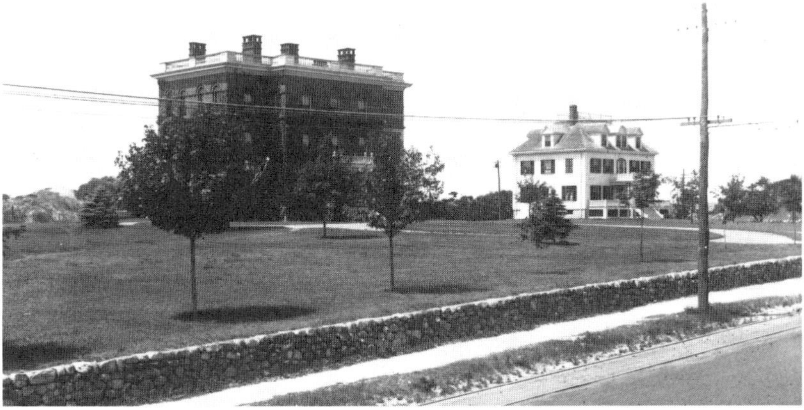

The white clapboard nurses' residence shown here in 1913 was repainted brick red a short time later to better match the hospital.

lecture room and two classrooms. On each of the two upper floors were eight bedrooms with a common bath; with some of the dormitory rooms able to take two beds, there would be space to house twenty-four nurses and students. A lack of shelter to and from the hospital was remedied some ten years later, when a tunnel was added to connect the basements.

When the bids came in, the low one by John W. Day exceeded the funds available by $276 and, with no money to spare, the committee was instructed "to make such deductions as will bring Mr. Day's figures to approximately $5,000." By eliminating the porch roof except for a canopy over the door and removing one of the two dormers on each end of the roof, thus cutting two rooms on the third floor, the figure was met.

In December 1901 the building was almost ready for use. It had been designated The Abbie L. Davis Home for Nurses, in memory of Mrs. Barker's mother, and was dedicated that month at a ceremony to which, through an inadvertent but dreadful faux pas, the Barkers had not received an invitation. Alfred Brooks recounts how they told him "with great merriment, of sitting quietly at home during the dedication," and we can only imagine the red-faced Trustee who must have delivered the apologies of the Board to the very proper Mrs. Barker. In any event, the breach of propriety was forgiven. Mr. Barker was elected a Trustee in 1903 and later served ten distinguished years as President, from 1914 to 1923.

It is perhaps appropriate here to put to rest two legends that have persisted through the years about the residence. One, that the old farmhouse was incorporated into the newly constructed building, is obviously apochryphal. The other, related to it, is the claim by some of its former residents that the ghost of Jonathan or Eben Brown stalked its halls with imagined bumps and groans. This can now be seen as highly unlikely, since the old house was some distance away and disappeared completely when it was no longer needed.

One other construction project was undertaken during these earliest years. By 1901 it had become evident that the laundry was too small. Without space in the main building to house a larger one, the Auxiliary promised the approximately $3,000 required to erect a separate building. Completed in December 1903 at a cost of $3,349 plus equipment, it was turned over to the Board at a special meeting at which "Mrs. Maria Bray, President, having been presented with the keys and documents, delivered them to Mr. Pew with her usual pleasing mien and apt remarks."

Medical Matters

The Medical Staff meanwhile was kept on a tight rein by its Medical Board Chairman, Dr. J. Everett Garland. A man of strong convictions who could be forcefully outspoken if need be, he had the respect of his colleagues as a skilled physician and surgeon. With his Harvard and European training, he would have been an asset to the staff of any hospital and, had he chosen to practice in Boston, would have been a prime candidate as professor at any of the area's medical schools. Under his leadership the Staff and Trustees maintained a mutually supportive relationship throughout this critical period.

The equipment they were given was simple, but reasonably up to the state of the art for the times. Roentgen's 1895 discovery that a mysterious variation of cathode rays could penetrate flesh to make shadowy pictures of bones and the body's inner structure was still a medical novelty. Medical science took it seriously from the beginning, however, and once it had been proved out in Boston Dr. Garland made sure his hospital had it. The first such device here, battery powered, was in service shortly after the hospital opened, but by 1901 the Trustees were made aware that "the physicians are anxious for a new X-ray machine, the present one not being adequate at any time." Early the next year a new machine, paid for by the Auxiliary, was installed and met the need for the next several years. Diagnosis of tumors, gallstones, kidney stones and tuberculosis; barium examination of the intestinal tract; and, of course, study of fractures were then made more accurately, although

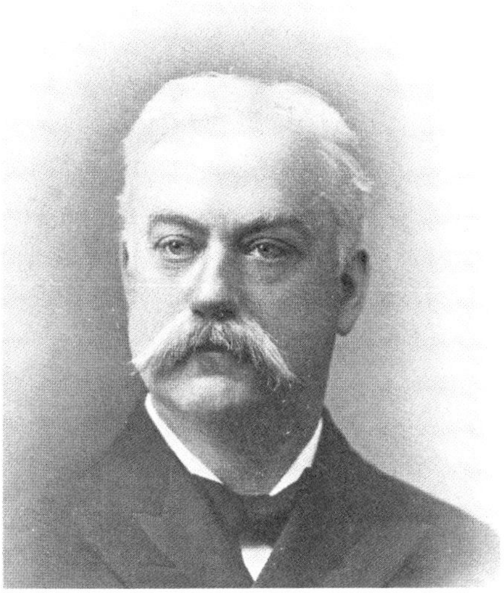

Dr. J. Everett Garland was a key figure in the early years of the hospital. His death in December, 1907 was a turning point in the institution's history.

those early machines, requiring long exposure times and often offering fuzzy pictures, were a far cry from modern radiology.

The outpatient department was elevated to a more formal status, with rules for its use issued in 1901. These established parameters for treatment there and set fees ranging "from 10 to 50 cents, according to work done or circumstances of patient"; an X-ray cost $2. A pathology laboratory was installed in 1901, but since its work was handled by out-of-town consultants, it remained a small and ineffective operation, relying on their attendance and on their home hospitals for study of the specimens.

The hospital had its own ambulance service, begun in 1898 with the purchase of a horse-drawn enclosed wagon for $545. David Hilton was appointed to "take care of [it and be] ready night and day for any call . . . without expense to the hospital." The operation was underwritten by a special Ambulance Fund established by ten donors and added to by others over the years, and except for upkeep, its only problem seems to have been heating it in the winter. Hilton and Frank H. Walker, (another volunteer, who replaced Hilton on his death in 1904) were good recruiters and as many as ten drivers were involved during the period. Among them these volunteers logged between 100 and 150 trips a year.

The 1902 request of the Medical Staff for a tennis court at the hospital comes under the subject of "doctors at play." In May of that year the Trustees "voted to grant to Drs. Logan, Egan, Moore and Cook the priviledge

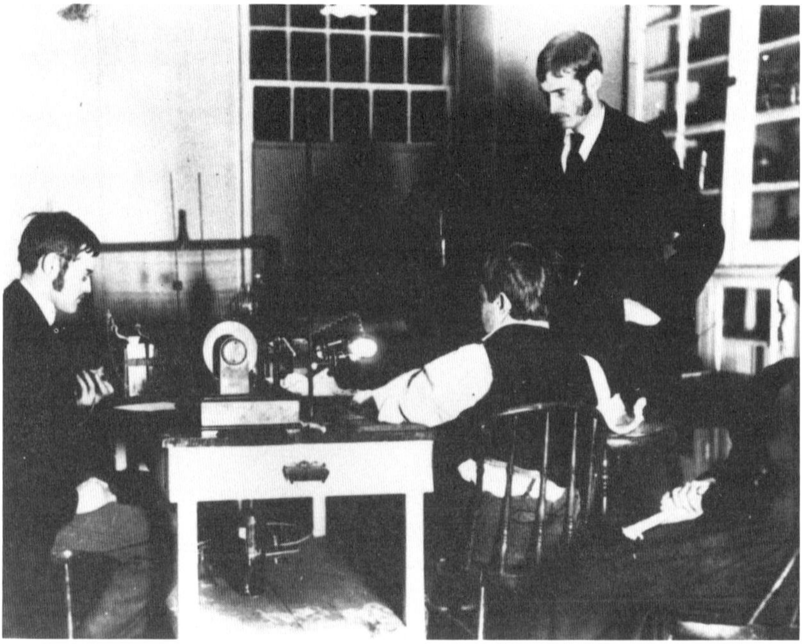

The first diagnostic X-ray in the United States was taken at the Dartmouth Medical School on February 2, 1896. The earliest equipment at AGH was similar to that shown here.

[*sic*] of maintaining at their own expense a tennis court at rear of hospital for use of physicians and nurses associated with the Hospital exclusively." The court, located in the shadow of the large rock formation west of the hospital, remained for many years until expansion required the space.

Early statistics show that in the hospital's first full year there were 113 patients admitted, with another sixty-three treated as outpatients. By the end of 1907 the hospital had admitted a total of 2,331 and treated 1,138 in the outpatient department. Surgical cases were dominant during the first seven years, but by 1905 medical cases were being cared for in almost equal numbers. Men outnumbered women on a 3:2 ratio during the first few years, but by 1905 women had caught up.

Patients unable to pay were placed on the wards, a term used universally at that time to reflect their status as wards of the Trustees while in the hospital. Ward Service by the physicians was given gratis, and, though each doctor rotated on and off the service every six months and served only two months at a time, it was not popular. Those doing the most surgery perhaps accepted it best as it helped them to keep their skills sharp, but by and large Ward Service was another ongoing headache.

Records also show that 328 of those admitted during the first ten years were fishermen – not surprising in a town where that was the principal industry. Only the records for the first five months, July through October 1897, are such that diagnoses can be tied to occupations, and we therefore cannot determine what brought them to the hospital after those months. Three of the eight admitted then had fractured ankles, two of which were broken ashore. There were two with severe respiratory problems, one suffering delirium tremens, an ulcer case and one with a congenital condition. It is hard to make a case that fishermen suffered more or even different ills from the rest of the population; if they did, the facts are not revealed by the published statistics. Another fifty-two admissions were of quarrymen, an occupation where accidents could be assumed to be common, but again there is no record to permit connecting the occupation to the diagnosis.

Although the illnesses treated in-house covered a wide range, many types appeared only infrequently. Typhoid was the most prevalent, followed by pneumonia, rheumatism and neuresthenia. Since only problem obstetrical cases were admitted, maternity was not a major factor, with sixty-six births during the ten-year period, although as forty-six of them occurred after 1904, it appears likely that there was some pressure developing to admit such cases. Under hospital rules no chronic or contagious cases could be admitted. A death rate of under 10 percent also belies the then-common characterization of hospitals as the last resort, a place to go to die.

Surgically, the treatment of fractures and lacerations was the most frequent reason for admission. Cancer was treated almost solely by surgery, burns and scalds were often seen, and surgical treatment of tubercular bones, joints and organs appears with some regularity. Appendicitis was not well understood medically until about 1900, evidence of which shows in the record; during the first three years eighteen cases were diagnosed and treated, while thirty were operated on over the next two years. Many appendicitis victims before 1900 had already been ill for several days before seeing a doctor, but after that, with prompter diagnosis, the recovery rate improved markedly. By 1907 appendicitis led the list of nonaccident surgery.

The use of ether in surgery was standard by 1897, with chloroform also sometimes used. After 1897, with all major surgery being done at the hospital, doctors had been made responsible for anesthesia. Those administering it, called "etherizers," were hampered by a general lack of understanding of pulmonary physiology, with the result that "ether pneumonia" was a frequent postsurgical complication. It was not until the bronchoscope and

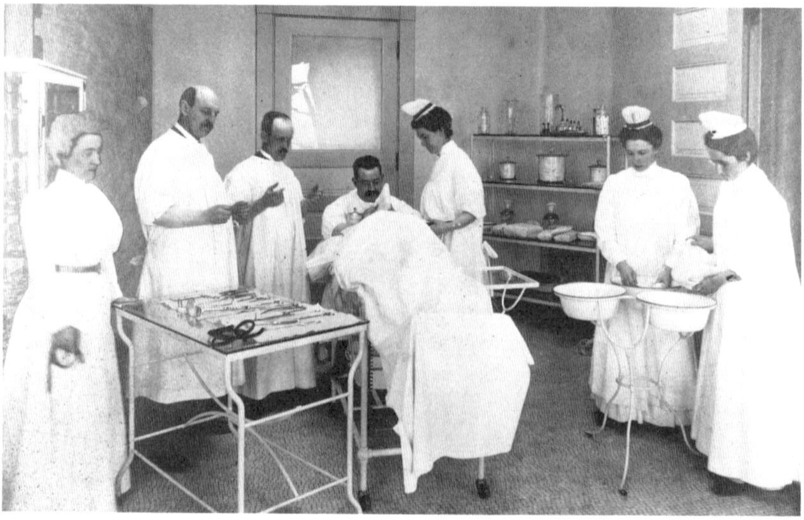

The original operating room in 1901 with doctors Hallett, Rowley, and Proctor at center stage. The stern nurse at the far left is believed to be Matron Pillsbury, and nurses Laura M. Hubley (class of 1899), Carrie W. Davis (class of 1901) and student nurse Cora A. Bassett (class of 1904) are at the right.

the use of endotracheal tubes several years later that this problem was eliminated.

The Addison Gilbert also had competition on Cape Ann during its early years from other hospitals established in Gloucester and in Rockport. In 1905 the Gloucester Emergency Hospital opened in a coverted boardinghouse on Short Street. It had a medical staff of four: Drs. Marie Benoit, Herbert Clough, Grace Harcourt and Charles M. Quimby, the latter later joining the AGH Medical Staff. It was purchased in 1909 by Dr. Alton J. Choate, who changed the name to the Gloucester Hospital and issued stock in that name and as the Cape Ann Therapeuterion for sale to Gloucester residents, who were also issued "life membership stamps" in lieu of dividends. Dr. Choate had an associate, Dr. William Hale, who maintained a Gloucester practice from 1902 to 1925, and the hospital operated until 1920, when Dr. Choate closed it suddenly, although he remained in the area until 1926 as Veterans' Bureau physician.

Choate lived and practiced in what was later rebuilt as the Lorraine Apartments. He is best remembered locally as an entrepreneur whose bubble burst when his hospital proved too small and unattractive to compete, and he could not raise the funds required by a more ambitious plan to convert the apartment building to a hospital.

Of considerably more significance, and perhaps incorrectly termed as competition, was the hospital in Rockport. The Trustees' insistence on a literal interpretation of the Gilbert will had rankled since Mrs. French first raised the question in 1899, and it came up again at a Board meeting on February 11, 1901. According to the record: "Mr. George R. Bradford came in and made some remarks about a proposed hospital in Rockport, desiring to know whether anything could be arranged in connection with this hospital so that a fund raised by Rockport people could be utilized in building a ward to this hospital and Rockport patients accommodated. . . . It was the sentiment of the Trustees that under the peculiar requirements of Mr. Gilbert's will and the conditions of the charter no such agreement could be made."[2]

Rockport's six physicians were on record in support of a hospital for the town. At the negative response by the AGH Trustees, they and other citizens obtained a charter for its establishment, even though funding it was uncertain. But Rockport also had a benefactor in the person of businessman Leander M. Haskins who had died in 1905 leaving his residence and seventy acres of land at the top of Summit Avenue to be used as a hospital and public park.

Against some opposition – including that of the Haskins heirs, who only reluctantly gave up the property – the project was approved at town meeting in 1906. The town-supported Haskins Hospital opened that October after extensive repair and rebuilding. Its small Medical Staff was headed by Dr. Augustus M. Tupper, and Mary E. Clarke, an Addison Gilbert Training School graduate of 1905, was appointed Head Nurse. Miss Clarke was at Haskins for three years, leaving to enter Tufts Medical School, where she received her degree in 1913. As Dr. Clarke she practiced in Malden, Massachusetts until her death in 1965, a fifty-year member of the Massachusetts Medical Society.

Like its larger counterpart in Gloucester, the Haskins Hospital had the support of an active Women's Auxiliary and Board of Trustees. It too suffered from financial difficulties, compounded by its small constituency, although that was partially offset by higher patient fees. But small as it was, it provided Rockport people a place to go when ill. By 1909 it was caring for about eighty of them each year.

An Era Closes

The entire community reacted in concern and grief on December 16, 1907 at news of the death of J. Everett Garland, MD, at age fifty-six. The Trustees spoke for all connected with the hospital in eulogizing him as "responsible for the harmony that has characterized the administration of the hospital, and . . . though not the elective head, he has been justly recognized as the directing head of the institution." Gloucester's Mayor decreed a day of mourning for his funeral as a mark of the community's respect for a man who had served his hometown as a member of its School Committee and a dedicated and respected physician-surgeon. The First Parish Unitarian Church was filled to capacity for the funeral, with an overflow of mourners on the grounds outside and along Middle Street.

Dr. Garland's physician son was convinced that his father died of overwork. Chronic cardiorenal problems and the morphine, he like many others of his time, used to sustain himself through arduous days, plus his intensity and forceful personality were, his family believes, also factors in his premature demise.

And with this sad event the hospital's first decade of operations came to a close — some successes, some disappointments, and at its end grief at the loss of a valued friend.

NOTES

[1]Osman Babson, a farmer dwelling a few hundred yards north of the hospital on Washington Street, was the father of veterinarian Dr. Elmer Babson and the grandfather of Dr. W. Warren Babson.

[2]G. R. Bradford was a prominent Gloucester businessman holding offices in several local industrial concerns and banks.

PART II
CONSOLIDATION AND EXPANSION 1908-1948

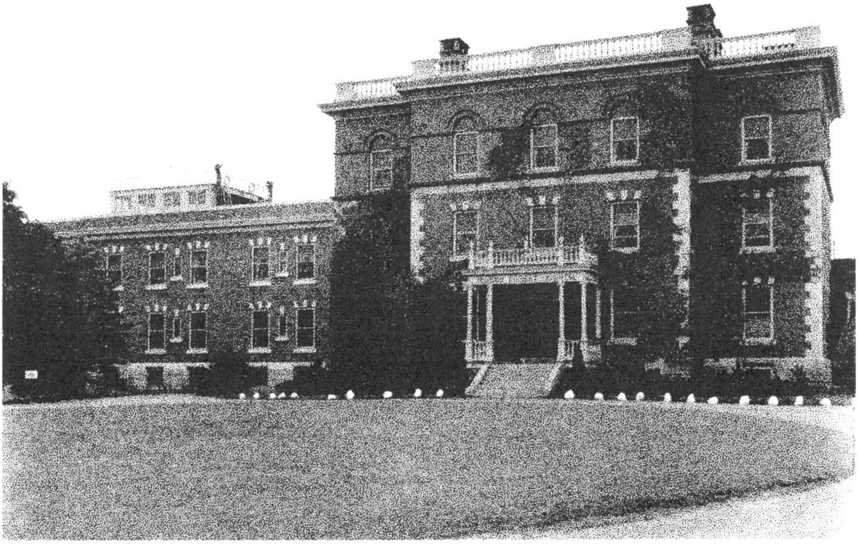

3

A Time of Testing

THE HOSPITAL entered its second decade with a changing cast of characters. By 1910 of the original Board of Trustees only Allan Rogers remained. John Dustin, his only remaining colleague on that Board, died July 1, 1909 at the age of sixty-six. In that death, said the Trustees in their tribute, "the Addison Gilbert Hospital met with the greatest loss in its history." He had served as its first President during the planning years and "then as Treasurer at a time in its management when a clear hand [*sic*] and sound judgement were greatly needed. . . . He did a man's work and earned a man's rest."

The membership of the Corporation, the equivalent of stockholders in a commercial enterprise, was being expanded also. Its only members had been the Trustees until six were added in 1900, but these had no function and never attended the Annual Meeting held each June (after a 1907 change in the bylaws, each January). Annual Meetings during those early years often failed to draw a quorum, with some adjourned as many as four times before they could be officially recorded. By 1910, however, with fourteen Trustees and twenty-six additional Corporators, this situation had been largely solved.

Medical Staff Unease

Dr. Garland's death as 1907 came to a close required new leadership of the Medical Staff. To be Medical Board Chairman, the Trustees appointed Dr. Thomas Conant, who had served as its Vice-Chairman from the beginning. A homeopathic believer, and thus of a different approach to medicine than the surgeon, Garland, he also lacked the controlling personality of his predecessor. With his appointment problems held in check earlier began to surface, most of them involving Medical Staff discipline.

One example of this can be seen in the possessiveness that physicians felt regarding their patients when the Trustees approved posting a notice in May 1908 which requested Staff members "to refrain from examining or talking to patients in the wards without the consent of the attending physician." Another disciplinary point in the same notice requested physicians "to refrain from talking over cases in the halls or corridors [since] a loud voice is readily heard by patients in the rooms." It further reminded the Staff of the regulation that called for medical rounds to be completed by 11 AM, an ongoing sore point that surfaced again in 1915 when the Medical Board once more admonished the Staff as to scheduled rounds and directed the Matron (by then known as Superintendent) to report infractions to it for follow-up.

On another occasion, when the Trustees had the temerity to suggest that additional Staff appointments might be helpful, the Staff's protectiveness led to a refusal and the promise that they would take care of the need for coverage by revamping schedules. Use of the low-cost outpatient department by those deemed able to pay a private physician at his office was another problem the Staff directed at the Medical Board, which opined that the hospital should "discourage such a practice."

These teapot-tempest issues were less important than the maintenance of medical records, a never-ending problem in hospitals everywhere. As long as Dr. Garland chaired the Medical Board, however, this had never been the case at Addison Gilbert. The handwritten ledger containing these early records is complete and well kept, consistent with standards of the time, but after his death negligence in record keeping became a problem. In December 1908 the Matron advised the Trustees that no records had been kept since August "on account of the unwillingness of the attending Physician to dictate notes to the Matron or nurses, notwithstanding the rule that requires them to keep the records of cases themselves [and] you are aware of the necessity of accurate records should any of our cases come to litigation." In strong reaction to this revelation, the Trustees directed that a letter be sent to each Staff member and to the Matron to remind them of the need for complete records. Dr. Charles H. Morrow offered his services to the Medical Board and was appointed keeper of records at a stipend "which in our opinion should be at least $100 a year."

A further Medical Staff issue involved a doctor who joined in 1905 and served off and on for the rest of a long life. The story of Scott W. Mooring,

MD began to take shape almost from the day he was appointed as a promising young surgeon, and facets surfaced at intervals thereafter. A native of Gloucester, he had been brought into this world by the senior Dr. Garland in 1877. Some twenty-eight years later, after Harvard Medical School and the still customary European study, he joined the Medical Staff headed by Dr. J. E. Garland, the son.

The newcomer was very similar to his chief in many ways. Both were outstanding physicians; both were totally confident and outspoken in their opinions. They clashed almost from the first until finally in September 1907, perhaps influenced by Dr. Garland's increasing physical problems, it was obvious that something had to give. Dr. Mooring resigned but was quietly reappointed to the Staff early in 1908, after Garland's death. He didn't get along any better with Dr. Conant, then well along in years and practicing a medical method doubtless scorned by the self-assured young Mooring.

The problem soon became obvious to others as well as Dr. Conant as on February 25, 1909, the Trustees called a special meeting with Drs. Conant and Egan "for the purpose of considering certain matters relative to the alleged misconduct of Dr. W. Scott [*sic*] Mooring at the hospital." Discussion revealed that Dr. Mooring was complaining that his orders were not carried out and that medicines were not being properly administered by the nurses. They countered that Dr. Mooring was sometimes unwilling to come to the hospital when called and gave orders by telephone that they could not legally carry out, among them the injection of salt solutions.

A frustrated Dr. Conant told the Trustees; "Dr. Mooring is a sorehead. He's looking for satisfaction and he may have his patient sue the hospital. He defies the Medical Board and even told us to go to H-- l.[*sic*]" Dr. Egan defended the nurses, who were not, he explained, experienced in giving salt solution, nor did he believe that any nurses anywhere should do so except under a physician's direct order and supervision. Dr. Conant and Trustees Dustin and Babson were appointed a committee to confer with Dr. Mooring.

They reported back a week later that he "admitted practically the charges and promised to obey the rules and conduct himself properly." Apology to the Medical Board, the Matron and the nurses was also promised, and he further agreed to send no more chronic cases to the hospital. Vice-President Barker was requested to talk to Dr. Mooring about the apologies, and nothing further was recorded about the issue. He was, however, dropped from listing as a Staff member in 1910, an ostensible loss of privileges obviously honored only in the breach, as he continued to admit and treat his patients at the hospital. In 1916, still unlisted with others of the Medical Staff in annual reports, he was again reprimanded for removing the medical records of his patients from the hospital and a year later for violating the rule requiring morning rounds between eight and eleven o'clock.

A term of service with the Army Medical Corps in World War I, during which he is said to have performed brilliantly with front-line surgical units, took him away during 1917 and 1918. He returned as a local hero, but it was another five years before he regained full status as a listed member of the Staff, in 1924. Attitudes had perhaps softened on both sides by then, but, more practically, a more formal Medical Staff structure made further disaffiliation impossible. In any case, when he applied in October 1923 for reinstatement, he was accepted. Election to the Medical Board the following year sealed the reconciliation but didn't end the controversy that constantly surrounded this fine, but enigmatic, physician and surgeon.

There were also positive aspects of the post-Garland Medical Staff. The addition of a dietitian was suggested by the Staff in 1908 although it was to be another three years before one was employed, at $400 a year. The Staff also reorganized so that the work of the Ward Service and Outpatient Department was more equably shared. The Training School curriculum was expanded and the school was operating smoothly, with good Staff participation. The rules and regulations were modified in 1908 to meet Staff requests.

One such change permitted the Staff to nominate the Medical Board for guidance of the Trustees, who retained appointive power. Fees for Outpatient Department use by doctors' private patients were raised to $5 a visit, a move designed to discourage such use and encourage visits to the physician's office instead. And, greatly to the Staff's credit, a system of peer review was initiated in 1909, which required Staff members to appear before the Medical Board periodically to report on their hospitalized cases and respond to questions about them.

Surgical consultants were recommended by the Staff and authorized by the Trustees in an effort to upgrade that service in late 1909. Drs. Charles C. Scudder and Daniel F. Jones of Boston were appointed as the first of a long line of eminent physicians and surgeons. But even this foresighted action met with criticism. A few days later the *Times* carried a long anonymous letter condemning the move as depriving local doctors of their rightful work and going so far as to imply that AGH patients would be the losers. The writer, using the name "A BOOMER," described himself as a Gloucester booster and showed considerable knowledge in suggesting reorganization along strict medical and surgical lines, "as there is at all well managed hospitals such as the Massachusetts General and Salem Hospitals [so that ward patients who] deserve as good treatment and care as private patients [could

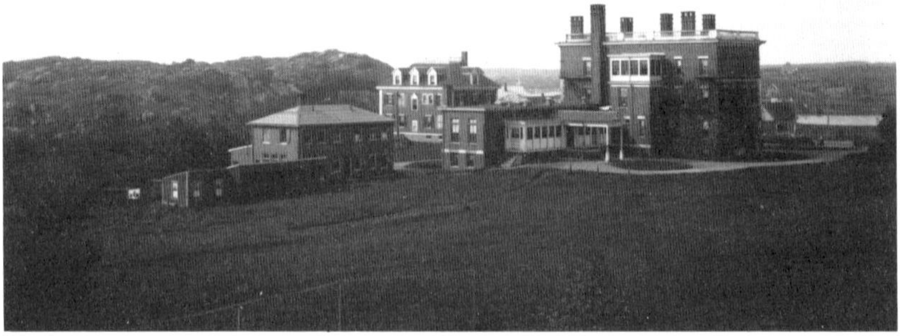

General view of AGH prior to 1915.

be] attended by our own local surgeons." The letter closed by questioning what Dr. J. E. Garland would have thought of this move, suggesting that further questions might well be raised by prospective donors in the future.

To the Trustees and Staff the letter must have sounded like the grumblings of one of their own. In any case, Trustee Nathaniel Babson appeared before the next Auxiliary meeting to defend the action, and Dr. Conant wrote a letter to the paper explaining that the appointments were made to improve local service by bringing a wider range of skills to a small community. A statement of editorial support by the newspaper concluded the exchange.

By 1915 the Medical Board had concluded that, despite improvement in Staff discipline and performance, further changes were necessary. Drs. Scudder and Jones had been asked in December 1914 to share "their ideas as to the improvement of the medical and surgical services of the A.G.H." Dr. Scudder attended the next meeting and presented some ideas, and by mid-1915 the first major change of organization was in place. The Trustees followed the Medical Board's recommendation "to divide the Staff into Medical and Surgical [so that] the efficiency of the Hospital would be greatly increased." The Medical Board met frequently that spring as it adjudicated the assignment of Staff members, all of whom were required to resign and be reappointed in July when the division was completed.

In addition the Medical Board was enlarged to six, three older doctors were designated consulting physicians, and a third Boston consultant was named for the medical side. Five were assigned to the medical side and four to the surgical service, and these would all share the ward service and do the bulk of the work. The others not otherwise designated would take special duties such as etherizer and assistants to the Staff, and in an early move toward specialization the longtime Medical Board Secretary, Dr. Snow P. F. Cook, was named Oculist-Aurist. At the year-end election of Staff officers, Dr. Cook was also made Chairman of the enlarged Medical Board.

The first dentists were added to the Staff in 1919, with the appointment of Drs. Allen Burnham and George H. Taylor. The latter, one of our sources of recollections of these early days, served for sixty-three years before retiring in 1982, and holds the record for the longest term of continuous service on the Medical/Dental Staff of the hospital.

By 1919 the moves the Staff had made could be seen as part of a national trend. Such steps were being encouraged by the newly established American College of Surgeons (ACS), whose goal was to set standards for medical practice. Its program of accreditation of medical performance, formulated during its first year, became the guide for hospitals wishing to attain approved status, and under it medical staffs were to be organized with bylaws and hold regular monthly meetings and clinical reviews. Staffs were further to restrict membership by excluding any who did not meet standards of competence and reputation, and were not to engage in fee splitting or other questionable practices. Medical record keeping and other hospital performance standards were also to be overseen as part of the voluntary accreditation program.

Not all hospitals or their medical staffs took kindly to such oversight of their work, and the Addison Gilbert was among these. Although it had already met some of the criteria, the Medical Staff resisted formal affiliation with the ACS and the consequent acceptance of its control and went its own way, facing problems as they arose and writing its own rules. But during all the discussion the disputes and unrest that had simmered for several years surfaced in 1919. Although almost nothing appears in the records of the time, the Staff was considerably reduced in number by year end, when several members resigned in a dispute over ward service and differences of opinion as to the desirability of following the precepts of the ACS.

On the Management Side

The Board of Trustees through much of this period was led by Fred Barker, although the presidency from 1910 to 1913 was held by investor-philanthropist John Hays Hammond. Mr. Hammond called Gloucester his home but was almost constantly on the move, overseeing his far-flung properties or at work for the State Department, and consequently had little time for local affairs. Elected hospital President in January 1910, he is on record as attending only one meeting during four years in office, and even then he turned the meeting over to Fred Barker to conduct.

Mr. Barker had also been Vice-President under Sylvester Cunningham and chaired the meetings during the year following the latter's death in January 1909. He was unwilling, however, to be nominated President the next year, and with no one else wishing the responsibility, the Board chose Hammond, who gave the office his name but little else, until the Annual Meeting of 1914 when Barker consented to take an office whose duties he had already performed for five years. He filled the position with distinction until 1923.

Relations with the Medical Staff were conducted at "arm's length," and the Matron was the emissary between the two bodies. She was the highest-ranking hospital employee and of all her duties trying to please these two groups of men must surely have been the most difficult, responsible as she was to the first for running the hospital effectively while doing her best to see that she and her staff of nurses kept the second satisfied. Five Matrons in the twelve years following 1897 would seem to attest to the hazards of the job.

Emma Gordon stayed only a year, resigning in 1898 to marry a Boston doctor. Her place was taken, not very successfully, by Head Nurse Vida McLean on a temporary basis. It then took until early 1900 before Grace E. Pillsbury was recruited from service at the State Mental Asylum at Danvers; she came in April at a salary of $65 per month (which suggests that inability to pay an attractive wage was part of the problem). Her tenure was fairly long and trouble free, however, lasting until her resignation in April 1909.

She was replaced by Abbie A. Bliss in June 1909, but contrary to the implication of her name, the next few months appear to have been anything but happy for her. In November, after she had been only six months on the job, the Medical Board wrote the Trustees that "the best interests of the hospital would be served by [her] resignation." No explanation was offered, but the fact that her resignation was tendered and accepted on the same day the Trustees received the Staff's letter suggests a mutual lack of regard and affection. Her replacement, Josie Mahoney, also had a short stay; she lasted only until September 1910.

Dita McKinney followed the short stay of Miss Mahoney. Arriving that same month, she was the first to be designated Superintendent. Her starting salary of $1,000 per year, increased to $1,200 a year later, was higher than that of any of her predecessors except Miss Gordon and perhaps was intended to reflect the new title. But by 1912 her problems became too much for her, and she resigned in May because of "poor health and the increased work and worry necessarily imposed upon the Superintendent."

A month later Julia May Leach arrived on the scene from the hospital at Amherst, Massachusetts. She had been a charter signatory when the Massachusetts Nursing Association was founded in 1905, and her activist bent made her the first really effective Superintendent. Miss Leach proceeded to work for the next three years without a vacation and only an occasional day off, a hard pace which by November 1915 brought her to what she called "the breaking point." In a letter requesting six months' leave without pay plus the two months of vacation she was due she told the Trustees: "The work here is more wearing than any place I was ever in and I am about at the end of my strength, both mental and physical. For the last year I have felt I was not doing all I should but it was all I could do and I can do very little more without a long rest and change. . . . I must think of myself as well as the work here."

She returned a year later, her place having been filled by her assistant, Martha J. Avard, who at some point during the year had put in place at least one work-reducing reform in hiring the hospital's first clerk-bookkeeper to perform a job traditionally done by the Superintendent and her nurses. Miss Leach returned in time to see the hospital through the two years of United States involvement in World War I, a period that only added to her other problems. Her readjustment following her absence was made easier by her now-experienced assistant who, on replacing her permanently in June 1920, was to bring new meaning to the title of Superintendent.

As the Trustees faced the second decade of the new century, their gravest problem remained that of financing the operation. The early enthusiasm that had spurred the community's philanthropic interest was diminishing; as it did so, the need for increased income from service to patients was becoming greater. As a consequence, a recurring theme over the next several years echoed the mutual concern of Trustees and Medical Staff over the ability of patients to pay and the collection of overdue accounts. There was still an extreme reluctance to raise rates, and the first modest increase did not come until 1908, when the Trustees voted a $5 charge to "private patients in the operating rooms and the Surgeon shall provide his own etherizer and assistant Surgeon." Also that year the State Board of Charity accepted a $2 increase to $7 weekly for its patients. A room rate increase was voted in 1910 but never put in effect.

The much needed adjustment finally came in a late 1913 vote. Ward rates stayed as before, but private patient rates rose to $21 weekly from the previous $15, obstetric cases were set at $25 per week and a new intermediate category utilizing two-bed rooms was initiated at $14. Nonresidents requiring care were to be charged $28, with $35 the fee for a nonresident requiring obstetric service. A further small correction was made in 1917 when a minimum charge of $5 was set for stays less than forty-eight hours, with a $5 delivery charge established for maternity cases.

Five years passed before another increase was deemed vital. Reluctantly, the Trustees voted that as of January 1, 1919 the cost of a private room would have to be $28, with maternity at $35 and the intermediate rate at $21. Ward rates, unchanged since 1897, were finally increased to $14. Nonresidents were expected to pay $35, with $42 the rate for their maternity cases. That year also saw operating room fees double, to $10.

We need only look at the financial reports of the period to understand the severity of the problem. After a period of reasonably comfortable balances, the Trustees were told in July 1911 that there was $27.07 in the cash account; six months later there was $134.02, with $1348 owed suppliers; a year later the account was overdrawn by $344. Things continued in that vein, and by the close of 1919 had hardly improved, with operating expenses for the year at $26,445 against $21,094 received from operations. The fact that $17,700 had been received from investments, about half of which was from rental property, helped, but with receivables of $3,000 and notes plus invoices payable of $24,334, it was not an easy time.

When expenses exceed income it is obviously difficult to pay bills, a position the hospital found itself in all too often during this period and beyond. The solution tore the Trustees between the inability (and possible reluctance) to collect what it was owed and the resulting failure to meet the demands of the merchants who supplied the goods required to serve patients. Pending needed rate increases together with a positive collection procedure, about the only way to meet bills was to borrow or to sell off assets. The former was the obvious first choice, and in January 1912, for the first time except for a $3,000 line of credit in 1909, the Treasurer was "authorized to borrow $2,000 to be used toward the payment of outstanding bills." Similar decisions followed until by March 1913 the Treasurer reported total notes payable of $11,000.

Free care continued to absorb much of the hospital's resources. The extent of the Trustees' concern is evidenced by the 1911 request for a monthly report of the "free care days" each month, and with 622 such days during a year that totaled 4,765 patient days, this concern was obviously justified. Although the ratio varied widely over the years, it averaged about 10.5 percent of total patient days. Perhaps in justification, the President's report for 1918 noted "a larger percentage of what is called 'free hospital treatment' . . . than in any previous year," but went on to point out that "the intent of the founder is by so much carried out." That it was being so "carried out" even as costs were rising and the free-bed funds no longer produced sufficient income to cover the cost of being charitable surely frustrated the Trustees, but they at least kept faith with their consciences and what they interpreted as Addison Gilbert's wishes.

Gifts and Bequests

Public giving was hardly a factor during these years. Gifts were small and intermittent, and the Trustees appear unwilling to press too hard for them. Some evidence of their reluctance is found in the President's report of 1912: "Gloucester is a city of many charities and some one or more of them are constantly before the public asking for assistance." But they also recognized the need for support, as the report went on to question "as to how long [the Trustees] could be justified in running the institution at a yearly loss."

Only two gifts stand out during this span. In July 1918 Ethel H. Bradley, Sylvanus Smith's granddaughter, gave two $1,000 Liberty Bonds to establish the Martha A. Bradley Fund in memory of her mother. And in 1914 Edward H. Haskell of Boston made the first of a series of annual $300 donations to fund the William H. Haskell Bed. Colonel Haskell described W. H. Haskell, his father, as "an esteemed citizen of Gloucester . . . and an intimate friend of . . . Mr. Addison Gilbert." This contribution continued until the donor's death, in 1924.

Bequests were somewhat more encouraging. Trustee Sylvester Cunningham left $10,000 at his death in 1909, and four other benefactors provided $5,000 each for free beds. Another bequest, only $700 but challenging in its terms, was that of Eleanor W. Rowe, whose wish was that the sum "be invested . . . and neither the principal or interest therefrom . . . used for any purpose until both together amount to $7,000. And thereafter the interest only may be used for the personal benefit of in-patients in said hospital, and said $7,000 shall be held as a permanent fund to be called 'Patrick Relief.'" Mrs. Rowe's fund did eventually reach $7000, and as the Patrick Relief Fund it continues to benefit the hospital and its patients today.

But all these were overwhelmed by a bequest of which the Trustees received notice at their March 1910 meeting. The 1896 will of Rev. Jeremiah J. Healy had, they learned, left $5,000 "to our Gloucester City Hospital,

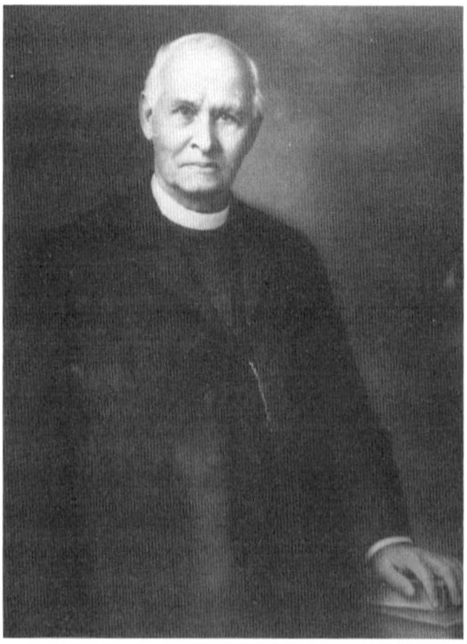

Father Jeremiah J. Healy left a bequest in 1910 which remained the largest single gift to the hospital for many years to come.

now in process of erection, [plus] all my pictures and paintings." A final clause further provided "to our Gloucester City Hospital, allready [*sic*] remembered in item 15, all the residue of my estate and property, real, personal and mixed."

Jeremiah Healy had been pastor at Gloucester's St. Ann's Church since 1871, when he was assigned there, a newly ordained priest sent from Salem, to replace the aging Father Luigi Acquarone. He came to the small, impoverished parish determined to make it over, a task to which his persuasive personality was well adapted. He succeeded nobly as despite parish doubts and opposition he began to accumulate property around the Park (now Pleasant) Street area, gathering funds along with land for the construction of the handsome granite edifice which, since its ceremonial dedication in 1886, has stood as a monument to his imagination and leadership.

Father Healy was a unique priest. His beginnings were humble as, born January 30, 1835 in Bantry, County Cork, Ireland, he emigrated to America in his teens to escape his poverty-stricken homeland. Employed first as a newspaper proofreader in Baltimore, he abandoned secular life at age thirty to study for the priesthood at St. Mary's Seminary. After coming to Gloucester he sought out and became the friend of many of the city's foremost residents, among them John Hays Hammond and Addison Gilbert, combining their counsel with his own astuteness in accumulating a sizable personal fortune in securities and real estate. Such friendships undoubtedly influenced his later interest in Gloucester's nonreligious institutions such as the hospital.

His estate was large for those days, and the will provided for several specific bequests totaling $128,000. Among these was one for $10,000 for books to be selected by his Archbishop for "our Gloucester public library" or, if not accepted by the city (which had some years before declined an offer of a library building), for a St. Ann's Parish library. It also established "The Father Healy Fund for the Poor" with $50,000 left to the city, the nucleus of today's Father Healy Fund now jointly administered by representatives of the church and the community. In all thirty-six individual bequests were designated for relatives, Catholic charities and other institutions.

The estate was soon found to be more valuable than perhaps even he had ever realized. An initial inventory filed in June 1910 listed personal property and securities of $260,476.76 and real estate in Boston, Gloucester and North Brookfield, Massachusetts, where he had relatives, valued at $17,300. In Gloucester, five dwellings, all on Prospect Street and Pleasant Street, totaled $11,600. It was probably inevitable that with so many legatees and such a large estate there would be contests, especially among relatives. Several were indeed soon filed, and there were also other problems such as that stemming from his failure to designate the hospital by its legal name. These and other issues were to mean years of adjudication, and their eventual settlement was further delayed by the dilatoriness of the executor, Dennis Healy of Hardwick, Massachusetts, the testator's brother and also a beneficiary.

Anticipating contests, the Trustees appointed a committee of three Trustees, Fred Barker, Nathaniel Babson and Benjamin A. Smith, "to take such action as they may deem proper." They also voted thanks to his housekeeper/niece, Agnes Healy, "for the gift of the large portrait" of their benefactor. This portrait was loaned to St. Ann's Library in 1921 for display at the fiftieth anniversary of Father Healy's assignment to the parish and was returned to the hospital two years later by Father Myles J. Kiley, then the pastor. It now occupies a prominent place in the hospital, not far from that of Addison Gilbert.

The hospital received the $5,000 direct bequest in June 1913, which was then Trustee designated to fund two Father Healy Free Beds. Then, in April 1915, the executor filed a supplemental inventory listing previously unrevealed, though hinted at, real estate in Washington, D.C. that Father Healy had purchased from the Diocese there some years earlier. This was described as "a block of apartment houses known as 'The Worcester' and 'the Norfolk' situated at the corner of Second and D Streets" along with two vacant lots, totally valued at $72,000. With this adding substantially to the residual estate, all of which was designated for the hospital, litigation became a serious matter. Much of it was directed against Dennis Healy, who had delayed five years in filing the accounting in which the Washington property came to light.

By 1919, with probate finally complete, the gross estate had been valued at $287,804.82. The hospital had received the residual cash, $125,238, to be credited to its General Fund and there to become the keystone of its unrestricted endowment. This and the Washington real estate created a bequest destined to remain for almost seventy years the largest made to it. It also encouraged the Trustees to seek endowment more vigorously, as they foresaw that complacency over such sudden wealth might influence others. A special appeal in the 1919 *Annual Report* sought further endowment of free care, the reduction of which, they said, "could not for a moment be thought of [and] was the intent of the founder and . . . should be the real purpose of the hospital."

There was considerable perplexity at the time as to how a supposedly humble priest could accumulate such a fortune. It is, however, not the place of this story to do more than speculate that it resulted from sagacious counsel by Father Healy's wealthy and influential friends and his own native intelligence. It would seem that his wealth was not a matter of concern to his superiors, since his Washington holdings had been acquired directly from the Church and were bounded by a church and parochial school. What he had he shared with others, during life and after, spending little on himself.

The Washington property was considered well located and consisted of four three-storied brick buildings with a total of thirty six-room apartments. The Trustees, impressed by their potential, decided to hold them as an income-producing asset and to retain Daniel Shea, a Healy nephew, as manager. He took care of most of the maintenance himself and collected the rents which, at just over $6,000 annually, were not the highest believed possible but were considered not unreasonable for the time.

By 1922, however, the problems in being an absentee landlord were becoming evident, and an offer to buy the properties for $115,000 was accepted that October. Fate intervened before the sale could be consummated as a fire severely damaged the larger Norfolk unit on January 15, 1923. With the sale thus negated, the Trustees decided to use the insurance to restore the building for another try, appointing N. C. Phillips, Fred Shackelford and Lincoln Simonds a committee with full power to sell at a minimum price of $100,000. In early 1925, after a year during which the apartments were again fully rented, a buyer was found. The hospital went out of the housing business, and fifteen years of litigation, frustration, and excitement were history.

Other Matters of Health and Health Care

In addition to the hospital and its physicians two other agencies were and are concerned for the health of Cape Ann's people. The Gloucester Board of Health, established by state law in 1881, antedates the hospital. A municipal body, it is responsible for oversight of the community's general health, although it has no power over the hospital or the doctors. Its function is best described as preventive and statistical through its annual reports which, during the early years at least, are the source of data unavailable elsewhere.

The Board of Health has done significant work to improve the well-being of the city's people. In its general oversight of sanitation, for example, it took steps early in establishing the city's garbage collection and thus eliminated a major health hazard. It was a factor in getting the first sewer system installed so that, at least in the central city, the use of cesspools ceased. Typhoid fever, already under better control after the inside "water closet" replaced the outside privy, almost totally disappeared following the sewer installation in the early 1930s. Its clinics and school health programs not only detected problems early but were also effective dispensers of information to assist in understanding the principles of sanitation and the prevention of illness. The administrators of its many health programs, the City Physician and the School Nurse, were Board of Health appointees and reported directly to it.

For the most part its relations with the hospital and the private physicians have always been positive. The Chairman has usually been a physician and thus a member of the hospital Medical Staff, as is the City Physician. Among its Chairmen, it might be noted, the Egans, father and son, served for a full quarter-century, with Dr. John J. Egan, Sr. in the post from 1926 until his death in 1944 when he was succeeded by his namesake son, who served until 1950. Both also served as the hospital's Chief of Staff during part of their terms as Board of Health chairmen.

The other agency, the Gloucester District Nursing Association (now integrated with the Visiting Nurse Association of the North Shore), was first suggested at a meeting of the hospital's Women's Auxiliary Executive Committee on April 9, 1908, when it was recorded that the Matron, Miss Pillsbury, "advocated district nursing in Gloucester." The matter of this newly developing concept was further "discussed and warmly supported" at a meeting of the Auxiliary on June 11 that year, but it was left to others to advance it further.

Eugenie Heller, a Rocky Neck artist, took up the cause in 1912, and the next year the thirty-member group she organized employed its first nurse. By mid-1914 there were three nurses making eight hundred visits each month at 50¢ a visit, and in May of that year it became the Gloucester District Nursing Association, a private nonprofit agency supported and governed by a membership drawn from among the city's residents. It filled a long-standing need and rapidly grew to the point where a year or so later it was recognized as the largest membership organization in Gloucester, boasting over a thousand associate members.

In keeping with its charter purpose of "providing skilled nursing for the sick and the teaching of hygiene as applied to homes and surroundings," it early established a tuberculosis clinic and a dispensary, following these with infant care and prenatal classes and other clinics as the need arose. It pioneered the concept of industrial nursing locally when in 1918 it established a program to carry its mission of home health care and instruction to the workplace; the success of this program inspired many of the larger industrial plants to install their own full-time plant nurse. Over the years it has maintained a close and effective cooperation with the hospital, recognizing with it the need for good nursing care, whether at home or in the hospital. Its earliest credo, stressing prevention as well as care, remains as true today as it was then, and it has well proven itself an essential element in the community's health care.

Illnesses remained much the same, although respiratory problems such as bronchitis, influenza and pneumonia were being seen more often while the epidemic diseases, typhoid and malaria, were occurring less frequently. Arthritis, rheumatism and cardiac problems were recorded in growing numbers, but the greatest increase came in maternity admissions. By 1910 births were approaching thirty a year, a figure that held true through 1919, with 292 recorded during the ten-year span. Finding space for obstetrics was becoming a major problem by then, however, and in 1919 only six such cases were accepted.

Surgical cases continued to dominate the treatment lists, with appendicitis by far the admissions leader; fifty cases a year was the norm by 1913. Earlier diagnosis had by then reduced the likelihood of peritonitis to assure a much lower fatality rate. Abscesses and hernias were also fairly common, and there were five to ten operations for cancer each year. Accidents of all sorts were inevitable and contributed to the surgical workload.

The state of the art was still primitive by today's standards. Ether dripped through a gauze cone remained the basic anesthetic, and its distinctive, clinging odor continued to permeate the hospital for many years before it was replaced by other techniques. Anesthesia procedures were formalized with the appointment of Dr. Philip Moore as etherizer in 1910, a year that also brought the introduction of silver nitrate solution as a prophylaxis against newborn eye infection and of standard urinalysis testing of all ward patients upon admission. Typhoid fever vaccination was common by 1912 and, together with a better understanding of public sanitation, was a major factor in the dramatic reduction of the disease and the need for its hospital treatment.

Laboratory work was becoming a growing part of the hospital function, and in September 1914 the Medical Staff recommended the appointment of Dr. Harper E. Whitaker, a new Staff member, as the first bacteriologist-pathologist. Although he did not replace the consultant pathologists, he was at least an in-house presence for the performance of such simple testing as was being done.

The major health problem of the period came just as the Great War, as World War I was known, was drawing to a close. Except for the general shortage of nurses, the Addison Gilbert had felt little effect from the war, but it and the entire Cape Ann community were involved in the influenza epidemic of 1918. The flu began in Europe and rapidly spread to this country with returning servicemen. Before it was over it would be worldwide – in the words of Winston Churchill, "it looks as though this epidemic may kill off more people than the war has." No area escaped its ravages. On September 6, 1918 the *Times* reported the first cases in Boston, with more than three hundred naval personnel at Commonwealth Pier stricken. Four days later it reported the first Gloucester death, and before the month was out there were so many cases here that outside assistance was required.

The Board of Health, the District Nurses and the Red Cross had by then established an emergency hospital at the G.A.R. Hall, where some fifty men and women were crowded into the open ward. Miss Leach from the AGH had been put in charge with one other nurse and such volunteers as could be enlisted to help. There was little she could do until the arrival of a fourteen-nurse unit from Canada, and by the end of September, despite occasional slackening and optimistic reports, the situation had reached crisis proportions. Other treatment units were opened, one even in the district court over the old police station, but still more space was needed for the increasing numbers falling ill.

Isolation and fresh air were recommended, and a tent hospital was suggested as the best way to gain these and the needed space. The month ended as plans were being made to establish such a unit on the hospital grounds, the Trustees having authorized the state "to erect and maintain temporarily . . . at their own expense, such portable buildings as [they] may desire." They also stated "that should the Hospital be called on to furnish nurses, physicians and other necessary care and attendance that it would be whol-

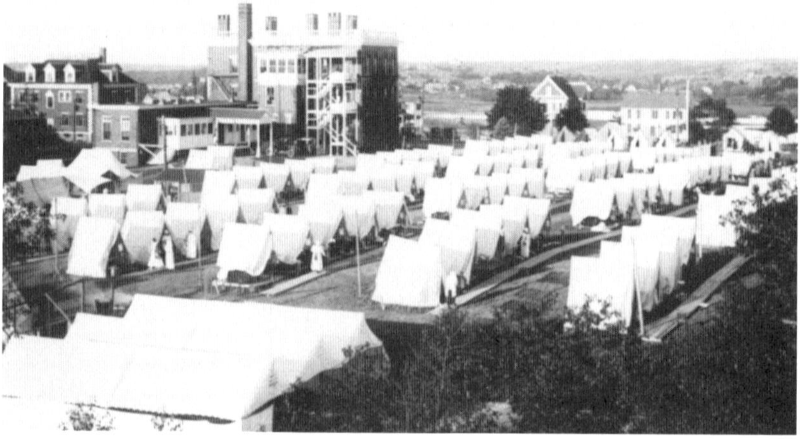

The influenza epidemic of 1918 brought a massive tent hospital to the grounds of AGH operated under the direction of the Massachusetts State Guard.

ly impossible not only as a matter of increased expense to the Hospital, but also the inability to obtain additional nurses." (In defense of this position, it must be remembered that this was a time of desperate financial problems and that nurses were indeed in short supply nationwide.) The State Guard took on the task, and, except for such help as could be offered by the hospital's physicians and nurses, it became an independent operation.

The epidemic ran its course until finally in late October the tent hospital was closed, with its last three patients transferred into the hospital itself. The weeks it had run had taken a terrible toll. Cape Ann lost more than 250 people, with hardly a family spared. It had struck all ages and all walks of life, but without the selfless assistance of hundreds of volunteers it would have been worse. The women especially gave hours of exhausting labor alongside the staffs of the various agencies involved. It was a community effort beyond the capability of any single institution, and, except for services rendered by its physicians and nurses, the use of its laundry by all the sites, and the fact that its grounds were used for the State Guard tent hospital, the AGH had but little direct involvement. It had been a fast-developing, overwhelming epidemic beyond the ability of a thirty-bed hospital, already filled with regular patients, to manage.

An incidental result of the flu epidemic was the establishment in 1919 of a city-operated hospital for the treatment of contagious diseases. This was located in the residence owned by John Estabrook at 531 Essex Avenue and purchased by the city following his death that year. Its formal name, Braewood Hospital, was less often used than the cognomen "the contagious hospital," and it seems to have been used chiefly in the treatment of tuberculosis.

Under jurisdiction of Gloucester's Board of Health, Braewood was a fully staffed institution with a superintendent, nurses and a kitchen. It had its own Women's Auxiliary with some members drawn from the larger AGH group, all with the will to help. Other than that, however, it was largely ignored by the general public, the newspaper and the larger Addison Gilbert Hospital. The sole mention of it in Trustee records was in November 1920 in a letter to the Board of Health calling attention to "the unfinished condition of the new Contagious Hospital and . . . [we] respectfully suggest that the Hospital be equipped with the proper furnishings and that a suitable roadway be made to said Hospital."

After four years of marginal operation its Auxiliary voted in April 1924 to turn its treasury, then about $3,000, over to the city for use in a proposed health camp on the premises. Instead of accepting this offer the Municipal Council Committee on Summer Health Camp recommended sale of the property. The Council voted "without discussion" to do so on July 2, 1924, and Braewood Hospital followed the Gloucester Hospital and Rockport's Haskins Hospital into oblivion.

4

Too Small: The Hospital Expands

THE STORY OF the period from 1920 to 1934 primarily concerns a hospital that required more space. The Addison Gilbert had operated for almost twenty-five years with its original thirty beds, and, unlike the early days, it was becoming the place to go to be cured when illness or accident struck. In 1919 it admitted 458 patients who, staying almost fifteen days each on average, often taxed capacity. It had been forced to refuse almost all obstetrical work, acceptance of which would have added an impossible 2000 patient days to the 6755 it logged that year.

The Maternity Wing

A separate wing for maternity cases had been first suggested in 1905, when Mrs. Bray proposed and raised $500 toward a plan for Auxiliary sponsorship. The issue came up at intervals through the years following, but lack of funds and perhaps confidence subdued serious consideration of it. The Medical Staff gave little support to the suggestions, preferring to use what beds there were for acute illness while handling their maternity work in a nonhospital setting.

The great majority of births took place in the mothers' homes, and physicians were accustomed to home delivery and aftercare. For cases where the residence was not adequate or the mother required extra care until she could be up and about there were several maternity homes in Gloucester, among them one located in Riverdale near Gee Avenue with another on Main Street

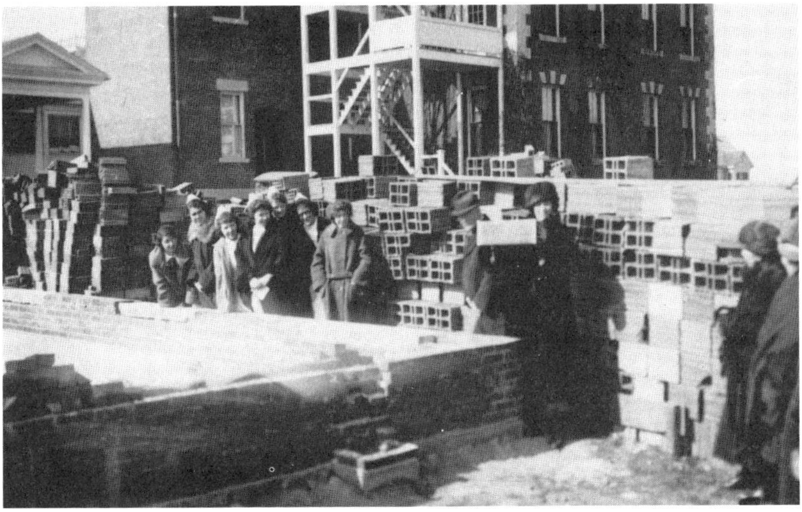

The Women's Auxiliary played a leading role in supporting construction of the 1924 Maternity Wing. Here they help lay the cornerstone and bury a time capsule.

where, according to legend, Howard Blackburn had been cared for while recovering from his ordeal on the Grand Banks.[1] Another, on Concord Street, was operated by Mrs. Ella Herrick, whose grand-daughter, Ellen Coull, a 1933 graduate of the hospital's nursing school, was a beloved maternity nurse at AGH until her retirement in 1976.

Fresh impetus was given the proposal for a new wing in March 1915, when the Trustees received a letter from the new Nurses' Alumnae Association, which had been organized at the training school the previous year. The letter advised that the group had "recently started a building fund towards a Maternity Ward. The nurses, more than others perhaps, realize the need for such a ward and with your approval and cooperation are ready and willing to help raise the needed funds." With this, a committee made up of Trustees Barker and Babson plus architect Ezra Phillips was appointed to investigate and report back.

Two more years passed without action until in 1917 the Auxiliary reentered the fray. That group, which almost succumbed after Mrs. Bray's presidency ended in 1915, revived in becoming a catalyst for support of a new wing. When Fred Barker met the women that April he brought with him cost estimates ranging from $18,000 for a single-story, nine-room ward to $26,000 for eighteen rooms on two floors. He also advised "that the Trustees were ready to carry out the wishes of the Women's Auxiliary whenever a sufficient amount was placed in the hands of the Trustees." A cynical interpretation of this suggests that the women, nurses and volunteers, were being told to "put up or shut up," but a more charitable view is that the Trustees were simply being cautious.

Discussions continued pro and con for another two years as the "urgent demand for a Maternity Ward" did battle with "a division of opinion as to whether this was an opportune time [post-war 1919] to go before the public and attempt to raise from $100,000 to $150,000," a figure which by then included enlargement of the Nurses' Residence.

Opportune time or not, Ezra Phillips was requested to draw plans, and at a December 1919 meeting with the Auxiliary, when the matter was "freely discussed," the Trustees, still somewhat reluctant, gave in. They voted to "approve the raising of a $50,000 Fund . . . provided, however, that no part of said amount shall be taken from any funds of the Hospital," and they agreed to commence maternity wing construction "as soon as $50,000 was raised or satisfactorily pledged." The women's cause was further helped when Colonel Edward H. Haskell, then President of New England Baptist Hospital, spoke to the Trustees in early 1920. Colonel Haskell, an Eastern Point summer resident and a generous donor, was already favorably known at the hospital. He suggested "that this extension of the hospital work would

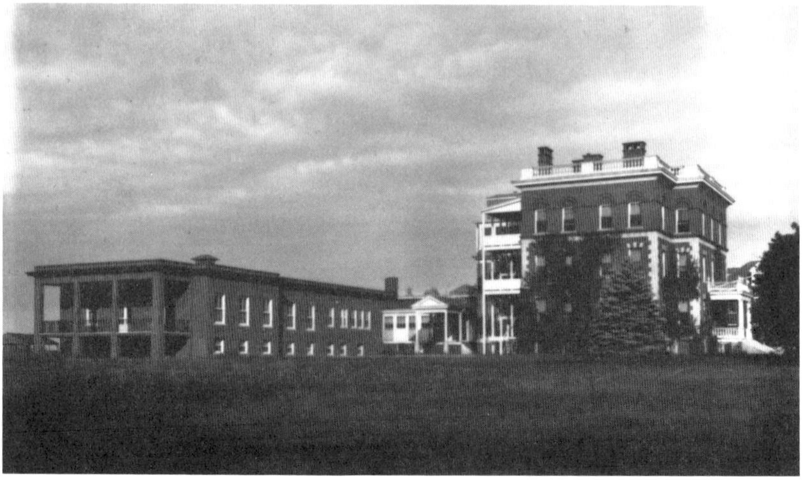

The completed Maternity Wing shortly after it opened in 1925. This was the first major addition to the hospital which, other than the fire escape added in 1915, had remained essentially as originally constructed.

not only increase earnings, but would be of great benefit to the entire community."

Before the year was out the Auxiliary and the nurses were organizing for a fund drive with an immediate goal of $40,000, confident "that when building operations were actually begun . . . additional money could be raised." The Board accepted this and insurance man William E. Kerr was appointed drive Chairman. The work got under way with male leadership and female labor, and by year's end the *Annual Report* indicated the campaign to be well along, with $26,000 on deposit and a further $4,000 in pledges.

The initial effort raised $35,203, and a second drive for $40,000 more was mounted in 1924. This, under the direction of newly elected Trustee N. Carleton Phillips, was more formally organized with captains and teams of workers, and, under the slogan "You owe your ALL to Motherhood, Help the Gloucester Maternity Ward Drive," its goal was reached.

During the period of uncertainty as to funding availability plans had been drawn and redrawn with advice from the Medical Staff. In 1923, still moving cautiously and determined to use only publicly raised funds, the Trustees took bids "for building walls of Maternity Ward and roofing in the same, [proceeding] towards completion of the building as far as money is available for that purpose, building operations to be started not later than the Spring of 1924." Bids ranged from $28,155 to $37,750, and the low bidder, E. S. Griffin of Gloucester, was given the job to go as far as possible before the money ran out.

August 1924 found the Trustees sufficiently confident to contract with Griffin to complete construction for a further $35,945, with L. E. Smith & Company to install plumbing and heat for $9462. The following month, with construction under way, they voted to open the hospital to maternity cases "with the provision that such cases must not be allowed to interfere with the regular work of the hospital," a move followed by an immediate and sharp rise in maternity admissions. Late the next spring $14,830 worth of equipment was on hand, and in September 1925 the Superintendent was directed "on account of the pressing need for rooms" to open the wing for use. The formal opening with an Open House was held October 1, and ten years of struggle vindicating the determination of the women of the Auxiliary and the Nurses' Alumnae Association came to an end.

The new building visitors saw on tours guided by members of the two organizations justified the long struggle. A two-story wing (today called West Wing) to the west of the main building contained six private and two semiprivate rooms plus a six-bed ward on its main floor. A nursery held fourteen bassinets, and there was also a delivery room, a sterilizer room and a kitchen. New X-ray and laboratory space was provided on the ground floor, which also held seven more small rooms for overflow or for live-in nurses, as needed. One of these rooms was allotted to the Alumnae Association to be furnished by its members as a meeting room, serving thus for the next twenty-five years. An office for writing and storing medical records completed the lower floor.

When all accounts were in, in 1926, the Auxiliary, with justifiable pride, summed up the results. The hospital had raised $75,892 plus special gifts of rooms by bequest or as separate gifts. To this the ladies added, through their Ways and Means Committee's special events, a further $15,397. They had more than met their goal and paid almost the entire $95,794 the construction and equipment had cost. And they had proved, as they would again many times over the years to come, that one should never underestimate the power of determined women!

Trustees and Management

The most severe problem the Trustees faced continued to be financial. Although income occasionally exceeded expenses after 1919, that being the happy outcome of five of the fourteen years to 1934, in only two of those years was the margin sufficient for comfort. It exceeded $7000 in 1921 and achieved a peak that remained a record for many years at $17,400 in 1927. A year later red figures again appeared and after 1929, with an economic depression settling in, matters grew worse. The deficit of $26,166.85 in 1933 had become typical.

Borrowing also became common, continuing throughout the period with occasional interludes when notes were reduced but never eliminated. The patience of Gloucester's bankers reached its limit in 1920 when they demanded collateral in the form of the hospital's precious endowment securities to guarantee the previously unsecured loans. By 1933 some $35,000 of these had been pledged, and, making matters worse, interest rates had risen to an unprecedented 5.5 percent. Endowment funds were reluctantly invaded in 1925, when the Treasurer was authorized to sell "294 shares, or any part thereof, of stock in the N. Y. Central & Hudson River Railroad . . . proceeds to be used to reduce the amount of notes . . . now outstanding."

Since 1909 investment of endowment had been a function of the Finance Committee with full power to act but with advice, if it saw fit, from Old Colony Trust of Boston. In meeting its responsibility the committee followed prudent investment rules and held generally to popular investment trends. At first this had meant railroad bonds, but by 1910 electric utilities and telephone bonds were beginning to show as part of the portfolio. By 1917, with the Healy cash requiring investment, gas utilities and municipal transit issues were being added, with 85 percent of the new acquisitions in bonds. A small amount was also ventured into industrial issues such as a United States Steel 5 percent bond to mature in 1963. This was a long maturity; most were selected from the ten-to twenty-year range.

Bonds were to remain the leading choice through the next several years as older issues matured or were sold, and as the 1920s passed the committee moved increasingly into the industrial sector, with such stocks as General Electric, Bethlehem Steel and Copper Export Association joining the list of holdings. In 1925 real estate mortgages apparently were considered worth a small venture. Six, totaling $57,000, were written that year, all in Brookline or the Newtons. Some $16,000 was thus invested in 1927, and of the total $75,000, some was repaid on schedule with some to be rewritten during the hard times of the 1930s. All were closed out by 1940, not without some losses, although most were paid off satisfactorily. Such residential mortgages would not appear to have met the "prudent man rule" most often used by the committee, and one can only speculate as to why they chose to enter that field.

It would seem that the persistent financial problems would be enough for the Trustees to endure. Thus we can only imagine the torment they must have felt when they assembled for a special meeting on February 18, 1925. The record of that session is terse and to the point: "It was reported that a shortage existed in the accounts of the Treasurer [and] the resignation of Horace A. Smith as Treasurer of the Hospital was presented and accepted." They went on to elect a new Treasurer, architect Ezra L. Phillips, and to instruct the Finance Committee "to cause a complete audit of the Treasurer's accounts for the past six years . . . and check up and list all securities of the Hospital." A colleague, in a position of trust since 1904 when he replaced his father, Captain Sylvanus Smith, in the office, had betrayed that trust.

The news became public knowledge the next day with a front page headline in the *Times* – "BANK TREASURER RESIGNS; AUDIT SHOWS SHORTAGE." The Gloucester Safe Deposit & Trust Company's share of the problem had been uncovered when a routine bank examination revealed a shortage in personal loan collateral given by Mr. Smith totaling $5,000; this was immediately made good by means of a mortgage lien on his West Gloucester residence. Less simple was the hospital's shortage, first announced as $17,000 and later found to total over $19,000.

Subsequent examination revealed the entire shortage to have been in cash funds with uncredited interest, uncredited cash from sale of matured bonds, and outright cash withdrawals. Public sympathy was expressed for Mr. Smith and the hospital, sympathy that proved justified when, on April 10, the Trustees received a letter and certified check for $19,484.94. In his letter Mr. Smith stated his concurrence in the course of action taken by his former colleagues, admitted having erred, and said he was ready "to take such further punishment as may be necessary." He recalled his twenty-five years as Treasurer and his feelings of comfort "working for a worthy object and being of service to [his] fellow man," closing with an expression of regret "for the pain I have caused you who have been my friends . . . and assuring you that I will always be glad and willing to help the hospital and its work in any way I can." The Trustees voted to make news of his repayment public, which they did in a formal statement published in the *Times* the next day.

On April 21 he was bound over to the grand jury in $20,000 bail, and the trial was held in Salem in October. A guilty plea resulted in a sentence of one year in the House of Correction, but because of public sympathy, his repentance and complete repayment, the case was placed on file and no time was spent in confinement. In 1934 he presented the hospital with a portrait of his father, which suggested that he also considered the matter closed. The community apparently agreed, and he became a bookkeeper in Gloucester until his death following a coronary thrombosis at his Essex Avenue home on May 23, 1958. It was a sad affair in which no one was hurt except Horace Smith and his family.

Following the defalcation the Trustees made adjustments in their own protocols, the first being appointment of a special committee to include the entire Finance Committee "to revise bylaws and look into our method of keeping accounts." They also voted to bond the Treasurer for $10,000 and the Superintendent for $5,000. One of Mr. Smith's comments had been to the effect that he had labored for no compensation. Possibly with the thought that a stipend for those who bore the burden would reduce temptation, late in 1925 the Trustees voted "to establish the salary of the Treasurer at $500 per annum."

Funding: An On-going Problem

The Smith affair was little more than an interruption in the business of running an already financially troubled institution. The Trustees had borrowed, hypothecating their capital to do so, and, to a smaller degree, they had disposed of some of that capital, but through it all they had never seriously faced up to one of the root causes of the problem. They were still extremely reluctant to raise rates, but except for stricter collections, this was the only remaining solution.

The increase of 1919 was followed in April 1920 with a $1 a day increase in private medical-surgical room rates and a $12 weekly rise for a private maternity case. Nonresidents using such rooms were hit somewhat harder, at $12 and $21 per week respectively. Ward and intermediate bed rates were reluctantly increased by $3 and $3.50 weekly in January 1924, and there matters stood for many years. By the 1930s the Great Depression had precluded further consideration of increased billings, which in large measure were by then uncollectible in any case.

The Trustees' determination to give as much free care as possible began to wane as financial problems worsened after 1927. In 1928 they canvassed other hospitals to ascertain their policies on the subject, finding a diminishment of such care, with many suffering the same financial trauma. They were also aware of Medical Staff concerns that some patients, knowing they could be treated free in the hospital's Outpatient Department or in a bed, used that method to avoid a doctor's office or home visit charge. The question of cutting back became moot, however, by 1931, when public charity became an essential of the raging Depression. That year the number of "free bed days," at 2,154, was double those of 1929. By 1933 they had leaped to 3,116 and covered almost 22 percent of total patient days.

Another kind of free care the Trustees were less willing to accept took the form of uncollected patient accounts. They had first faced up to that problem in 1912 and again in 1916, when they ruled that if intermediate bed rates were not paid in advance, the patient would be placed in the ward. In 1924 the matter of collections was given to the Committee on Accounts, which was told that it "should be as active and prompt in collecting as in approving bills against the hospital." This move to make the committee that spent the money also responsible for collecting it was only another unsuccessful step in seeking a solution to a classic hospital problem of those days before health insurance.

Total unpaid accounts reached $6,434 by mid-1926 and the problem had been shifted to the Committee on Abatements, which theretofore had played the more beneficient role of adjudicating reductions. In March 1927 that committee was "instructed to use all means to collect even to the extent of bringing suit if thought advisable." A year later, with receivables at $9,198, a decision was reached "that after two months, accounts should be given to William J. MacInnis for collecting and if in his opinion the accounts appear to be uncollectible, to be returned to Committee on Accounts for further attention." Mr. MacInnis, "Billy" to his many friends, was then a young attorney, who would become a Trustee some twenty years later, but he was no more successful as a bill collector than the various committees before him.

Fred A. Shackelford, the next choice for the thankless, seemingly hopeless task, replaced Billy MacInnis six months later, with overdue accounts then approaching $10,000. Fred Shackelford, a Gloucester real estate specialist with an office in the Savings Bank Building, is remembered as a quiet, unassuming man somewhat set in his ways. He was a willing worker on the Board of Trustees, to which he had been elected in 1906, and served as its Clerk from 1909 until 1923, when he replaced Fred Barker as President. Refusing reelection to that office in 1926, he became Vice-President until 1932, when he was chosen Treasurer, a post he held until 1939. He was an early Life Trustee, his tenure as such lasting from 1949 until his death in 1956, after a full fifty years of Board service.

He must also have had a persuasive streak, for by the end of December 1928 receivables had been reduced to $7327, a feat in which he had Medical Staff support which, perhaps at his suggestion, voted to give each physician a monthly list "showing his patients for past months who did not pay hospital bills." Further Staff support came in the form of a questionnaire first proposed by Dr. Mooring, by then a member of the Medical Board, to have physicians determine the financial status of their patients before admission. This was, probably fortunately, one of those decisions that was never enforced and, once the Depression hit, couldn't be.

By late 1930, with uncollected accounts in excess of $12,000, whatever positive effects Shackelford had wrought were gone. When they reached $15,504 in 1932 he was enjoined as Treasurer "to be in intimate contact with the credit of patients entering the hospital and upon their discharge and afterwards." As encouragement and in recognition of the work entailed his annual stipend was increased by $700 to $1,200. The frustration level reached its peak the next year, with receivables of $16,152 and cash on hand at $213.14. And certainly no one was happy with the February 1933 decision to reduce all wages and salaries by 10 percent.

Philanthropic Support: 1920—1934

Philanthropy was not a major support factor during this period. Most gifts were designated to fund special needs rather than operations, as typified by that in 1928 by Mr. and Mrs. John H. Hammond, $5,000 "for the benefit of underprivileged children." A gift of $704.20 by the Shriner's Club of Cape Ann in 1924 "to establish a fund for the purpose of supplying children patients . . . with necessities and appliances not usually included in the Hospital treatment" further suggests a special concern for sick children and their welfare in the third-floor Children's Ward.

Another special-purpose gift was publicized in recognition of Nathaniel Babson's ability as a fund raiser. The tribute written upon his death in 1927 described how "through his efforts a great many were led to take an interest in the hospital and in one particular case, that of Mr. George W. Pulsifer, late of Chicago, Mr. Pulsifer was led to look over the institution and expressed himself as highly pleased with everything he saw there. On his return to Chicago, his home, he forwarded . . . his check for $5,000 to be used for the benefit of a free bed fund."

Other summer residents began to take more notice of the hospital, especially the regulars, families who viewed Cape Ann as their second home, who voluntarily offered support for special projects as well as general operational purposes. Those with large gardens also kept the hospital amply supplied with flowers all summer, delivering them by chauffeured limousine or occasionally on a personal visit.

Endowment funds also received attention during those years, with almost $100,000 added through bequests. Notable among the dozen who thus remembered the hospital was Fitz W. Winter, a retired Main Street merchant and the late Dr. Garland's neighbor on Pleasant Street, whose 1933 bequest of $25,000 plus residue became $31,000 a few years later. George W. Upton, owner of the Oceanside Hotel in Magnolia and a long-time booster, left $10,000, as did Colonel Edward H. Haskell of Boston, whose earlier gifts and his counsel regarding the Maternity Wing had familiarized him with the institution. Two that brought back memories of George Marsh came from Jennie S. Moxon and her niece, Helen Davis. Miss Davis lived on Leonard Street in Annisquam and had been secretary and very close personal friend of her summer neighbor there, Mr. Marsh. The Moxon bequest established the Helen Davis Fund, and a few years later Miss Davis herself left $3,640.

Nat Babson left $5,000, as did Fred W. and Helen Tibbetts, both in the form of named endowments. Mr. Tibbetts, although never a Trustee, was a leading Gloucester citizen well known for his leadership qualities; he had been Chairman of Gloucester's 1923 Tercentennial celebration. Mrs. Lucy Brown Davis left $15,000 and was later memorialized by her daughter, Catalina, via a gift of landscaping; a plaque on a stone in the front parking area continues to offer testimony to that gift. Miss Davis died in 1933, leaving a general-purpose endowment as well as a trust of which the hospital has ever since been among the beneficiairies.

The Rockport Problem Is Resolved

A bright spot of a different nature occurred in 1923, when the people of Rockport were finally declared equal in becoming able to use the Addison Gilbert on the same basis as their neighbors in Gloucester.

The Haskins Hospital, too small to be efficient, was only minimally endowed, and the town's residents were unable or unwilling to finance it adequately. But it did have a good, though small, medical staff, and for a decade after it opened it had served to the best of its ability. The end came on a cold night late in January 1918 when its heating plant broke down, and, unwilling to use funds voted for its repair, the Selectmen chose to close the hospital down. Except for a brief reopening during the flu epidemic that autumn, the Haskins would not again function as such, despite several special Town Meetings during the fall and winter of 1918 and 1919 that sought to find ways of reviving it.

So once again the community's sick had to remain at home or, if hospitalization was needed, come to Gloucester on an emergency basis or hope for acceptance at Beverly Hospital or the new Cable Memorial Hospital in Ipswich. Pressure was once again brought on the AGH Trustees, now thirty-five years away from their initial interpretation of the founder's will. On June 11, 1923, without fanfare or advance notice, they quietly voted "that citizens of Rockport should have the same status as those of Gloucester in regard to privileges at the Hospital." The only publicity given the decision was a single paragraph in the Rockport section of the *Times* ten days later, which called it "pleasing information." It was a decision with mutual advantages, as Rockporters added to patient census figures and gradually became loyal supporters of the institution, sharing today in its governance and contributing to its general well-being.

The move also benefited the Medical Staff, with Drs. Ezra Cleaves and Augustus M. Tupper immediately invited to join, the latter as honorary consulting physician. They were followed in 1926 by Dr. Harold N.Baker, and all became valued members of the Staff.

We can only speculate as to what brought on the AGH Board's change of heart. It is difficult today to justify their long-held interpretation of the founder's wishes. There is no record of any public discussion, nor apparently did they seek guidance from the Probate Court at Salem regarding a change in what they had so long accepted as a restriction in the will. Addison Gilbert may not even have considered the possibilities of such an interpretation, and he certainly did not specifically exclude anyone from his hospital. All involved, Medical Staff as well as Trustees, must have discussed the matter over the years as they did in 1899 and 1901. Conjecture suggests that the Board, contemplating a larger hospital in 1923, simply decided that they had been needlessly literal and that, in finally making the change, the less said about it the better.

That step taken, further relaxation of the nonresident policy came more easily. Visitors to the city had long been accepted, as had summer residents, with employees of the latter admitted to the ward at $15 per week if the employer guaranteed payment of the bill. When in July 1926 Essex residents were given equal privileges the Trustees had finally freed themselves from what must have been a long-term embarrassment.

The old Haskins residence, though no longer a hospital, was reopened for care of the sick in June 1933. A three-year lease was given Clement K. Heberle, MD, who used it as a private sanitarium for the treatment by natural means of chronic disease, emphasizing fresh air, sunshine, simple foods and round-the-clock nursing care. The building, which meanwhile had been renovated under lease by Gloucester banker Arthur B. Sewall during the 1920s, was further improved by Dr. Heberle, with new plumbing and general renovation.

Heberle, a native of Taunton, Massachusetts and the son of Charles T. (Cap) Heberle, had spent most of his youth in Gloucester. Following his medical study and an internship in Boston, he opened a practice in Gloucester before establishing what he called "Restcroft," more popularly known as "Dr. Heberle's Sanitarium." It was open to anyone, but was specially equipped for the treatment of rheumatoid arthritis. It remained in operation until June 1935, when a second three-year lease expired.

The Probate Court, in response to a petition by the Rockport Selectmen, decreed in 1950 that the remaining Haskins Hospital trust funds and proceeds from partial sale of the land could be used for the "hospitalization of worthy and needy inhabitants of Rockport at the Addison Gilbert Hospital . . . or at some other like institution." This decision, incidentally, would also seem to have laid to rest any lingering doubts as to the legality of the 1923 decision at the AGH. The old building had by 1950 fallen into disrepair, and its remains were bulldozed into rubble and burned by the Rockport Fire Department on April Fools' Day ten years later.

Superintendent Avard

Martha Avard first came to Salem hospital from her native New Brunswick in 1904 and thence to Addison Gilbert as assistant to Miss Leach in 1912. She soon became known as a strong hospital person – supportive of it and those under her, respected and loved by her nurses and students,

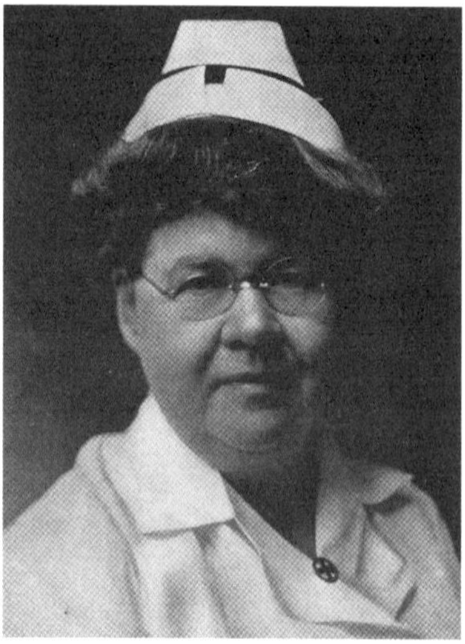

Martha J. Avard, RN brought new meaning to the title of Superintendent when she was appointed in 1920.

who learned early her high standards of neatness and deportment – and something of an enigma to those outside the hospital who didn't understand her unswerving loyalty and somewhat stern demeanor. She stood in awe of neither Trustees nor Medical Staff, keeping after the former until she got what she wanted for her beloved hospital and its staff and standing up to the latter when she felt they needed it or were not following hospital regulations or their own rules.

As Superintendent she was also director of school operations and the chief recruiter of its students, many of whom came from New Brunswick or Nova Scotia; during her early years the Maritimes brogue was more frequently heard in the classrooms and dormitory than the New England twang. Indeed, for many years after she left her fellow Canadians were a source of strength on the nursing staff and gave it a unique character.

One of them, nurse Muriel Walker of the Class of 1929, now retired to Rockport after almost fifty years of nursing at AGH, recalls Superintendent Avard well, as does Madge Brideson Noble, Class of 1916. As Mrs. Noble describes her, she was "very strict, very fussy, but a fine person and a good teacher. When she told you something you never forgot it – and she was meticulous! Uniforms clean and starched, shoes *really* white, and – oh, my goodness – absolutely no short hair! The nurses loved her, though."

Mrs. Noble recalls the day she was operating room nurse under Dr. Scudder, himself "a bit of a tease," when he spotted Miss Avard behind her. "He sternly protested my sponge count, but I knew I was right and stood up for myself — I didn't realize Miss Avard was there, and we argued back and forth with her getting all upset because one of her girls was in trouble and arguing with a doctor. Well, he knew I was right all along and he was just teasing her. Finally he said, 'Well, I have to compliment you on your ability and gumption,' and he winked at me so I knew it was all right. But Miss Avard was about to die until she saw him wink at me."

Miss Avard's deteriorating health made it necessary in 1937 for the Trustees to suggest her retirement, at age sixty-two. This she accepted in a typically loyal letter of appreciation in which she gave thanks to the Trustees, the Medical Staff and the Women's Auxiliary for their support, interest and cooperation. And to her from the Trustees: "Your long and happy period of connection with the hospital has made bonds which are not easily broken; twenty-five of the best years of your life have been given to this institution. During that time, in a way, Addison Gilbert Hospital has been your life; under your care it has grown in size, in scope, in value of its services, and you may well take pride for your important share in its present success and its promise for the future." This outstanding hospital personality had only a short time of life left to her. She died in her native New Brunswick six years later, in 1944.

The School of Nursing

The growth of the training school must be counted among Miss Avard's accomplishments. During her time here it improved its course of study not only "on campus" but also through affiliation with other hospitals at which the students could gain specialized experience. These outside ties began in 1913, when each student was expected to spend three months at St. Luke's Hospital in New Bedford learning obstetrics. By 1933 the school had worked with such institutions as Boston Floating Hospital, New York Nursing and Child Hospital, and the Children's hospitals of Boston and Portland in pediatrics. Obstetrics was by then being learned in affiliation with Boston Lying-in and the Manhattan Maternity hospitals. In the mid-twenties joint courses were established with Beverly Hospital and its school to better utilize the faculties of both. The Medical Staff continued its interest, giving regularly scheduled lectures and conducting rounds for students. It had become a three-year course, with a total of twenty or more students enrolled much of the time.

The training was rigorous, with twelve-hour days the rule. Miss Walker's reminiscences and those of Mrs. Dorothy Oleson, Class of 1934, are valuable sources of insight into school life which, besides study, ranged from doing the hospital laundry and scrubbing floors to singing carols for the patients at Christmas. Morning prayers and formal capping and graduation ceremonies were the rule, and Miss Avard's own course in ethics would be forever remembered by every graduate. Dottie Oleson's journal recalls seven days of work a week with a few hours off on Sunday "if you were lucky," with some of the work by the time they were seniors including home care at patients' residences.

By 1933 the school had contributed 152 nurses to service around the nation. Since 1924 its graduates had been eligible to become Registered Nurses under a state program of examination and registry. The Commonwealth had assumed regulatory power over nurses' training in 1922, and among its requirements was meeting high standards for accreditation. The well-run AGH school came under its scrutiny early that year, and in March Trustee Elmer W. Babson, DVM, reported that he had been in contact with the Massachusetts Board of Education. He was able to state that the school "was rated very high and I am assured that the Hospital will experience no difficulty in complying with the necessary requirements."

The small size of the hospital, still with only thirty beds, was the most difficult hurdle. The need for a minimum of fifty beds for Class A rating of its school had been a factor in the decision to add a maternity wing in 1924. With that in place, despite what Miss Avard described as "the new severe regulations and conditions now being imposed by the State Board of Registration which makes it extremely difficult, if not impossible, for small hospitals to continue to operate training schools," the school was fully accredited and remained so for many years. With accreditation, its graduates, formerly designated simply as "Trained Nurse," could now bear the prized designation "Registered Nurse."

Direct gift support was never a factor in the school, which throughout its life remained dependent on the hospital and small tuition fees for operating funds. One gift was made to it, however, and is notable for its origin and inspiration. On March 29, 1929 Clement S. Houghton of Boston made a gift of $10,000 to be designated the Susan B. Tracy Memorial Fund. Susan B. Tracy, RN, had been a faculty member at the school from about 1921 as instructor and practitioner of occupational therapy. She had other teaching affiliations in the area, but the Addison Gilbert school, where she had taught first, was always her favorite. With her easy, outgoing personality, she was also a great favorite here. Her death in 1928 was a great shock to the hospital family.

In Mr. Houghton's letter of transmittal he stipulated its purpose as "training nurses in occupational therapy and/or the practice of this art in the treat-

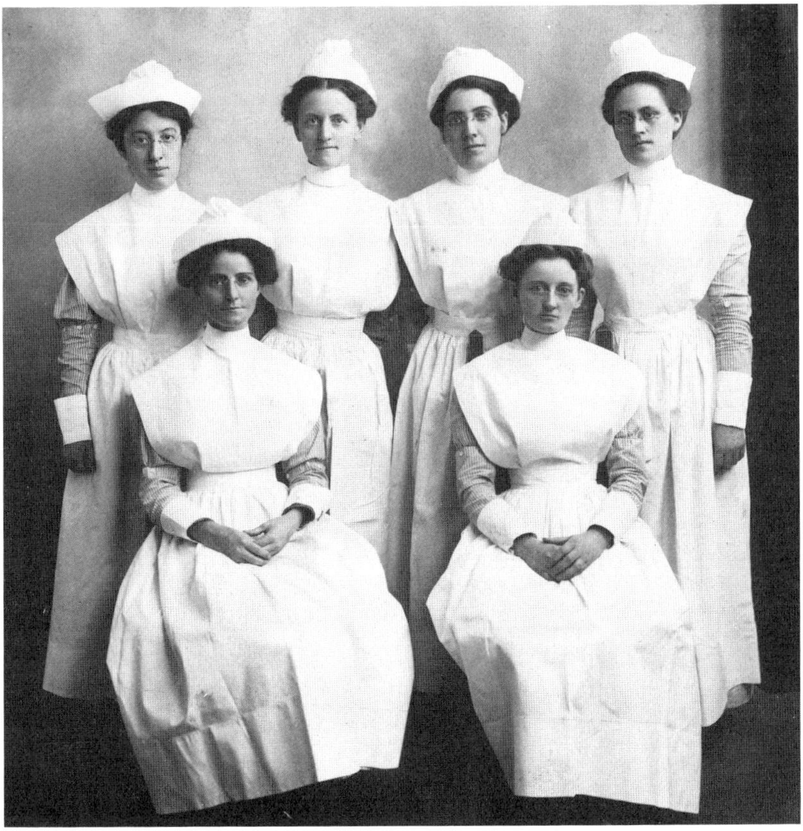

The Class of 1913 which founded the AGH Nurses' Alumnae Association in October of 1914. From left (standing) are Catherine C. Mealey, Emily Rogers, Isabella B. Belshaw, and M. Estelle Shields. Margaret Ryan and Anna H. Scanlon are seated.

ment of patients." In closing he explained his gift simply and to the point: "My son, William, undoubtedly owes his life to Miss Tracy's devoted care during his infancy, and we all have held [her] in affectionate and admiring regard for many years; therefore we delight to honor her and perpetuate her memory."

No story of the School of Nursing would be complete without the story of its Nurses' Alumnae Association, founded in 1914. With some fifty graduates by 1914, about half living and working either on or not far from Cape Ann, Miss Leach and Miss Avard suggested unifying past and future graduates as friends of the hospital. The Class of 1913, largest of the six graduating classes to that time, recruited assistance from past graduates and on October 28, 1914 established the Addison Gilbert Hospital Nurses' Alumnae Association with provision for each subsequent graduating class to join. Katherine MacDonald Fanning, Class of 1901 and then Superintendent at Haskins Hospital, was chosen its first President. Chartered shortly thereafter by the state, its loyalty and activities have been closely tied to the hospital ever since. It became a liaison between its members and the hospital, maintaining a relationship even for those whose careers took them far away. It played a part in every major project the hospital undertook after 1914 and has even, as in the case of the original maternity wing, taken the initiative in promoting some of them. Some of its members have been honorary, one such being Martin Lofquist, who through it maintained a lifelong interest in the hospital. Others, graduates of other schools, have been made members through long service at Addison Gilbert.

Its gifts, large and small, in support of hospital programs have been many, most often taking the form of equipment for which its members could professionally perceive a need. One of a different nature followed the First World War, when the several AGH staff nurses in the service were recognized by the planting of a small grove of spruce trees on the hospital grounds. Most of these have succumbed to expansion, storms and time, but a few survive on the Washington Street side of Prentiss House.

Meanwhile the Medical Staff . . .

The formation of the American College of surgeons, despite early resistance to its dictates, meant that after 1919 a new influence had entered the picture. No longer could hospital medical staffs govern their own affairs with the same independence as before. Coupled with a slowly developing confidence on the part of hospital trustees, this meant changes in relationships. The AGH Medical Staff was no different from others in this regard, and after the shake-up of 1919 it began to adjust to the changing times.

With nine resignations that year the Staff had been severely reduced. Despite the addition of Drs. Cleaves and Tupper from Rockport, in 1925-26 it had only twelve members on active status. There were, however, twenty-eight doctors on Cape Ann, some of whom affiliated with hospital Medical Staff members in a group reminiscent of the old Gloucester Medical Association. Calling itself Physicians of Cape Ann, it at least kept the local profession on speaking terms as they met to discuss fees and other conditions of practice.[2]

The requirement that hospital Staff members serve without recompense

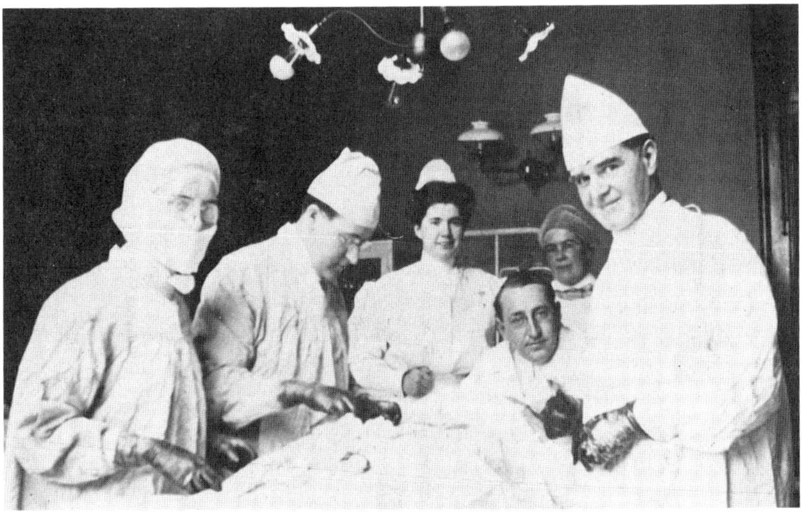

Action in the original operating room in the early 1920s. Regrettably, none of the staff are identifiable.

on the ward was a factor in keeping the others from joining it, and they were only too happy to be allowed to treat their patients at the hospital as nonmembers. This and other issues festered for several years, during which the Trustees as well as the Medical Board chafed at the inefficiency of the situation. Bickering between Staff and Trustees was obvious on the outside and would keep membership low until almost the end of the period, when steps toward correction and reconciliation, plus the prospect of a new wing, gave the Staff the growth it needed.

One source of argument lay in the matter of the Trustees' right to admit patients, private as well as ward. Feeling that the Trustees catered too much to patients of nonmember physicians, in March 1925 the Staff through Dr. Mooring openly challenged them "to define in detail the function and powers of the Medical Board." At a meeting with the Trustees shortly thereafter the Medical Board went further and openly questioned "what authority, if any, the Trustees have over private patients." In a stopgap compromise in November the Trustees adopted a Staff proposal to limit treatment of patients at the hospital to members of the Staff, with new applicants for membership to submit credentials and make formal application before being granted privileges.

This did not solve the issue, however, and in 1927 the Medical Board requested a modification to the new rule in which it would "grant the privilege of treating private patients at the Hospital to Physicians who are eligible to and have applied for membership in the Massachusetts Medical Society or the Homeopathic Medical Society [and that the physician] then follow regular rules for admission to the Hospital." Staff membership was even then not a requirement, however, and while this step recognized the basis for the problem it did nothing to effectively rectify it. This fact finally brought the Staff to the realization that the accreditation power of the ACS, so long resisted, could help them.

In January 1928, with Dr. Cleaves' motion to procure a copy of the ACS *Manual of Hospital Standardization*, the matter came to the point of resolution. With the manual in hand the Staff and Trustees set out to meet the requirements for accreditation, the most stringent of which appeared to mandate a more formal Staff organization with bylaws, regular meetings, better record keeping and the employment of a laboratory technician. At a full Staff meeting in February Dr. Mooring's motion "that as soon as a Technician is employed we proceed to fulfill all requirements of the American College of Surgeons, and as soon as possible qualify for admittance" was carried. The request went to the Trustees, in whose hands it languished until December, when, under Medical Board pressure, they accepted Dr. William Irving, a new Staff member, as pathologist. Two months later the appointment was complete, with Dr. Irving to work in cooperation with the pathology consultant, Dr. F. L. Burnett of Boston.

Meanwhile, in January 1929, Dr. John J. Egan, a member of the original Medical Staff and a fine physician-surgeon, was Chairman of the Medical Board, and under him the reformation was completed.[3] Despite all the struggle the records of the Medical Staff are strangely silent, but the Trustees recorded at their April meeting their approval of the Staff's recommendation to accept the proposal for "recognition of the Hospital by the American College of Surgeons [after] adoption . . . of the minimum standards of requirements . . . effective May 1, 1929." The first ACS survey for final acceptance took place a year later, but with that vote the matter was finally resolved and another milestone passed.

In August 1929 the new "Rules and Regulations of the Staff," which restated many of the prior rules but added several more and described the new form of organization, were given the Trustees for acceptance, and were put in force the following May. They met all ACS requirements and, most important, made it mandatory for a doctor to be a member of the Medical Staff before he could admit or treat patients at the hospital. The Trustees were apprised "that the Medical Board was no longer in existence and that the newly organized staff had assumed the duties and activities of the two previous bodies, the Medical Board and Medical Staff." Dr. Egan was elected Chairman of the Staff and its Executive Committee, which consisted simply of the old Medical Board under a new name. Dr. Ezra E. Cleaves was made Secretary.

These changes, important as they were, did not overcome the long-standing need for better communications between the Trustees and Staff. For years the two bodies seem to have operated almost in separate worlds, with communication confined to memos and letters delivered by the Superintendent and occasional forays by emissary or committee from one to the other. Dr. Cleaves, who remained as Secretary for many years with his meticulous records, gives wry insight into this situation as he describes for his colleagues one such interchange on the subject of the new rules and regulations in early 1930:

In accordance with the vote of the Staff, your Secretary repaired to the Sanctum Sanctorum of the Trustees at the Cape Ann Savings Bank. . . . Here, at the Stronghold of Finance, he was joined by the Chairman of the Staff, Dr. Egan. The two representatives of your organization, after a short wait, were admitted to the meeting where they were courteously and cordially received by the President and the large number of members who were gathered there; and it is gratifying to note the fact that a spirit of friendly interest and cooperation was manifest on the occasion of this joint meeting.

Without further ceremony, the President, Mr. Phillips, who, may I add, impresses one as being unquestionably a dominant figure in the affairs of the Hospital, requested your Secretary to read the Regulations one by one.

Not long after this, in a refinement that appears to have been intended to bring the two bodies into closer cooperation, the Trustees voted to appoint "a contact committee of five Trustees" and request that the Staff also appoint five of its members "to meet in joint session at regular stated dates to confer in matters of importance concerning the operation of the hospital." Just how well this forerunner of the later Joint Council performed can be questioned, since subsequent formal communication with the Trustees suggests that the Staff's Contact Committee met separately and conveyed their findings and opinions to the Trustees via the Staff Executive Committee. This move to better interchange seems to have expired altogether by 1932, when the Medical Staff recommended its abolishment. The two most important groups in the efficient management of the hospital, although their members were socially friendly and met regularly on the golf course or tennis court, maintained this arm's-length stance for many years.

But at least things could calm down and both sides look with hope to better times ahead. The hospital was ACS accredited and consequently had a laboratory with a full-time resident technician to assist Dr. Irving while also operating the X-ray equipment. It also had two consultant Roentgenologists and a Medical Records historian. The Medical Staff, bolstered by the new membership requirements, grew to nineteen, plus consultants and two dentists.

There were still cliques among the Staff whose members remained jealously protective of their private patients, and even with the addition of the historian, some doctors continued to neglect their record-keeping responsibilities. And there was surely continued grumbling about the requirement that all share in the Ward Service. Adding to the lingering discontent, the Trustees inexplicably caused a near bloodletting when, in November 1931, they adopted a rule that they could "for any reason by them deemed sufficient" allow nonmember physicians to care for private patients at the hospital. After an exchange of letters that rule was amended and rendered harmless, with the Staff retaining its new role as arbiter of hospital admissions.

Staff control of admissions carried with it the concomitant responsibility for granting privileges, a power by which it could determine who should or should not treat patients within the hospital. Its power to deny recommendation to the Trustees for acceptance of new members was crucial to a newcomer's ability to practice. The ACS standards were also strict on the subject, and the Staff took its responsibility seriously.

An example lies in the practice of Dr. Lester C. Feener, whose case came up about the time the issue first surfaced. Dr. Feener had opened an office at 40 Middle Street in late 1925 and applied for Staff membership and hospital privileges in December 1926. He was appointed assistant physician in June 1927 with a further stipulation permitting him to perform surgery, but only with an assistant approved by the Medical Board. He was especially interested in gynecological work and in 1928 had enlisted the surgical support of Dr. Edward M. Hodgkins of Boston, under whom he had done his residency. Dr. Hodgkins, although not a member of the local Staff, was nonetheless approved as Feener's assistant, and by the end of the year the pair, apparently with little notice, had performed ten hysterectomies. Three of the patients died. It was the eleventh case, in January 1929, that brought them to the Staff's belated attention.

That patient, twenty-five years old and pregnant, also died. Dr. Hodgkins' report of the operation was read at Staff meeting, and Dr. Feener was ordered to appear before the Medical Board for questioning not only on that operation but also on the others performed the previous year. With the realization that his work had not been reviewed earlier, the Board knew that a full investigation would be required to avoid the unfavorable publicity attending what could be perceived as an illegal operation.

Dr. Feener's testimony held that the woman had a history of heart trouble and that he did not feel she could deliver her child safely. But with further evidence and opinion to the contrary, he was charged with "continued disloyalty to the Hospital, gross negligence in obtaining information, and poor judgment in evaluating obtained data to the end that cases have been operated on to their great harm and thereby the Hospital has become a subject for severe criticism." His case was not helped by Dr. Hodgkins who, although he had agreed with the decision for the operation, told a Staff meeting in January 1929 that he had "known Dr. Feener some years and that he was crazy or nervous at times and that to be charitable, call it eccentric."

Dr. Feener was asked to resign, Dr. Hodgkins' surgical privileges were withdrawn, and presumably the Staff had received some valuable experience in peer review and its importance. Feener continued in local practice for a short time by referring his patients to Beverly Hospital and then moved to Texas, where he is said to have developed a cardiological practice.

Another physician's problems during this period caused far more anguish among the Staff and Trustees and in the community itself. It involved a popular and highly talented physician whose roots were deep in Gloucester's life as a member of one of Cape Ann's foremost medical families.

Dr. Roy Garland was the son of the first Dr. Joseph Garland and a half-brother of Dr. J. Everett Garland. A 1905 graduate cum laude of Harvard Medical School with further training at Massachusetts General and Boston Lying-in hospitals, he was considered a fine physician and brilliant diagnostician. He came home in 1908 to take over his deceased brother's office and practice and soon gained a wide respect and affection among the people and his colleagues. Applying soon thereafter for Staff membership, he was appointed by the Trustees in March of that year. Following the Staff realignments of 1915 he was assigned to the surgical side and later that year was named to the new six-member Medical Board. This outstanding and popular doctor would seem to have been on the way to a fine career.

But he soon began to miss Medical Board meetings and was occasionally recorded as missing or being tardy for morning rounds, and his medical records began to fall behind, a failing in which he was not alone. Soon stories began to circulate concerning what were "his escapades while drinking." Worse, rumors of illegal operations, a euphemism for abortions, began to circulate. Eventually his case reached the powers at the Massachusetts Medical Society which, after a hearing, deposed him as Fellow and Member in

1923. On May 21, 1924, under mounting pressure from all sides, he requested and was granted a six-month leave of absence. The leave became permanent, and he never again was listed as a member of the Medical Staff.

He maintained a practice in Gloucester, however, referring his patients to Beverly Hospital when necessary and all the while retaining professional acceptance as a member of the Physicians of Cape Ann group. He also remained popular socially, which may have been a factor in the 1931 vote by the Trustees to permit non-Staffers to treat private patients at the hospital.

The final blow came in March 1932 when a case was reported at Staff meeting listing "general peritonitis" as the cause of death from "a criminal abortion" performed outside the hospital. Dr. Garland was charged and tried at Salem Superior Court in a case that received little or no public mention. Although no jail sentence was imposed, he was placed on probation and deprived of his medical license. The latter was restored in 1938, and he maintained a small practice in Gloucester until his death in 1956. Dr. Roy Garland's story was, and will always be, a note of sadness at the hospital and among his many friends. He could have been one of the great ones.

Intra-Staff problems continued to include the ongoing saga of Dr. Mooring, who can be seen to have viewed himself as a cut above his colleagues, their rules and what he evidently regarded as their petty reproaches. An example lies in his consistent refusal to don gown and mask in the operating room. Although sepsis had long been controlled by O.R. sterility, he insisted on his right to enter the immediate surgical area in street clothes and without mask or cover for his grey-streaked black hair. His persistent violation of a 1930 Staff rule requiring proper gowning led in 1932 to a confrontation with the Trustees in which he told them he would not take his surgical service rotation "if the present O.R. supervisor is retained on duty." Miss Eglenton, the supervisor, had been guilty of insisting on his proper dress if he was to enter the area for which she was responsible. The Staff, divided as usual pro and con on the subject of Dr. Mooring, was ambivalent and not wholly supportive of her. She left of her own volition shortly thereafter, and Dr. Mooring eventually gave in to peer pressure for proper O.R. decorum.

Mooring was without doubt a brilliant man with little patience to suffer gladly those he considered fools. A constant smoker with brown eyes deep-set in a ruggedly handsome face, he used a quick wit and sharp tongue to put down pomposity and what he considered inept medicine; it has been said of him that he would have made a good lawyer, and surely many of his colleagues must have wished he had chosen that profession. In the words of one of the long-retired nurses who remember him, "he was a man you either loved or hated," a judgment shared by his patients, one of whom said "he loved to collect your money, but he'd cut you dead on the street."

But for all his quirky personality traits, he had the good of the hospital at heart and did much to improve its standards. He introduced the Schick Test, a method for determining the need for immunization against diphtheria, in Gloucester in 1924. Its subsequent use in the public schools by the Board of Health was a major factor in the almost total elimination of that childhood scourge here. In the early 1930s he was the first to urge appointment of chiefs of service as a way to improve Staff efficiency. He introduced blood transfusion to the AGH and donated the first equipment for performing the procedure, and although his proposal for a prenatal clinic was voted down, he was simply ahead of his time on that subject. His fight for quality is also apparent in his 1931 "scathing criticism of the Staff Clinical Conferences," which, according to the minutes of yet another meeting at which he spoke his mind, he called "a waste of time . . . of no benefit to anyone . . . not properly prepared [and lacking] discussion." He was also responsible for the 1932 appointment of a new Staff Efficiency Committee "to oversee for incompetent or inefficient work" by members.

He was a natural leader, quick to give his opinion but finding it irksome to listen to others. As he grew older he is described as loath to adapt to new developments such as intravenous treatment and nasal gastric suction during surgery. His failure to maintain his own medical education left him behind the newly appointed younger doctors of the 1930s, whose use of more modern methods he scornfully derided. At his peak he had been an effective, though prickly, proponent of the hospital and the medicine practiced therein. On the decline he was still a factor, but his bark would have less effect as the medical world passed him by.

Prentiss House and Nurses' Residence

The enlargement of the Nurses' Residence, first suggested in 1919, had become urgent following completion of the Maternity Wing. More nurses on staff and a growing school meant that its capacity was taxed, with twenty-nine residents; another eleven were housed in the six basement rooms under Maternity. More classroom space was also needed.

Within the hospital itself the Staff had long chafed at the lack of sufficient medical-surgical beds, and the ACS, in its 1930 accreditation survey report, had urged serious consideration of reducing overcrowding. The Trustees had been aware of the condition for at least ten years, with census figures often counting more acute-care patients than there were beds. In 1925 the hospital exceeded 10,000 patient days for the first time, in part because of the new wing but chiefly in the acute-care section. When 1930 logged just over 17,000 patient days and an 85 percent occupancy rate, often with beds in the corridors and twenty-seven beds on a floor designed for seventeen, expansion could be delayed no longer. The decision was also helped by demographic figures showing the AGH with two beds per one thousand population, at a time when the national average was five.

The older proposal for expansion of the Nurses' Residence was given priority, and the Trustees, with N. C. Phillips as President, commissioned plans in late 1929, with fund raising scheduled for the following year.[4] Ezra Phillips, N. C.'s brother and by then in partnership as Phillips and Holloran, was asked to prepare the plans with guidance from hospital building consultants. His directive called for him "to use the present Nurses' Home as the basis on which to add and construct the proposed Nurses' Home."

A building fund campaign was launched in the summer of 1930 with President Phillips as General Chairman. The goal was set at $175,000. With such a massive effort facing them, the Trustees retained outside fund-raising counsel, a move that brought Dwight Folsom of the New York firm of Will, Folsom & Smith to Gloucester for the first of many campaigns. It also marked the first entry of Rockport people into an effort in support of what was now also their hospital; three teams under Everett R. Wilkinson covered the Sandy Bay side of the Cape. The work got under way in late June with the first newspaper announcement of the plans. Folsom established a "by the book" organization of divisions and teams still used today, and the campaign brochure designed by his firm and describing both projects was a model of its kind. The campaign itself ran the last two weeks in August, cannily utilizing the presence of the summer population.

Success is the only word for this first all-out effort, despite its early Depression start. Its roaring climax came at the Victory Dinner at City Hall when Dr. John J. Egan, Sr., Chief of Staff, rose to announce "that Mrs. Margaret Brady Farrell of Bass Rocks has established a memorial to her late brother, James J. Brady, in the amount of $23,000." This was not the first generous Farrell gift nor would it be the last, but it was one of the most exciting, coming as it did at the climax of a well-executed campaign. The Farrell name, which still ranks high among the list of the hospital's supporters, was inscribed on the first of many recognition plaques bearing the name, and what later became Prentiss House still remains a focal point of the family's interest in this Gloucester institution.

The August 26 issue of the *Times* carried a banner front page headline: "OBJECTIVE NOT ONLY ATTAINED BUT OVERSUBSCRIBED – TOTAL IS $253,187.50." The lead paragraph read: "$253,187! When these fig-

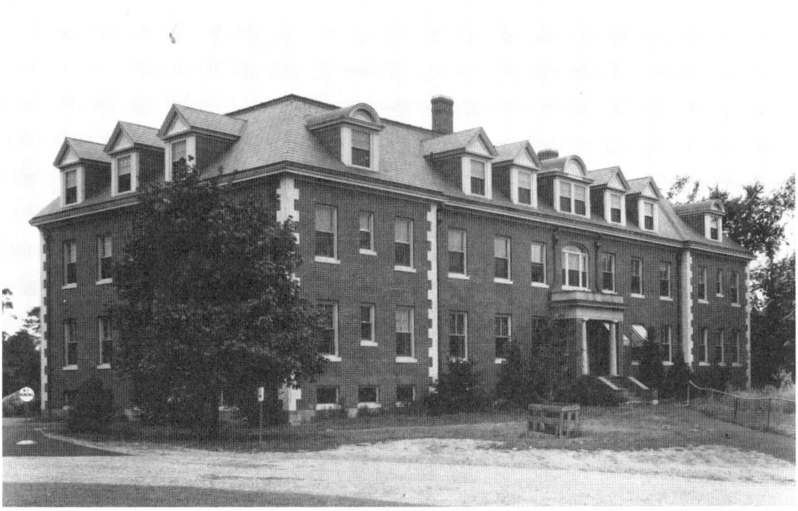

The Nurses' Residence just after completion of the additions in 1931. The two new wings and the original building were brick veneered to match the hospital.

ures were shouted above the tumult in City Hall last night, the very rafters of the sturdy old building shook." By the time the books were closed, the drive had obtained 2,647 outright gifts and pledges, with the latter accounting for about two-thirds of the total.

With funds in hand or pledged there was no hesitation about getting construction started. The foundation for the residence addition, built by J. S. Pomeroy of Gloucester, was in place by February, and the rest of the work went out for bid. R. E. Runels Construction Company of Lowell came in low at $51,000 and was awarded the contract subject to a proviso, added with an eye to local business conditions, that Runels "make every effort to give preference to local labor, also to make every effort to buy all materials from local dealers." The architects were empowered to enforce this ruling. Subcontracting was kept local, with L. E. Andrews Company doing the plumbing and heating. Faulk Brothers, in the first of that firm's many jobs for the hospital, brick-veneered the entire building replacing clapboards in place since 1903. The nurses and students, displaced during construction, were assigned quarters in a house rented from Trustee Elmer Babson for $50 a month.

The new construction added wings at each end of the old building, with two large classrooms in the north end of the basement and a large room on the Washington Street side becoming a kitchen classroom for teaching dietetics and cooking. On the first floor were four new single bedrooms with toilet facilities, plus a classroom in the north end; seven bedrooms plus facilities occupied the south end, four of which were later converted to an apartment for the Superintendent. A library, living room and reception room, dubbed "The Date Room" by the nurses, took over the old section of this floor. Upstairs, the second and third floors were entirely dormitory with forty single rooms, which appeared, together with those on the first floor, to be sufficient to meet the most ambitious plans for the years ahead.

The first-floor living room from 1901 had been endowed by a gift of $2,500 by Patrick M. Longan in memory of his wife, Georgianna. Mr. Longan, also donor of a room in the Maternity Wing in memory of his mother-in-law, Delphinia Morrisc [*sic*], was a native of Gloucester and had been chauffeur to John Hays Hammond in his younger days. Like so many of Hammond's associates, he had benefited from his employer's investment wisdom to become independently wealthy himself, and, although he had moved to California and his oil holdings there in 1912, he never forgot Gloucester and its hospital.

The Longan Room was, in his words, to be used for the "comfort, recreation and enjoyment of the nurses." It was to become a comfortably furnished

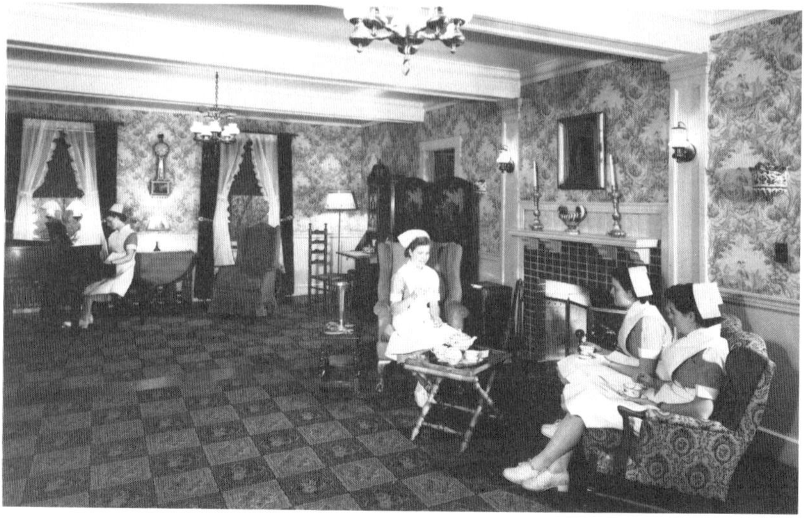

The Longan Room, endowed and furnished in 1931 by Patrick Longan, became a popular gathering place for nurses and for meetings of the trustees, the auxiliary, and others.

room for many purposes involving the school and the hospital. Among its furnishings was a Steinway grand piano, a fine instrument described several years later by the *Times* as "the best piano in town." The room with its piano was the inspiration for another gift by Mr. Longan in 1936, when he gave $1,500 as an endowment to support a musicale each year on his wife's birthday, a tradition that was followed faithfully every October 19 for the next thirty years, always with a bouquet of roses on the mantel, as he had directed. Although the concerts are no longer held, the room remains as he gave it and is the only surviving interior feature of that building. The Auxiliary, which had met almost from the beginning at the old G.A.R. Hall on lower Washington Street, transferred its meetings there and assumed responsibility for its maintenance and decor.

The construction and facilities of the enlarged residence required about $85,000 of the funds raised, leaving some $168,000 for the building of the new wing, which had already been designated as Prentiss House. The name derived from a major gift in August 1929 shortly after initial planning had begun. This gift, which gave significant encouragement to the then still hesitant Trustees, was announced in a letter from summer resident Colonel John W. Prentiss: "Mrs. Prentiss and I would like to contribute $50,000 to the new building. If you and your Trustees agree to accept this gift, our only conditions are that the new building be of fireproof construction, and that it be called 'Prentiss House.'" Needless to say, acceptance came quickly, — Prentiss House it would be. The gift also proved the fund-raising theory of the value of such leadership giving, as N. C. Phillips pledged $5,000 and Trustee Isaac Patch $1,000 the same evening in challenges to the rest of the Board.

Colonel Prentiss was a self-made man whose life's rule was "get the job you like and work like hell." He found his place with the Boston-based Hornblower & Weeks brokerage as a young man and, after establishing a New York branch of which he was manager, rose high in the business. Not long before his bellwether gift to the hospital, he had also astounded Wall Street by offering to buy the Ford Motor Company for one billion dollars; he didn't win that one, but the offer was typical of the man. He and his wife loved Cape Ann and made themselves and their summer home, Blighty, available for various community projects.

Ezra Phillips' plans for Prentiss House were ready in August 1931, and the project, which by then also included a new boiler house, was put out to bid. Because of its size no local contracters wished to undertake it, and the job went to R. E. Runels, who simply carried on from the Nurses' Residence project. Subcontracts were awarded to Gloucester firms, with L. E. Andrews again doing the plumbing and heating and Charles E. Pew the electric wiring. The work was completed in August 1933 for just over $120,000, exclusive of furnishings.

What the people of Cape Ann got was considered impressive – eighteen private rooms plus a four-bed tonsil ward; solaria, some years later enclosed as six-bed wards, on each of the two floors; a new Accident Room and, on the ground floor, eleven small rooms described as help's quarters. In the old building the surgical area was rebuilt and across the corridor, where today are located the administration offices, doctors' and nurses' lounges were added. On the ground floor of the revamped ell was a dining room for doctors and nurses directly across from a new kitchen made possible by the relocation of the boiler plant. The Trustees took over the old Nurses' Dining Room on the first floor and their old room became the Medical Records office. Except for the lobby, the old first floor front became office space; the Superintendent had her private office in one of the rooms of her former apartment.

The new wing was well and tastefully furnished with private baths between each pair of rooms with the latest lighting, radio and telephone outlets, plus other features such as lounge chairs contributing to the ambience. There was even a silver service for each room, with sugar bowls, creamers and coffee pots all engraved "Prentiss House." And, as the *Times* dutifully noted, the rates remained the same as for other private rooms at $6 a day. Of primary importance, however, was the fact that the hospital finally had sufficient beds in which it could properly care for the people of its service area.

One feature not originally planned was made possible by the Hammonds who, as the 1930 drive wound down, made a gift of $10,000 "for the development of a Roof Garden where patients can enjoy air and sunshine." This evolved into plans for a nautical motif and became the Hammond Deck, atop the new wing. It was fitted out as a ship's wheelhouse with wheel, bell and binnacle, and there was a raised hatch outside on the caulked deck with the wheelhouse roof, complete with rail and life-rings, reached via a ship's ladder. Although there is no record of the origin of the cabin fittings, a chronometer added in 1934 is known to have come from the schooner *Natalie Hammond*. The Hammond Deck received acclaim and much use, especially by the occupants of the adjoining children's ward, until the 1950s, when further construction of bed space put the third floor of the old building out of service for patients.

A troublesome problem soon surfaced as the economic depression began to have an effect on pledge collections. The situation simmered until mid-1932, when the Trustees faced "the matter of pledges on which no pay-

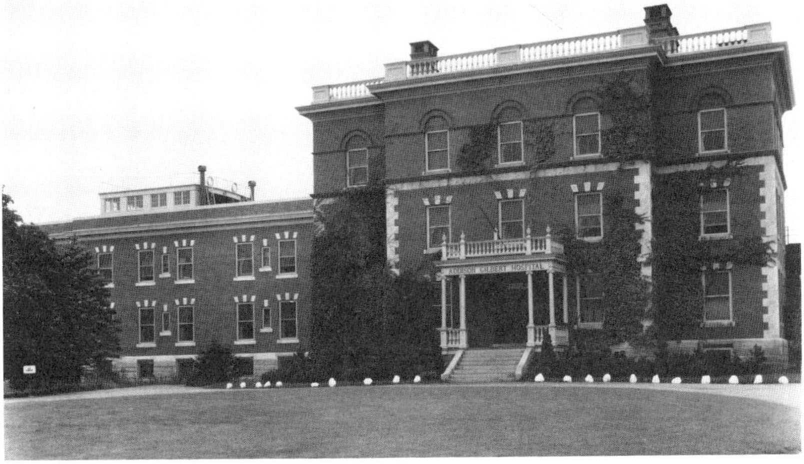

The facade of the AGH post 1934 with Prentiss House at the left and the Hammond deck on the roof.

ments have been made." President Phillips suggested employing someone "to interview those who have made such pledges," and the matter was left to him and the campaign treasurer, Trustee J. Hollis Griffin of Cape Ann National Bank, as a committee with the still customary "full power" to act. Their efforts met with but slight success, and by September 1933 it was necessary to invade unrestricted endowment to meet construction bills.

The problem dragged on as the nation's economy worsened, and in 1936 the committee had to report that "some will be eventually paid . . . some cannot be paid as they have lost their money; some can be [traded] for labor or materials; some, if interviewed, will give all or part of pledge; some can be collected by the committee, through pressure or by suit." There was no desire for the latter course and, given the times, it probably wouldn't have been effective. The lost pledges were seen simply as another facet of the financial problems, to be borne as stoically as possible.

Other Plant Improvements

Large events naturally dominated the period, but some smaller matters deserve mention. The construction of a separate boiler house at the time of the Prentiss House construction was the culmination of discussions that began at least as early as 1923 when the Trustees, hoping to minimize the need for constant repairs to the obsolete original equipment, first considered combining several separate boilers into a single central plant. In early 1932 L. E. Andrews Company completed installation of up-to-date coal-fired equipment in a new building which, although the boilers have long since been replaced, still serves today.

The need for a portable bedside X-ray machine not only led to an improvement in that service but also eliminated a problem that had plagued nurses and patients from the start. Use of the X-ray located on the ground floor required transporting patients down two or three floors over the main building staircase. This back-straining operation was hard not only on the often seriously ill patient but also on the nurses who did the carrying, sometimes assisted by a physician or two. The same route was of course required to and from the operating rooms as well.

A portable X-ray had been the subject of long and often vigorous debate, but such equipment was heavy and could not be moved between floors without an elevator. And so it was that when, in 1921, the Staff got approval for "the purchase of a new Campbell Coolidge Clinette X-ray Unit, portable," the issue was forced. In April 1922 it was voted to install an elevator at an estimated cost of $13,483, of which $10,000 had to be borrowed. The Medical Staff had its new X-ray and, surely just as important, after twenty-five years of carrying patients up and down stairs the nurses were relieved of one of their more arduous, if not downright dangerous, chores. That elevator with its heavy hand-operated latticed gates, located just off the front lobby, would serve for more than fifty years.

The horsedrawn ambulance went out of service in 1917 when the city purchased a motor vehicle for the Police Department. The Medical Staff suggested "the desirability of some arrangement whereby the Hospital patients might be conveyed in that ambulance," and not long thereafter the old ambulance, then handled by a taciturn, somewhat difficult driver named Allen, was retired. The city arrangement worked well for the most part, although the doctors were soon complaining that "the police ambulance is uncomfortable and hard on very sick and injured patients." A new city ambulance after 1931 resolved that issue while leaving a chronic problem concerning charges for its use for later city councils and hospital Trustees to work out.

One of the more dreaded possibilities at any hospital is fire. The Addison Gilbert, whether through diligence or simple good fortune, never experienced that crisis, even in its earliest days when fire protection was crude and dependent on in-house fire buckets and the horse-drawn, coal-fired engine operated by the city. In 1915 fire-hose stations were installed and portable hand extinguishers were placed on each floor later that same year. Outside stairways were added at the rear of the main building shortly thereafter and, with the establishment of a state Building Inspection Department and new state regulations, further steps were later taken to prevent fire and its spread.

Gloucester's Fire Chief, Homer R. Marchant, whose department was largely motorized by 1916, also began the practice of careful and regular examination of the hospital. In 1920 he recommended installation of the first in-house fire alarm box to augment the nearest one out on Washington Street. With a box exclusive to the hospital, he promised to send extra kit: two ladder companies, one steamer, the hose wagon and a chemical truck with thirteen men instead of the seven who normally covered a first alarm. The hospital box was pulled for the first time during the morning of May 9, 1928 when a fire in the laundry was extinguished with minor damage. The sounding of the alarm on the waterfront horn caused considerable concern throughout the city before Chief Marchant sounded the "all-out" on ascertaining the limited nature of the incident.

When the hospital was first built a cesspool sufficed for disposal of wastes, but after 1925, with additional beds, this system soon became a problem. A septic sewage system, something new in those days, was deemed necessary and was installed in 1928, at a cost of $1,099. It served its purpose adequately until 1939, when the city sewer was extended up Washington Street so the hospital could be tied in.

Improvements were made in other areas as well. The kitchen was upgraded with equipment acquisitions, including electric refrigeration, in 1927 and with new stoves following the move after 1934. A central telephone switchboard was installed in the early 1930s when the front lobby area was given over to office space. In 1933 the Trustees voted to erect "a suitable shelter adjacent to the street for the accommodation and comfort of visitors and others from the hospital" while waiting for Morris Katz' Gloucester Auto Bus, which had replaced the old trolley line in the early 1920s. Even the tennis court was improved in 1921, with a new bluestone surface donated by Dennis C. Ballou, but the purchase of a power lawn mower, requested in 1926, was deferred.

When the first expansion period ended the hospital boasted seventy beds and had managed reasonably well to keep up with the times. The Trustees had gained a greater measure of recognition as the ultimate authority while the Medical Staff, although still protective of its prerogatives, was slowly becoming more willing simply to practice the best medicine it could. The

Superintendent had become a more effective manager with the result that the post of Visiting Trustee, since the earliest days the eyes and ears of the Trustees within the hospital, had given way in 1929 to the powerful House Committee.

NOTES

[1]A near fatal incident which is well-described in *Lone Voyager* by Joseph E. Garland.

[2]See Appendix C for listings.

[3]The only other member of that Staff still serving was Dr. Snow Cook.

[4]N. Carleton Phillips was one of Gloucester's industrial leaders as head of the Russia Cement Company. "The Russia," as it was familiarly known, became LePage's, Inc. in 1941 in order to better identify it with its best-known product, LePage's Glue.

5

The Hospital Comes of Age

THE YEARS BETWEEN 1934 and 1948 saw many changes – social, political, industrial and in the health care field. Dominated first by the continuing effects of the Depression and interrupted toward their close by the second major war in twenty all-too-short years, they were the precursor of more dramatic changes to come.

Cape Ann was a microcosm of the rest of the nation in facing layoffs and heavy unemployment by 1934. The case load of Gloucester's Board of Public Welfare grew from 1,380 in 1930 to 2,484 in 1932, and by 1934 25 percent of the population was being supported by some form of benefit program. As described in the Welfare Board's report for that year: "Lines of applicants and recipients fill all City Hall corridors."

The fisheries suffered along with everyone else and, except for a good year in 1935, remained depressed until the opening of the redfish industry in 1939. This new fishery, plus the opening of the State Fish Pier that year and the outbreak of war in Europe, combined to bring the fisheries back, but only after a decade of personal and corporate suffering.

The federal government under the administration of President Franklin D. Roosevelt was doing its best to alleviate the nation's economic problems. The Works Progress Administration (WPA), a program to provide work via government-supported projects put in place in 1935, kept many men and women off the welfare rolls. Although geared mostly to public works such as street repair and building construction, it also supplied workers to hospitals and other such institutions that requested them. By 1937, as reported by Dr. Elmer Babson in his January 1938 Mayoral Inaugural address, the people of Gloucester were receiving about $600,000 annually from it and other government programs.

The hospital endured the tight financial situation along with everyone else. The collection of unpaid building fund pledges and of patients' fees for services, already slow, grew more difficult as the years wore on. Room rates, low even by the standards of that period, could not be increased, and payment of them in any case could not be enforced on people already in danger of losing everything. Staffing was kept at a minimum, which made it possible to avoid wage cuts beyond that of 10 percent across the board in 1932. City employees volunteered a similar cut that same year to help offset the increase in tax delinquencies.

Doctors' bills, like those of the hospital, were all-too-often uncollectable. Many physicians recall being paid in kind, with vegetables, services or fish and shellfish, which at least kept food on the table. Although many of their patients would eventually pay their bills, some would never be able to afford the appendectomies, the broken bones, the children born or all the illnesses treated free by their family doctors during those years. Cape Ann was fortunate that everyone who needed and requested it got medical treatment and hospital care, with or without payment.

By 1936, two years after Prentiss House was opened, the hospital was operating at a rate of 20,000 patient days a year, with a 70 percent occupancy average. Although this required more employees, it also made for a more efficient operation and eliminated overcrowding. Management, although seriously hampered by ever-present financial problems, was easier.

The Superintendent

Martha Avard remained as Superintendent during the first three years of the period, retiring in 1937. With the approach of her retirement another of those chronic quarrels between the Medical Staff and Trustees flared as the Board pondered the appoinment of her assistant, M. Louise Sanford, as her replacement. The Staff, at a special meeting that July, drafted and presented the Trustees with a formal resolution of two "Whereases," one to praise Miss Avard and the other to protest that "the Staff is without information regarding [a] successor — a matter which very much concerns the Staff." The resolution, passed with only one dissenting vote, recorded opposition to Miss Sanford's appointment "on the grounds that [she] has demonstrated her unfitness for the position and that her appointment . . . would be prejudicial to the best interests of the Hospital."

Louise Sanford was a young women with a good background of experience, impatient with the old way of doing things and eager to move the hospital into what she saw as a better world. Her quick mind and outspoken attitude had alienated some older Staff members, while the Trustees, on the other hand, welcomed her view of the future and her ability to speak up to the Staff. After a joint meeting of the two bodies, at which the Staff remained unconvinced of her worth, the Trustees, holding to their contrary opinion, voted unanimously to appoint her in August.

Miss Sanford served as go-between for the Board and Staff over the next three years. Although there is no evidence to suggest continuing antagonism on the part of the latter, neither were there the customary encomiums when she resigned in December 1940 "to take a few months rest before accepting the Directorship of another Hospital." The Board's judgment of her ability was vindicated not only by her proven ability but by her subsequent career, as she later became Administrator of the Children's Polio Hospital of Kentucky (she was dubbed a Kentucky Colonel by that state's Governor in 1954) and a consultant on children's diseases to the Federal Public Health Service.

Her replacement, Marion L. Jackson, was appointed without fanfare in February 1941. Miss Jackson was Director of Nurses at Winchester Hospital at the time and before that had had twelve years as Superintendent at two other Boston suburban hospitals. Like Miss Avard she was a strict disciplinarian, carefully formal in her relationships, and is remembered as a gracious lady with her pristine white uniform and precisely folded cap. She was among the first to be named a Fellow of the American College of Hospital Administrators, in September 1947; her thesis, "Public Relations in a Community Hospital," was appropriate to the times and to her experience here.

The Governing Body

The Board of Trustees and the Corporation had expanded in many ways from the original "Gilbert Five plus Two," the exclusive group which directed the early years. The Corporation, composed only of Trustees for the first several years, was part of the evolution.

That body, from which members of the Board are drawn, broke with its early WASP banker-businessman tradition in 1924 when it added three clergymen: Albert A. Madsen of Trinity Congregational, Myles D. Kiley of St. Ann's and Francisco G. Martins of Our Lady of Good Voyage. Although a small attempt to broaden the membership base, it had no effect in stimulating interest or attendance at annual meetings, which continued to be so sparsely attended that lack of a quorum almost invariably caused two or three adjournments.

This situation was further addressed in 1929 when a committee was appointed "to revise the list of Members of the Corporation." Its report, delivered at the twice-postponed Annual Meeting in March, advised that a list of prospects had been drawn up but then recommended tabling the matter to the 1930 Annual Meeting. In April 1930, after three adjournments, ten new Corporators were elected. They were the first additions since 1925 and included the first Italian and lay Portugese members: Benjamin Curcuru, Manuel Domingos and Manuel Viator.

Twelve more new members were elected in 1934, then nine years passed during which only nine were added. In 1943 – obviously a vintage year – thirty-three were chosen, after which the subject was again dropped. In any case, by 1948 there were eighty-two residents of Gloucester and Rockport listed as Members of the Addison Gilbert Hospital Corporation. They were, however, members in name only, selected as representatives of the community but without significant function to keep them involved or interested. For the Trustees it remained business as usual by an exclusive group giving lip service to the outside world.

Attendance at annual meetings did not improve. Only the Trustees appeared interested in them, an assumption borne out by the fact that during the entire period from 1934 to 1948 a single non-Trustee Corporator was in attendance only four times. The lone Corporator surely felt out of place, but perhaps his lack of company is explainable also by the fact that the meetings were still being held in the late afternoon at Cape Ann Savings Bank, where there was barely enough room for even the Board, and notice of them consisted of a single paid ad in the newspaper – legal, but hardly stimulating.

The Board itself grew in fits and starts, setting its number at will and as it perceived a need. Its members served one-year terms and were, barring death, almost invariably reelected each year. Its committees were largely ad hoc to fill special needs although by the mid-thirties, under President Phillips, five standing committees, abatements, accounts, finance, house and training school, were being annually appointed.

Of these only the Finance and House committees, the latter the equivalent of today's Executive Committee, kept records that have survived. The House Committee, which at its creation in 1935 had been "empowered and instructed to take steps to increase the efficiency and economy of operations," met at least once each month prior to the monthly Board meeting, and its recommendations seem to have carried considerable weight. The Abatement and Accounts committees, having outlived their usefulness, were discontinued in 1943, but a Publicity Committee was added in 1944.

The Board, which at first had no guidance beyond its own instincts, also could by then rely to a greater degree on outside guidance and the experience of others. The American College of Surgeons, for example, although primarily a physician-oriented group, had been influential in hospital affairs since 1919. There was no strongly effective affiliation specifically supporting hospital governance and management, however, and the need for such an organization was becoming more apparent as hospitals grew in size and complexity of their management problems.

Thus it was that the American Hospital Association came into its own. It evolved from the Association of Hospital Superintendents, which had been organized in 1898, changing its name to American Hospital Association (AHA) a few years later. It remained essentially a superintendents' club until the 1930s, when its role in the development of health insurance gave it credibility and a sense of purpose. The increasing involvement of government in hospital affairs gave it further impetus to expand, with consequent involvement of Trustees and others. Its $100,000 budget of 1942 was a far cry from today's multimillion-dollar operation, and it is today an effective voice for the more than 5,500 hospitals and other patient care institutions that comprise its membership.

The AHA is first mentioned in AGH records in 1907, when the Trustees declined an invitation to join. It next appears in 1922, when Miss Avard was "authorized and requested" to attend its Atlantic City convention, even though the hospital was not yet a member. Three years later, however, the Board voted to join the American Hospital Convention (Institutional), an offshoot of AHA, at $10 a year, and on June 4, 1925 it became member #849 of the Association itself. It did not hesitate to avail itself of the AHA's experience, as the Board voted the next May "to ascertain . . . just what service [it] is prepared to render the member hospitals, especially in regard to survey of buildings, equipment and method of operating hospitals." By 1948 the AHA had expanded as a very real factor in the life of its members, and would continue to grow in guidance skill and political power.

The Massachusetts Hospital Association (MHA) performs the same basic function as the AHA, with its strongest influence at the state and regional level. It was formed in 1936 and today enrolls two hundred hospital and other institutions statewide. This hospital's first affiliation with it was early in its history, when in December 1936 the Board contributed $10 "towards the expense of handling legislative matters concerning hospitals."

Another outside affiliation nearer home is found in the rather loose ties that developed in the mid-1940s to Salem Hospital. Although there had long been a working relationship between the two hospitals' medical staffs consultatively and through shared services — laboratory and X-ray, for example — this had not extended to the Board or administration prior to 1945. In March of that year, spurred by the possibility of a Rockefeller Foundation grant, Salem's Board met with representatives of the AGH, Hunt Memorial of Danvers, Mary Alley of Marblehead and Cable of Ipswich. Harold Maddocks, the AGH President, had already been made a member of the Salem Board and represented this hospital.

Out of this meeting came the North Shore Plan of Coordinated Hospital Service, financed by a tempting $20,000-annual five-year grant. The proponents predicted cooperation in pathology, radiology, anesthesia, medical records, social services and the hospitals' medical libraries, and under it Salem would make available certain of its scientific and technical services to the four smaller hospitals. The *Times* called the idea "unique in hospital history and [attracting] nation-wide interest." Interhospital cooperation did not come easily, however, as six months later the AGH Board severed relations with the Salem Hospital Community, thus designated by the leadership of that institution, "including Trustee representation on the Board of Salem Hospital."

Some enthusiasm for rejoining the coalition returned with the January 1946 invitation by Salem to again name a representative. Mr. Maddocks and later President Carroll K. Steele were thus designated, and although the latter advised the Board in 1947 that he had attended the Salem Annual Meeting and "had found it helpful," no real progress was made. By March 1948, when the House Committee reported "unsuccessful attempts . . . to find a way to determine our obligation to the Salem Hospital [and] agreed to let the matter rest for a time," the four-hospital effort was disintegrating. Sporadic attempts were made over the next several years to keep the coalition active, but today, although relations are friendly and several areas of shared services remain, there are no formal ties.

Financial Problems Persist

Financial problems continued to plague the Trustees, and the Depression only made them worse. Patients' payments, always slow, became worse with additional beds after 1933. Early in 1934 Superintendent Avard was authorized "to make use of promissory notes in settling patients' accounts," and the Medical Staff Executive Committee went on record as urging physicians to "impress the patients that they should endeavor to pay the hospital something even though it is a very small amount."

By 1936 the Trustees concluded "that it would be desirable to make a settlement of some kind with many of them, and the employment of some suitable person to engage in this activity was referred to the President and Treasurer with full power to make arrangements." In August that year Robert F. Thompson, a Gloucester native, was "engaged to collect outstanding accounts at $30 per week including use of auto." Payment in advance for all nonemergency maternity cases was required after 1937.

In 1938 the Board voted to place certain accounts in the hands of its attorney, a drastic approach, though not a new one, and, judging by the Treasurer's reports on the subject, not very effective. The charge-off of $15,728 in accounts receivable in May 1941 was probably inevitable, and the only consolation the Board had was the knowledge that their dilemma was not unique to them.

The hospital's creditors also suffered. In April 1938, with the Depression still raging, accounts payable were $11,383 and growing. When they reached $12,608 in June the Treasurer was authorized to transfer $7,000 from uninvested capital, a move that stemmed the tide only temporarily. By August 1940 the hospital faced payables of $17,713, and $10,000 more was transferred from capital a year later, with payables at $22,437. Borrowing became necessary the next year – $15,000 to meet the most pressing of the $25,192 then outstanding.

Free care was fading into the past as "the welfare" took care of many of the previously unassisted poor. The Gloucester Board of Public Welfare informed the Trustees in December 1940 of its "appreciation of services rendered without charge in the past and [of its] complete willingness to compensate for services for which the city [is] legally responsible in the future." In 1943 the city budgeted $1,000 "to cover work done for recipients of Soldier's Relief in addition to the $4,000 received through the Board of Public Welfare." Old Age Assistance patients were not admitted to the Ward Service after 1944 but went instead into the intermediate category, a decision that helped the doctors as well as the hospital, since they too could then be recompensed for care that was given at no charge on the ward.

The Social Security Act of 1935 also provided benefits for the ailing elderly after September 1936 in granting an allowance for hospital treatment to those over sixty-five and receiving Social Security. Although but a small step, this was a foretaste of further benefits to come and was welcomed by hospitals and physicians alike. Even the American Medical Association, traditionally opposed to anything resembling compulsory insurance or what it labeled socialized medicine, accepted the inevitable.

Of equal importance to the attempts of government to ease the burden of health care costs was the emergence of health insurance during the 1930s. Such assistance had long been the rule in most of Europe and took its earliest form in this country in the ethnic benevolent societies introduced by immigrants. Some trade unions and businesses also established private plans even before 1900, and some private insurance companies had devised plans to cover specific diseases early in the century. But all found such plans expensive and difficult to control, and none except the benevolent societies really addressed the basic problem, coverage for the poor.

Programs for health benefits can be found locally as early as 1899 when the hospital's Trustees voted approval of "a proposed plan to interest the fishermen in the creation of a fund of sufficient income yearly to support such fishermen needing hospital treatment who are parties to the fund by regular contributions through the year of $2 each." The plan died unfulfilled and nothing was said about it again, although private charitable groups such as the Fishermen's & Seamen's Widows & Orphans Aid Society offered medical assistance from their trust income.

Ethnic beneficial societies established by the Finnish and Swedish people of the Lanesville and Pigeon Cove villages assisted their own, as did the Acoriana Beneficial Association among the Portuguese community. The latter association survived in Gloucester until about 1937, when commercial insurance and other assistance rendered it superfluous. It is also probable that subscribers to Dr. Choate's Cape Ann Therapeutarian plan at the Gloucester Hospital were at least given discounts at that short-lived institution.

The AGH established a plan to provide "suitable and adequate care for the nurses and employees" in early 1938, modifying it three years later so that free care would be provided only after a year's employment. This employee plan was followed by one allowing past and present Medical Staff members free hospitalization, giving members of their immediate families a 50 percent discount.

Employers generally were required by workmen's compensation legislation of the 1930s to provide funds through insurance to cover hospital and medical costs of work-related injuries. The larger employers of Gloucester people — Gorton-Pew Fisheries, LePage's and others — also had private broad coverage plans through commercial insurers before 1937, but most people on Cape Ann, as elsewhere, were essentially left to their own devices.

Out of their need came Blue Cross, once described as sired by the Depression and mothered by the hospitals. Groups of hospitals and even single institutions, first in Texas, then in California, New Jersey and Ohio, began by offering contracts covering hospital charges to employed persons. A New York plan in 1934 brought the concept further by broadening access and placing control under state insurance regulators, while leaving the operation itself under the hospitals. By 1937, especially where individual hospitals had established competing plans, the AHA had sensed a need for intervention for the protection of all, particularly for the small community hospital, which could not afford to fund a plan of its own.

The AHA formed the Hospital Service Plan designating competition-free territories operating under state insurance regulators. Within each territory all hospitals banded together under a central collection and management system, which assured premium payment by participating members. By 1939 the concept was nationwide, and the tax-exempt, hospital-managed plan had become Blue Cross. It was opposed, as might be expected, by the private insurers who by then were increasingly entering the field; they remained viable competitors, although on a smaller scale.

Early medical opposition to a perceived encroachment was allayed by the AMA, which convinced its members that if their patients' hospital bills were thus paid, the patient would have cash available to pay the doctor. With such justification the plans became acceptable as long as the hospitals didn't go further and encroach into medical practice, which some saw as a next step. And once the profession had accepted Blue Cross, it was inevitable that coverage of physicians' charges would follow.

Prepaid physician plans had emerged in the early 1930s, established usually by private industry and rural cooperatives, but their growth was limited by the old AMA bugaboos — fear of loss of independence, unethical contract practices and controlled fees. The gates were finally opened by a 1939 California plan, supported by Blue Cross and operated in much the same fashion, which soon gained wide acceptance. By 1945 Blue Shield was well established and operating as an adjunct to Blue Cross, independent but coming under the same umbrella of tax exemption and state control.

In September 1937 the AGH Board voted to participate in the Associated Hospital Service Corporation of Massachusetts, which had been established under the auspices of the AHA. Coverage, as described in a "Family Group" certificate issued to J. Stanly Thompson, his wife Natalie and sons John and James on June 1, 1938, was similar to that of Blue Cross, which soon succeeded it. By 1940 the Service Corporation had reimbursed the hospital almost $9,000, which suggests that it had been reasonably successful in enrolling participants.

It became Blue Cross about 1941 and more active in enrollment efforts. The hospital sponsored its employees for group membership that year, and in 1944 Blue Cross mounted a campaign among Gloucester individuals and commercial establishments. At year's close it was estimated that one in every eight residents had some form of Blue Cross coverage, and the hospital had received $23,415.17 for its services by 1943. But the record also shows that, then as now, there was argument and controversy over the amount and method of reimbursement.

There the matter rested for twenty-five years. Government plans were yet to come, and meanwhile the Blues, the private insurers, the Veterans' Administration and such limited coverage as was offered through Social Security helped not only to alleviate the cost of health care for the patient but also to assure payment for its providers.

Medical Matters

The precarious relationship between the Medical Staff and the Board of Trustees continued to hover, with little face-to-face contact. Other long-standing problems within the Staff also persisted. Attendance at Staff meeting was irregular, with consequent scant attention paid to the case discussions that were supposed to follow each business meeting. Peer review and such ongoing medical education as was available also was often overlooked, to the consternation of the more conscientious members. A more stringent bylaw amendment governing attendance helped, but didn't solve such problems as early departure from meetings.

Among the more positive aspects was the fact that some younger men were joining the Staff, bolstering its quality and strength while bringing a fresh viewpoint to its thinking. Drs. W. Warren Babson and John J. Egan, Jr. came in 1932, followed in 1935 by Dr. George M. Doyle. Thomas H. Odeneal, MD replaced Dr. Snow Cook as Oculist/Aurist in 1936, and Dr. David J. Cohen was appointed in 1937. Drs. George J. Pohas and Warren M. Poland arrived in 1938 and 1939 respectively.

All Staff appointments were subject to scrutiny, not only to meet standards set by the ACS but also because a conscientious Medical Staff wants qualified colleagues, and a hospital Board wants the best that can be had for the people of its community. Qualification thus was a major factor in granting privileges, but a lack of firm criteria as to what that meant sometimes led to disagreement. Membership in the Massachusetts Medical Society was deemed sufficient evidence of general aptitude, and without it privileges at this as at most other Massachusetts hospitals were not granted. Another essential was graduation from an ACS-approved medical school, plus, of course, reliable references.

This concern that only those judged qualified be granted Staff membership was intended to benefit the hospital as well as the people it served, but upholding it continued to lead to problems. Two cases further illustrate the difficulty of dealing with this sensitive subject which must sometimes differentiate between the desire of a physician to practice and the duty of a medical staff or board of trustees to assure competence and ethical conduct.

Dr. Milton A. Dexter had opened an ear, nose and throat practice in Gloucester and applied for privileges at AGH in September 1933. In processing his application it was noted that he had not supplied references, nor was he registered as a member of the MMS. Inquiry at Lynn Hospital, where his resumé indicated prior practice, turned up no Dr. Dexter but the suggestion that he was probably Max A. Dechter, MD who had been affiliated briefly there after leaving Noble Hospital in Westfield during 1932. His application was rejected with little discussion and action deferred for a year.

Without hospital privileges Dexter found it difficult to build a local practice and was forced to rely on Staff members to admit his patients, a situation as irksome to them as it was difficult for him. He had support, on the Staff, however, which was almost evenly divided pro and con even after negative responses had come from inquiries to his former colleagues at Noble. When he again applied for privileges the following year the Staff voted to send the matter of his appointment to the Trustees without recommendation, contrary to the rules of the hospital but indicative of the controversial relationship intra-Staff and with the Board.

In a written response by President Phillips in February 1934 the Board firmly rejected this approach and refused to act until the Staff met its responsibility for recommendation. Chastised, that body voted down a motion to appoint Dr. Dexter, and there the matter rested another year while he saw patients in his office but sent them to Massachusetts Eye and Ear Infirmary or Beverly Hospital when such treatment was indicated.

In April 1935 Dexter's application was again brought before the Staff Executive Committee and again rejected, but in a controversial split vote the full membership took the matter from the committee's hands and granted him Courtesy Staff status, equivalent to a probationary period but permitting him to treat private, but not ward, patients at the hospital. The Trustees, concerned at losing even a few patients to other hospitals, accepted the recommendation at their next meeting. The problem did not disappear, however, and when his reappointment came up the next year, accusations were made that he had been practicing outside of his specialty, taking patients referred to him by other physicians for ENT work and treating them for all their ills.

He pleaded his case in a long, impassioned letter, asking for acceptance and understanding but admitting to questionable practice. Despite his admissions of error the Staff, in what now seems like misplaced confidence, appears to have tried to help him. He was reappointed to the Courtesy Staff again in 1936 and 1937. His case had caused deep divisions within the Staff and certainly did nothing to ease the tension between it and the Trustees. To the relief of everyone the issue became moot when Dr. Dexter resigned in August 1937 ostensibly to move an ill member of his family to a better climate.

A later application had a happier ending after Morris J. Pett, MD, a native of Gloucester, requested privileges in 1942. His first application was turned down at Staff level because the small medical school from which he had graduated was not on the ACS-approved list. Again in 1944 rejection came for the same reason, but by 1948, when he applied for the third time, he had gained important support among the Staff. This support was further bolstered by the so-called Gallupe Plan, developed by Dr. H. Q. Gallupe of the Massachusetts State Medical Board to alleviate a wartime shortage of physicians, under which doctors without full training could practice under the supervision of a hospital's medical staff.

Further, in response to inquiry by the AGH Staff, the ACS clarified or relaxed its prior policy in advising that graduation from a nonapproved medical school need not bar a lower-level Staff appointment if the applicant otherwise met all ethical and other standards, confined practice to the scope of his competency and worked under general Staff supervision. Thus encouraged, the Staff recommended Dr. Pett for limited Courtesy Staff privileges that September, and the Trustees voted his appointment at their next meeting. In 1951, having been granted council status by the Massachusetts and Essex South Medical Societies, he gained appointment to the Visiting Staff with full privileges.

It was a popular decision. Dr. Pett, familiarly known as "Mo," was a well-liked general practitioner, always available, always affable. He was aware of his own limitations, and among his endearing features was the honesty of his self-appraisal and a sense of humility, a quality often absent among some of his better-trained colleagues. A popular public figure, he was accorded a rare honor a few years later when the people of Gloucester held a "Doctor Pett Day," during which they raised a considerable sum of money as a gift to him. This, in a gesture typical of his nature, he used to purchase pediatric equipment for the hospital. On retirement from active practice in 1973 he was awarded Honorary Staff status, which he held proudly until his death in 1976.

In other developments, the Ward Service remained a bone of contention. Almost everyone agreed with the hospital's policy that ward patients, some 10 to 15 percent of the total number, were entitled to as good care as was available to the private and intermediate patients who had a choice of doctor. However, the physicians on the medical side saw it as an uncompensated and confining chore to be accepted as a condition of hospital privileges, while those on the surgical side continued to see it as a not unwelcome assignment through which they gained experience.

Another irritant on Ward Service centered about arguments as to which patients should be entitled to it. Ward physicians sometimes balked at accepting a free-care case if they felt the patient was able to pay, and while this was understandable if it did in fact deprive the doctor of a fee for his services, it did not always sit well with the Trustees, who had to answer to a sometimes angry family which faced questions as to financial status. After one such case, in which an operation was held up by the surgeon who questioned the patient's right to ward treatment, the Trustees made it clear that they and they alone would make such determinations.

As the 'thirties advanced the ACS played an ever larger role in the lives of hospitals and their medical staffs. Its surveys were being made more frequently with the results anxiously awaited, for without approved status no hospital could long survive. Such a survey was made at the AGH in 1938, and the report that followed struck fear among the Trustees. Among citations of multiple failings were several of long-standing concern: poorly attended, infrequent and ineffective Staff Clinical Conferences; inadequate and incomplete medical records, over 200 with some dating back several months; too few routine laboratory examinations and autopsies. The report recommended "complete rehabilitation of the medical records," that surgery be better controlled so that "only those well qualified [are] allowed to do major surgery" and that a Department of Anesthesia be established to permit only specially qualified persons to give anesthesia. It closed with a warning that "under the present circumstances we cannot carry [the hospital on the approved list] much longer."

The sternly worded report was taken as an ultimatum by the Trustees, who advised the Staff that they intended to measure up fully to its requirements and that this could only be accomplished if the Staff immediately initiated the necessary action. Uncompleted medical records dropped to forty-three by September 1939, and the Superintendent was able at that time also to report to ACS that attendance at Staff meetings was up and that "very worthwhile Staff Conferences are [being] held." Of long-range importance, she reported that revised bylaws and "Rules and Regulations" were governing the Staff.

Astutely using as a guide the *Manual of American College of Surgeons* and *Hospital Organizations,* by Malcolm T. McEachern, MD, who happened also to be Associate Director of ACS, the Staff had undertaken several months of committee work and negotiation. The altered bylaws met ACS standards and reorganized the Staff into Honorary, Active, Courtesy and Consulting categories. The "Rules and Regulations" had also been rewritten to conform with ACS guidelines.

By 1942 further change was in the air, this time instigated from within by the Board of Trustees. Facing the retirement of senior surgeon Dr. Ira B. Hull and perhaps having in mind a similar problem in 1937 when Dr. Mooring retired, the Board requested deferment of action to replace him, pending development of stiffer standards governing qualification. The Staff acted promptly and sought advice from the Boston surgical consultants, Drs. George E. Leland and E. Parker Hayden, who together with Drs. E. Granville Crabtree and Roy R. Wheeler, consultants in urology and medicine respectively, met with the Staff and Board in joint session on March 5. The meeting, addressed by each of the four consultants with answers to a wide range of questions, was a turning point in the sometimes turbulent relationship and in the hospital's development.

From it came several new rules governing qualification for Staff appointment. Most significant was one stating that major surgical privileges would henceforth be granted only to doctors with three years of surgical training at ACS-approved hospitals who met all other ACS standards as well. Furthermore, surgical staff members would be required to analyze and summarize all surgical procedures performed and present a bimonthly report to the Staff. In another far-reaching requirement the entire Visiting Staff would henceforth be expected to spend at least two weeks each year in formal study at a teaching institution or at accredited seminars.

Anesthesia was an advancing art under the influence of the ACS. Although ether was still in use, nitrous oxide was more and more replacing it as an inhaled anesthetic. Spinal anesthesia, developed in the late 1920s, was introduced here by Dr. Babson, who had learned its use as a house officer at Boston City Hospital. Although its acceptance here was cautious, Babson knew it was approved when Dr. Mooring asked him to administer it in a pelvic-abdominal procedure. With these developments the day of the etherizer or the use of any available physician as anesthetist passed from the scene. Dr. George M. Doyle was appointed the first Chief of Anesthesiology, a further response to ACS requirements for departmentalization of the work.

The first professional nurse-anesthetist was employed later that year. She was Kate Blandford, RN, a former operating-room nurse who had left to train in anesthesiology in Philadelphia. She could do all but spinal anesthesia, which still required a physician, and quickly won over the Staff with her skill as she established a new standard of what good anesthesia could do for the confidence of the surgeon and the well-being of the patient during and after an operation. Miss Blandford remained until 1942 when she left to take a position elsewhere.

Laboratory and X-ray

The lab and X-ray departments remained primitive in their cramped quarters under the 1925 Maternity Wing, short of equipment and personnel. These factors, with a growing hospital and improving techniques, were becoming an embarrassment. Leona Mitchell, retired Chief Medical Technician, describes a state of affairs that could not be tolerated much longer.

When I arrived in 1940 the lab was in the basement under the old OBS, a large rectangular room with a small kitchen table with a center drawer. On one wall there was a counter on which sat a table-top incubator about a foot square where we incubated a few blood cultures and blood plates that we did for bacti. We made our own culture media and the O.R. autoclaved it for us, and our blood cultures were done in Ehlenmeyer flasks. We made our own blood plates and obtained horse and sheep blood from the state labs on a bi-weekly basis.

The old wood framed wing was not soundproof, and I can recall our concern the first times we heard groans from the floor above in OBS and were sympathizing with the poor patient in the delivery room until one of the nurses assured us that it wasn't the patient we heard but Dr. Greene "who always helps his patients in delivery by groaning with them."

The lab was equipped with a black soapstone sink with hot and cold running water. A door let us into the darkroom where we developed the X-rays. We planted our bacteriology with platinum loops and an alcohol lamp and had one small staining rack at one end of the sink where we did both hematology and bacteriology.

I can remember the pint glass urine bottles, 25 to 30 of them, that were always outside the door awaiting us every morning at 7:00; they had to be washed and reused. We did urines, common blood counts which consisted of a white-red count, a differential and a hemoglobin. We rarely did hematocrits in those days because we had to fill the hematocrit tubes and centrifuge them for a whole hour. We did hemoglobins by the Sahli acid-hematin method and Guaiacs on stools and occasionally parasites. We did non-protein nitrogens, not bound urea nitrogens, and boiled them with a micro-bunsen burner; we had no hood in those days. We did our blood sugars in a boiling water bath the Benedict solution and matched both the colors of our NPNs and our blood sugars in an old Dubosc colorimeter. A cou-

ple of years later we got a Leitz photo-electric colorimeter, really the height of instrumentation in those days.

The combined lab/X-ray unit had gotten its first full-time technician, Mildred E. Mattson, in 1930. Working under Dr. William R. Irving for lab work and Dr. Harper E. Whitaker, the Roentgenologist, she had her hands full. The lab pathology was supervised by Dr. Francis L. Burnett, a Boston consultant living in Manchester, who came occasionally to do autopsies, with most specimens sent to his Boston office for study and report.

By 1939 the Superintendent was able to show that X-rays had almost tripled in six years, with lab tests up more than four times from the 3,000 performed in 1933. Since these services were becoming vital to the operation of the hospital, she was able to convince the Board that three full-time technicians were needed, an argument strengthened by the ACS, which had been critical of the laboratory in its latest survey.

That survey also exposed the hospital's vulnerability in having an almost less than part-time pathologist, as the ACS insisted on better supervision and especially more autopsy work and routine laboratory examinations. Although Dr. Burnett was by then supposed to spend two days a week here, this schedule was seldom kept, and dissatisfaction with the arrangement mounted steadily on all sides. By 1941 the State Department of Public Health was adding pressure through its licensing requirements, and when Superintendent Jackson came before the Board that October and "reported that there was no supervision of the laboratory whatever [by Dr. Burnett]," the Trustees knew something had to be done. The situation, plus his refusal to do autopsies, also aroused the Medical Staff, which began to agitate for his replacement by a more cooperative pathologist. World War II, which created a shortage of doctors, frustrated these desires, and there was nothing to do but live with the problem until peace returned.

War Interrupts

The lab problems, along with almost all the others, became academic after 1941 as the United States entered World War II. Its effect was wide and deep across the nation and locally was primarily reflected in the absence of hundreds of Cape Ann's young men and women as they joined the armed forces. Those left at home did their part in the general war effort, in industry and as volunteers.

The impact was felt at the hospital in staffing and supplies, both of which suffered from shortages. The armed services required large numbers of physicians and nurses, men and women of experience who could only be found among those staffing the nation's hospitals and clinics. Vast amounts of material were required: medical supplies, bedding and other cloth goods, gasoline, food — indeed, everything that had been taken for granted in peacetime was preempted or at best in short supply and possibly rationed.

The Medical Staff was especially hard hit, as five of its eighteen active members — Drs. Babson; James F. Collins; Egan Jr.; Pohas and Poland — left during 1942 for the service. The loss of five young physicians was felt keenly in the Ward Service rotation and especially on the surgical side, where only those with specific training and experience were permitted to practice. The shortage was made more acute as two others, Dr. Hanford Carvell, on the Staff since before the previous war, and Dr. Egan, Sr. from the original staff, died before the war was two years along.

Two old-timers came to the rescue. The now mellowed Dr. Mooring, retired from Ward Service since 1937, rejoined the rotation list. Dr. Ira Hull, not long retired, joined Dr. Mooring in rebuilding a qualified surgical staff. Both served to the end of the war and in February 1946 were once again retired to Senior Staff status with encomiums from their colleagues and the grateful Trustees. Also performing yeoman service was Dr. David J. Cohen, described as doing almost all the maternity work and often staying all night at the hospital.

The concern of the Board over further possible losses led it to take what steps it could to prevent further Staff attrition. An August 1942 vote "that the President take immediate steps to prevent the loss of any further doctors to the service" was, given the tenor of the times, a desperate measure. It became more specific a year later in instructing him to consult with the local Draft Board and advise that body "that [the Trustees] felt that the services of Dr. Irving were essential to the operation of the hospital." No more doctors left, so whatever persuasion the influential President Phillips used was effective.

Dr. Pohas was assigned to the Army Air Corps Medical Service and saw duty stateside before being sent to England late in 1943. He was among the early landing parties on the Normandy beaches on June 6, 1944 and remained until the beachhead was secure before being returned to the base hospital in England. Dr. Poland was a United States Navy Medical Officer and went through the South Pacific island battles ashore and aboard ship which, as any veteran of that fighting knows, was traumatic duty indeed.

Dr. Egan also went navy and, after base duty in the states, served to the end of the war as Commandant of the Naval Hospital at Guam. Dr. Babson did not leave the country; his Army Air Corps duty took him from Grenier Air Base in New Hampshire to Langley Field in Virginia, where he served as Chief of Surgery and gained valuable experience in fracture and trauma management in treating the returning wounded. Dr. Collins did not return to Gloucester after his service, instead taking an administrative post at Boston City Hospital.

There are no records of others of the hospital family who went to war. We do know that one Trustee, John R. (Jack) Cahill, Jr., was young enough to be eligible, and he served as a Naval Lieutenant aboard *USS Macon* for two years. Leona Locke, later to become Mrs. Mitchell, left her new position in the lab to become a Navy Wave, much to the consternation of the Trustees as they contended with that department's troubled function. Four staff nurses, none of them AGH graduates, enlisted, and several others left for positions elsewhere. All twenty-nine graduates listed on the plaque dedicated by the Alumnae Association to its members who served were employed elsewhere when they joined the armed forces.

The Nursing Service thus faced shortages, as did those at other hospitals, with which the AGH had to compete for personnel. This competition naturally led to pay increases, and by war's end general duty nurses were receiving $95 per month and head nurses $110. Floor nurses not wishing to live at the Nurses' Residence were given an extra $20 monthly for expenses, a major step in ending the tradition that had always required nurses to live and board on the hospital grounds. Private duty nursing was another war-induced casualty, and remained almost extinct within the hospital after the war.

Replacing the departing nurses was not easy; they were in short supply everywhere. The American Red Cross, foreseeing such an emergency, had begun work late in 1941 to establish a program to train aides. These were to be enlisted as a corps of volunteers and although they could not replace nurses as such, they could give assistance with many of the less skilled tasks and enable those remaining to devote their time to their patients. Training was given at many hospitals, including the AGH.

In May 1942 Miss Jackson reported to the Board that the first class of twenty-three Red Cross Nurses' Aides had been graduated and were at work. By the time the program ended in 1945 the AGH had trained 146 local women who, in their blue pinafores and caps, rendered 18,684 hours of service without recompense other than the knowledge that they were doing their part in the massive war effort. As conditions slowly returned to normal after the war they were less and less needed. Disbandment came in June 1946 at a gala banquet at the Hotel Moorland, where they received recognition pins and high praise from President Harold Maddocks and their volunteer directors, Mrs. J. Fletcher Burnham and Mrs. W. Harold Otis.

It was an active time for other volunteers also. The Women's Auxiliary formed neighborhood bandage-rolling groups in various parts of Gloucester and Rockport. The Red Cross also organized a Canteen Corps, which assisted in the hospital's kitchen; established in 1944, it had at least twenty-five members who reported on a regular schedule for dietary service. Another group was formed after a three-man committee visited the Superintendent to see if the men of the city could also help. By April 1944 the Addison Gilbert Hospital Men's Volunteer Corps had been recruited by John H. Lovett and Carroll K. Steele and was at work under its captain, Edward B. Ely. The men helped with the heavy work in moving patients, assisting convalescents and replacing absent housemen (the housekeepers of that time), laundry help and maintenance workers. These groups joined the Nurses' Aides for recognition at the Moorland banquet.

A further attempt to alleviate the shortage of nurses was made by the U.S. Public Health Service in establishing the Cadet Nursing Program, a 1943 effort that was planned as a shortened training course at selected hospital schools of nursing. The AGH was among those selected with a course organized here late that year, but its two-year program precluded any possibility of its being of material assistance before the war ended. It was phased out in 1945.

Rationing of supplies and some medicines became a way of life. Penicillin was among the latter, and the hospital's monthly quota was distributed by a committee of three physicians representing surgery, medicine and the ear-nose-throat specialty. Food rationing forced cancellation of guest trays for those visiting patients and of the luncheon meetings occasionally held at the hospital by outside groups. But even with shortages some improvements were made during those years, with added lab, X-ray and operating room equipment.

With the end of the war in August 1946 the hospital began to return to normal. Doctors and other staffers returned, although there remained a general shortage of nurses for a few more years under conditions of competitively high salaries available elsewhere. Some of the wartime Red Cross Nurses' Aides were brought back to help alleviate that problem during 1947. Several memorial gifts were made, among them an operating table "in memory of our members who served in World War II," given by the Gloucester Lodge of Elks. A former Mayor proposed a new wing to honor Gloucester's veterans, a concept that died for lack of funds.

The war had a significant effect on the practice of medicine. There were new drugs and methods of treatment to supplement the older knowledge of biology and immunology and bring about decreases in incidence and death from contagious and infectious diseases. Gloucester Board of Health records indicate a low incidence of diphtheria, typhoid, tetanus and tuberculosis as all joined smallpox on the list of former scourges. Scarlet fever, for which there is even now no vaccine, was among the more prevalent of the contagious illnesses, surging in 1944 and reaching a high of 103 reported cases in 1947.

Not all noncontagious diseases were affected by the postwar advances. Cancer and cardiac-related problems were still not well understood, although cardiac surgery had begun to take its first tentative steps in Europe during the war. These two remained the leading cause of death in Gloucester, with cancer responsible for an average of thirty-seven deaths annually through the 1930s and 1940s. Larger by far was the average of 145 deaths annually attributed to coronary and arterial problems during these decades. A sharp increase in reported cardiac deaths after 1940 can be attributed to better diagnosis, as many deaths formerly reported as "cause unknown" or interpreted incorrectly were then being recognized as coronary in nature.

The wartime development of pencillin and antibiotics brought dramatic decreases in death from nephritis and respiratory diseases after 1940. Tuberculosis (TBC) had been on the decrease locally since testing of cattle and the pasteurization of milk became mandatory in Gloucester in 1929, but the real breakthrough came in 1947 with the introduction of streptomicin and para-aminosalicylic acid. Together with isoniazide, which made bacterial chemotherapy possible, these developments reduced the treatment period, with a 95 percent success rate. Tuberculosis has rarely been seen on Cape Ann since 1967.

The scope of medical practice, although advancing in the years just prior to the war, was still far from what is being done today. At the AGH gastrectomy (rarely performed anywhere before the mid-1930s), colorectal, gall bladder, common bile duct and pelvic surgery were being done with increasing frequency. The use of blood transfusion, intravenous fluid and electrolyte replacement, and nasogastric suction were major additions to the state of the art. Much of the credit for the introduction of these methods here must go to Dr. Babson, who in some instances put this hospital among the pioneers. His was, for example, almost the first use of bacteriophage in the treatment of blood poisoning in Massachusetts.

By 1946 further advances were being made, many of which stemmed from knowledge gained during the war. Gastro-intestinal and thyroid surgical techniques were among those improved, as were the handling of fractures and trauma. The use of penicillin and antibiotics was becoming routine in controlling infection, reducing that postoperative complication to a minimum.

Postoperative management was undergoing other changes. Better anesthesia, including endotracheal inhalation, reduced the recovery nausea common with ether, and the use of nasogastric suction minimized the hazards of gas formation which too often resulted in ileus, an earlier life-threatening complication. It all meant that the patient could return to activity sooner, even while still hospitalized. This dismayed some of the older physicians and the nurses. Some of the nurses of that time, accustomed to bed confinement of two weeks or more, recall their amazement when Dr. Babson began getting his patients ambulatory on the day following surgery. "It was talked about as if a revolution had occurred," one of them says — an observation with considerable truth to it.

While many of the earlier procedures like appendectomies, hernias, abscesses, cancers and fractures remained commonplace, one of the most frequent into the 1930s, tonsil and adenoid removal, was rapidly being phased out. Until late in that decade children who hadn't gone through a T & A were considered to have been neglected, and there were 343 done in 1930 alone. July and August were always the busy months, with three or more such operations a day performed in the special area set aside for them. With the advent of sulfa drugs about 1937 and penicillin in 1943 tonsillar infections became manageable without surgery, and today pediatricians rarely justify the operation, only if attacks persist despite medication.

Another medical advance resulting from the war involved the storage of blood. Although the use of human blood as a life-sustaining treatment dated back to World War I, its value was limited, since transfusion could only be made direct from donor to patient, and blood could be neither stored nor transported. Research prior to World War II had made it possible to separate the liquid blood plasma from the solid red and white cells so that when dried the plasma could be stored and transported, then reconstituted with sterile saline solution for use, but with heavy demands for plasma it became essential to find new sources of whole blood for civilian use. From this need came the formation of a donor plan by the American Red Cross, the forerunner of the blood-banking program so effectively operated today.

Although direct transfusion had been introduced here in 1930 by Dr. Mooring, it was several years before it was being done on any significant scale. It was a cumbersome procedure and required on-the-spot donors, many of whom seem to have come from the Police Department, which was then operating the city's ambulance service. In 1937, as blood use increased, the Gloucester American Legion organized a "Blood Transfusion Squad" whose volunteer members came to the hospital when needed. This service was further formalized two years later when Drs. Babson, Egan and Irving, together with two laymen, were appointed a transfusion committee to coordinate the effort.

The plan they evolved called for formation of a reliable list of donors to be recruited from among the city's residents; Police Officer Joe Legendre gained considerable attention as a leader among the recruiters. Under the plan donors received $10 per unit given and recipients were charged $15 to $25 for each transfusion, with any excess after expenses prorated among the donors. Typing was primitive, but, as Leona Mitchell tells the story, "most of our patients got better in spite of the treatment."

With better matching techniques and improved whole blood storage, blood banking at hospitals became possible in 1943. The Trustees, intrigued by the possibilities, offered to spend up to $10,000 for processing and storage equipment. The Medical Staff, rejected the proposal expressing a preference for cooperation with Salem Hospital through its already functioning but overburdened unit. In 1946 the Massachusetts Department of Public Health put in place its own distribution center to supply whole and fractionated blood at no cost to any community offering donor service under the supervision of local Red Cross chapters. With this the Staff reversed itself and recommended installation of a storage unit here.

The first local blood bank was in place early the following year inscribed by its donor, the Gloucester Sea Food Workers Union, in memory of its seven members killed during the war. Gloucester became the seventh community to store blood for the Massachusetts Blood Donor Service and was thus permitted to supply free blood to anyone needing it. In addition to handling the collection, the Red Cross assumed responsibility for transporting it from the central lab in Boston to each participating hospital. From this work came today's Red Cross Blood Program, and from Gloucester's early participation by its people came also a notably fine tradition of response whenever blood collection is done here.

The Medical Staff: Another War Ends

With the end of World War II and a return of the Medical Staff to full strength again, some of the problems that had subsided would once more have to be faced. To its credit, the Staff had settled down to do the job during the emergency, with improvements in meeting attendance and maintenance of records. With other things on their minds also, the ACS and state authorities had relaxed that pressure. The situation had lain dormant except for a brief flurry in late 1942, when Dr. Gallupe of the state's Medical Board advised the Trustees that "the appointment of a Chief of Staff [is] the only proper solution of conflicts and problems between the Staff, Trustees and Administration." It was a concept often discussed but, like the several proposals for chiefs of service, always spurned by the Staff.

Matters came to a head in July 1946 following receipt of a letter to Miss Jackson from Richard P. McKnight, MD, Massachusetts Department of Public Health Supervisor of Hospital Inspection. In it he referred to a recent personal inspection of the hospital and stated that "we were surprised to learn that no one had been appointed Chief of Staff [and that] there is no responsibility . . . for heads of Departments." A second letter from him on August 8 was devastating: "This is to inform you that your hospital license which expired August 7, 1946 had been withheld owing to the fact that there is no proper staff organization . . . as mentioned to you in my letter [of] July 22."

When these two letters came to the attention of the Board at its August 20 meeting the reaction was one of incredulous fury. Miss Jackson was summoned to the meeting, held as always at the Cape Ann Savings Bank, for an explanation. According to the record of that session she "stated that these letters had been presented to the Staff [and] that previous criticism . . . had been disregarded by them and that on account of the war emergency the criticisms were not pressed . . . that there were divergent interpretations of the letters by the Staff." Dr. Babson puts it somewhat more strongly, describing the Staff as obdurate and determined that the state could not tell them what they had to do.

The Staff had already taken steps to obtain a set of the Department of Public Health's licensing requirements, but the Trustees, furious at the ignoring of earlier warnings, demanded immediate action. A special Board meeting was called for the following week, prior to which copies of the Staff bylaws of Salem and Beverly hospitals were to be obtained for study.

That meeting covered only one subject, but it lasted from 7:30 PM until 10:40. Taking the matter completely into its own hands, thus effectively closing out the Medical Staff for the first time, the Board voted unanimously to appoint a Chief of Staff and chiefs of Surgery, Medicine and Obstetrics to serve together as the Staff Council. It repealed all Staff bylaws and rules "which are inconsistent with this action" and directed the newly appointed Staff Council to submit "at as early a date as possible a code of bylaws and Rules and Regulations." Meanwhile the Council was given authority over the Medical Staff. Dr. Harold Baker of Rockport was appointed Chief of Staff to serve with Drs. Babson, Poland and Ronald Hallett as chiefs of the three services.

The fractious Staff did not take this action kindly, and voted at its September meeting to lay the Trustees' letter on the table without action except to "invite a committee of the Trustees to meet with the Staff to discuss the matter contained [in their letter]." It also voted to ask Dr. McKnight "to meet with the Staff at his convenience." The Trustees – on advice of legal counsel, Judge Lincoln S. Simonds, who urged them "to firmly maintain the action taken" – decided to act as a committee of the whole in meeting with the Staff.

From that joint session, held October 8, came grudging realization by the Staff that it must act. Dr. McKnight could not come to Gloucester until November so, unable to wait longer, the members proceeded to make minor changes to the bylaws and rules without actually addressing the real issues. These proposals were passed to the Board which accepted them subject to changes and further amendment to bring them into compliance.

Dr. McKnight added fuel to the fire when he inexplicably told the Staff in November that while there must eventually be a Chief of Staff and chiefs of service, there did not appear to be an emergency requiring such unilateral action by the Trustees. The next night the Staff Council again appeared before the House Committee to advise that the Staff was "more antagonistic than ever to the idea of dictation from the Trustees in the matter of Staff appointments [and] that the Trustees would have to be realistic and practical and accept the advice of the Council which could not function with a non-cooperative Staff." Four days later the full Board gave a vote of confidence to the Council and asked its members to make "as satisfactory arrangement as possible with the Medical Staff."

This could be taken as an olive branch back to a Staff that knew that it realistically had no choice but to submit. At a momentous meeting November 21, 1946 the full Staff agreed to accept the new bylaws and rules demanded by the Trustees. The decision was taken by the Council back to the Board which then, going by the rules, voted to accept the recommendation of the Staff. The Council, much to the consternation of the Trustees, then and there resigned, considering its work done and wishing to let the Staff make its own choice of chiefs and Council. In the Trustee's view, these were four men they had worked with and whose judgment they respected, and they could not conceive of others who could do as well.

They need not have worried. At its next meeting the Staff received the report of its disbanded Council, giving it a standing vote of thanks for bringing the issue to a close. It then proceeded to name the same four, plus Dr. Earle Greene of Rockport as at-large member, for recommendation to the Board for reappointment. That body graciously, and surely gratefully, accepted the recommendation.

With that move years of contentious misunderstanding were over. The

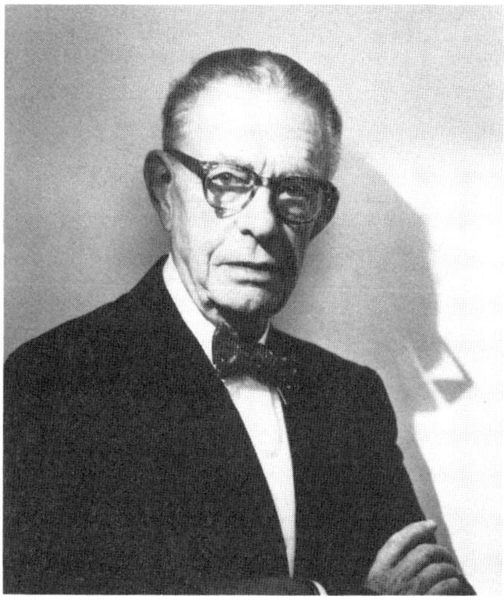

Harold Maddocks was president from 1942 to 1947, a period during which the hospital was sorely tried by the problems of World War II and in 1946 by a devastating clash of wills between trustees and medical staff.

Staff Council replaced the former Staff Executive Committee, and for the first time in almost fifty years the Trustees and Medical Staff were at peace in a working arrangement that has remained intact to this day. One of the casualties of the affair seems to have been Board President Harold Maddocks, who had inherited the problem from Carleton Phillips in 1941 and, to his great credit, had seen it through to a successful conclusion. He submitted his resignation as President in November pleading the need for "a complete rest." A young insurance man named Carroll King Steele was elected to succeed him at the Annual Meeting in January 1947.

Significant though it was, the 1946 dispute should not be viewed as more than the final encounter in a long search for identity between two strong-minded groups. Through it all both sides had maintained a common concern for the hospital's purpose and well-being, disagreeing chiefly as to the best course to follow. They had kept the conflict to themselves, out of the public eye and with very few, if any, employees knowing of it until it was over. With it the hospital can be said to have reached its maturity and was surely better prepared to face its future.

The Postwar Hospital

With peace on all fronts the hospital operation could begin to return to normal. Normal is, of course, a relative term sometimes meaning uneasy, and on that basis the financial situation was indeed normal. A postwar inflation merely made for a somewhat more severe "normalcy" than before.

In April 1947, with payables at $32,624 and "the cash balance inadequate to meet them," the Trustees approved transfer of the entire Maintenance and Capital Improvement Fund balance to the General Fund. A July report by an ad hoc committee of the Board called the situation serious, with cash on hand at $2,155. This amount and more was due on withholding taxes collected and not yet paid, and repayments were also due the government from the Cadet Nurse program. With those obligations plus overdue supplier and equipment bills of over $40,000, to say nothing of the need for $20,000 for urgent repairs, the Board voted to authorize sale of "such securities from the General Fund account as may be necessary." After several agonizing meetings the Finance Committee sold almost the entire bond portfolio and enough common stock to raise $27,000 with which to pay the most pressing bills. A final irony appears at the end of the October meeting, when Treasurer Robert Thompson stated that "he was not able by pressure of work to give the attention to collection of patient accounts that should be given to them."

A deficit of about $40,000 made for a gloomy close to 1947 as reported by Treasurer Thompson in a talk before the Gloucester Rotary Club. Over $50,000 had been drawn from capital funds, further reducing income. There was talk of possible closing or the need for the city to take over the operation as a tax-supported project. The knowledge that even the mighty Massachusetts General had used $735,000 of its capital and had closed 121 beds because it could not afford to pay the nurses did nothing to allay the gloom.

Increases in patient fees and appeals for public gift support were about the only options open to ease the financial pain. Although increased rates meant nothing if collection was impossible, more people were able to pay their bills with help from a growing Blue Cross and other third parties. Room rates had remained constant for eighteen years since 1924 except for spot adjustments in the Maternity Wing, and by 1942 the Board had come only reluctantly to the conclusion that an increase was needed. The new rates: ward beds to $3 a day, intermediate to $4.50 and private rooms to $7 in the main hospital and a dollar more in Maternity in each category. Once done it came more easily, and three more increases followed so that by 1947 ward beds cost $6.50 daily, semiprivate (formerly intermediate) $8.50 and private $11.50. Fees for X-rays, use of operating and delivery rooms, board of infants and laboratory tests were also periodically adjusted.

Employees faced the postwar inflation and the constant rise in the cost of living just like the hospital, which to the best of its ability must also offer adequate compensation. Nurses were best able to bring pressure to this end. With the war giving them influence they had not previously known, they found strength to obtain what meek compliance had never gained them. They were now less hesitant to speak up, especially where pay and living conditions were concerned. By 1946 a floor nurse was receiving $110 per month and a head nurse was at $120, with both categories paid an extra $30 monthly meal allowance and three uniforms laundered each week if "living out." In 1948 a further $10 monthly increase was granted, with the hospital laundering all uniforms.

More patients after the 1934 expansion required an increase in the work force at all levels. The first Admissions Office was established in 1944 to meet public criticism of delays in that procedure. An enlarged kitchen staff was placed under the supervision of the hospital's first professional chef that same year, prompting the resignation of his predecessor, who had run the operation for some twenty years. A larger housekeeping staff was required to do the chores once performed by floor nurses, relieving them for vital bedside care.

A paid vacation policy was put in place in 1936 under which nurses and other professionals were allowed four weeks per year; all other employees had two. Before Blue Cross was generally popular, employees needing hospitalization received it at no charge under a plan adopted in 1938. Wages, kept low during the Depression, had ranged from $12 to $30 weekly until the first minimum wage law brought the lower level to $16 in 1941, but after that wartime wage and price controls, together with operating deficits, combined to keep them low even after the war. Low pay could perhaps be justified by the tradition that working for a hospital, at least of the charity type, was a privilege offering the satisfaction of serving one's fellow man.

More patients also meant more medical records. Uncompleted records, a problem since the beginning, continued to be a source of irritation for the Medical Staff and frustration for the administration. But under increasing pressure by the ACS accreditation program, it was essential that they be maintained. In fairness it should be said that, although too many doctors considered record keeping a postponable imposition immune even from threats of suspension of privileges, not all were guilty; many did their best to keep their records current. For its part the hospital could only supply a good office staff in an effort to encourage the recalcitrants to comply, and a full-time historian (later called librarian) and clerk had been employed since the early 1930s.

A no-nonsense Records Librarian, Martta Somppi, first employed as an assistant in 1941, was put in charge of the office in 1944. Miss Somppi, later to become Mrs. Blanchet and a qualified Registered Records Administrator, ruled the department for the next thirty-two years, doing her best to keep things from getting out of hand. Her direct approach, often abrasive, sometimes irritated the doctors, especially those who were less than diligent in maintaining their records. She gained their respect if not their affection in a thankless behind-the-scenes post, but despite her diligence the records problem would never completely dissipate.

The laboratory situation, dormant during the war, also awaited correction. The Trustees feared offending Dr. Burnett lest he resign leaving the hospital without the ACS mandated Pathologist. A 1943 Staff proposal for a committee to supervise the work, deemed better than the one or two monthly visits by Burnett, had not been acceptable to the Trustees for that reason, but when, in early 1945, he requested an increase from $3 to $5 for each microscopic examination of tissue, they had had enough.

That spring a new Pathologist was recruited and with him came the start of a modern laboratory. Dr. Donald A. Nickerson, also Pathologist at Salem Hospital, brought in his Salem assistant, Dr. Geoffrey P. Keane, as part of his contract. Of greatest importance, the pair added regularity of presence with one or both making at least one visit each week, and often two. By 1946 Dr. Nickerson was coming every Tuesday and Thursday morning.

He insisted on equipment improvements. Mrs. Mitchell recalls:

With Dr. Nickerson's help and guidance we were able to purchase two binocular microscopes. We were able to get a spectrophotometer, and one of the doctors gave us a second photoelectrocolorimeter. We began to increase the number of tests we did here, and we developed quality control and standardized our equipment. We changed to international blood typing using A, B, AB and O. And we were encouraged to take courses at places like Harvard Medical or at Tufts.

But until the lab could expand physically, with space and equipment to do all the work here, the Pathologists had to carry most surgical specimens and nonroutine pathological work back to Salem for processing.

Like the lab, the X-ray Department had always operated under handicaps of space and staff, and one of the first changes Dr. Nickerson proposed was the separation of the two departments. The two arts required quite different skills, and, as the patient load increased, the need for separation of personnel was obvious.

Following Dr. Harper Whitaker's retirement as Roentgenologist in 1932, the post had been filled by a Boston doctor, Clarence N. McPeak, MD. Although the arrangement, similar to that with Dr. Burnett, was not entirely satisfactory, Dr. McPeak served until 1942. His replacement stayed two years before Dr. Stanley A. Wilson from Salem Hospital was retained in an arrangement that was to last for several years.

The department's scope and quality of work unquestionably improved during the Wilson regime. Some $12,000 was spent for new equipment in 1947, which included a fluoroscope to permit performance of some surgical procedures such as fracture correction more expeditiously and with excellent results. Having more equipment also required remodeling the room, although it remained under the obstetrical wing. It would appear that Drs. Wilson and Nickerson, colleagues at Salem as they were here, complemented each other's efforts as their respective departments here became increasingly essential.

Two specialized clinics that were established prior to the war are also of interest. The Cancer Clinic dated from 1934, when the Massachusetts Legislature called for the establishment of such clinics in various parts of the state, with funding available for X-ray and laboratory service plus clerical assistance. At the June 1935 meeting of the Medical Staff, Dr. Herbert L. Lombard of the State Department of Public Health explained that five such clinics were being formed and that the AGH was under consideration. He recommended that if one were opened here it should be under a Staff oversight committee, be staffed by three to five physicians as diagnosticians and be open at least once every two weeks.

The Staff recommended the proposal to the Trustees, who received it favorably. Drs. Babson, Burrell, Hull, Irving and Mooring were named by the Staff as clinic diagnosticians. The first clinic was held November 20 "under very encouraging conditions and . . . has proved its usefulness," according to Dr. Ezra Cleaves, its administrative Chairman and Secretary to the Medical Staff at the time. It continued successfully until 1942 when Dr. Cleaves reported difficulty staffing it with one of the clinicians in the service and the Staff already shorthanded because of the war. The problem was temporarily overcome by rotating assignments, but by the autumn of 1944 the situation was acute. Fewer cases, the unwillingness of physicians to serve and loss of both its paid staffers combined in its closing that November.

Revived after the war, it operated until the early 1960s, closing only after the state decided the program had served its purpose and ceased funding for it. The hospital, reluctant to drop it, continued it independently until 1965, when it was replaced by a Medical Staff Tumor Committee under Dr. Walter E. O'Donnell. Supplemented by a Tumor Management Group, which included regular cancer screening and examination at the hospital by some of Boston's leading specialists, it was the forerunner of the ACS-certified Oncology Clinic formed in 1976.

The Orthopedic Clinic was established to meet a perceived need for such specialized service here. A Boston specialist, A. Leo Brett, MD, had been on the Consulting Staff since 1937, making trips to Gloucester or seeing Cape Ann patients at his Boston office at the request of Staff members. These trips were becoming fairly frequent in both directions by 1940 and at his suggestion monthly visits were arranged, to permit seeing several patients each time. In 1940 he persuaded the Staff that Gloucester patients could be better served if he held regular clinic hours at the hospital, and what soon came to be known as "Dr. Brett's Clinic" was born.

Despite occasional doubts by the Trustees as to the added expense, the Brett Clinic served well. As the Staff pointed out, it eliminated the need for patients to travel to Boston and benefited its members who shared in the examination of their patients as they received the services of an eminent Boston orthopedist. Dr. Brett's Clinic operated to everyone's advantage until 1967.

Other hospital-based clinics in prenatal care and tuberculosis were briefly considered. The former was deemed unnecessary because the District Nurses already offered such a service. The TBC clinic would have duplicated one already operating at City Hall under the Board of Health. That public clinic closed in 1967 after the need for it diminished, but was reestablished briefly at the hospital for the benefit of the occasional patient.

Fund Raising and Bequests

As operating expenses rose and deficits went deeper, philanthropy and public support were gaining recognition as sources of badly needed assistance. Gifts had always been a source of funds, but earlier donors were primarily wealthy men and women whose gifts were relatively large and often made for a specific purpose. The general public had participated to some degree in funding the 1925 Maternity Wing and to a larger extent in the Prentiss House Fund, but these were capital projects. Except for occasional gifts in kind or small unsolicited monetary donations, most people stayed on the sidelines.

The local churches had traditionally depended on the gifts of their parishioners, and the Gloucester YMCA had conducted successful annual campaigns for several years, proof that the general public could and would help if asked. Indeed, at one point the Trustees went so far as to express the fear that the hospital would lose what donors it had to active campaigners for other causes, perhaps not an idle concern, as some of their fellow members could be found every summer working in the well-run "Y" drives. When the District Nurse Association ran its first public campaign in 1940, the Trustees knew that the hospital must also go to the public for additional funding.

Arthur S. Murch, Jr., then among the YMCA fund raisers and later to lead the hospital's efforts, recalls a meeting in 1941 requested by the hospital Trustees with the people at the "Y" at which the idea of joining forces was suggested. The "Y" representatives scorned the advances of the Johnny-come-lately hospital, suggesting that it come back after gaining experience, when they might consider the idea. The disappointed Trustees were left to face the chore alone and never had to return, for the hospital went on to become the most successful fund raiser in town.

At a special meeting in March 1942, citing the desperate financial situation, President Maddocks suggested a campaign "to assist the hospital in meeting its deficits." Mr. Maddocks took the chairmanship of the Campaign Committee and made some good choices to serve with him: Carleton Phillips, to whom very few ever said no; W. Harold (Bill) Otis, the Yankee banker from the Gloucester Safe Deposit and Trust; William H. Robinson, Jr., an Eastern Pointer; Jack Cahill, attorney; John Radcliffe, publisher of the *Times*; and Treasurer Bob Thompson. The committee selected Dwight Folsom, director of the Prentiss campaign, as adviser at a fee of $3,000 plus expenses.

Folsom's first task had been to survey the situation as to feasibility, and his hard-hitting report was submitted in July. Reminding the Board that "your present problems have been years in developing and cannot be corrected overnight," it went on to a detailed analysis of the hospital's difficulties, praising its devotion to free care while suggesting that too much of a good thing had led to low rates and disregard of hospital bills. He urged sharing the facts with the public, which he felt had the impression that the hospital was endowed and therefore immune from financial problems. "We are confident," he closed, "that [once] the people of the community . . . understand the facts about their hospital, [they] will rise to its support."

A well-organized campaign got under way in August, and three hectic and publicity-filled weeks later Folsom's prediction came true. The initial goal of $50,000 had been oversubscribed by $7,195, and almost two thousand of Cape Ann's residents and summer visitors had participated. It was a great beginning to a grand tradition and helped relieve the tight financial situation.

Not yet a firm tradition, annual campaigning almost faded away the next year when, contrary to the Board's June decision to hold a drive, the Steering Committee recommended "that in view of the absence of a vital financial emergency [this year], the multiplicity of appeals for funds in the community and the lateness of the season [we feel] it desirable to omit the campaign this year." This apparent complacency was not all the committee's doing, however, since most of the summer had been spent in discussions among the several charities as to the feasibility of combining in the new Community Chest concept. By the time all had agreed they could do better separately it was too late, for the hospital at least, to plan and conduct a campaign during the more productive summer season.

The concept of joint campaigning was revived the next year as the hospital and the Gloucester District Nursing Association combined in the first Joint Health Campaign. A one-week effort without fund-raising counsel was planned for May with a goal of $17,500 to be headed by Trustees Frederick M. (Fritz) Bundy and Harold Otis. It had none of the panoply of the 1942 drive and required more than the scheduled week, but in mid-July the committee could report that $22,089 had been raised from 3,739 donors. The hospital's share of the largely house-to-house effort was $15,505.

The Gloucester Chapter of the Massachusetts Society for the Prevention of Cruelty to Children joined the effort in 1945, again held in May with a still modest goal of $19,250. This one was under Trustee Arthur Murch as General Chairman and had the YMCA-experienced Carroll Steele as campaign director. Again a week was too short, but when it was over early that summer, $20,423 had been raised, with $13,262 for the hospital. A similar campaign the next year netted $19,558, with $12,770 for the hospital.

A lack of enthusiasm in 1947 that even the dynamic Mr. Steele could not overcome brought failure and a mere $10,000 of the ambitious $25,000 goal. And with that unhappy result came the end of joint campaigning, as four years of effort had netted less than the single campaign of 1942 and offered only slight relief to the still burgeoning financial problems.

Thirteen bequests during the years from 1934 to 1948 totalled $57,500, including $10,000 under the will of John Hays Hammond. Real estate netting $15,000, another $10,000 outright bequest and two of $5,000 plus the smaller ones rounded out the relatively small addition to endowment, another effect of the Depression. The hospital was also designated beneficiary of two trusts established, one in 1945 by Mary E. Winter and the other in 1947 by Alice V. Kidder.

Investment of the endowment funds, a gratifying exercise when times are good, became frustrating during the prewar years. Throughout the 1930s the banker-dominated Investment Committee watched values fall steadily as bonds, still the primary investment choice, dropped below face value, or worse, defaulted entirely. By 1939 the emphasis was shifting to common stocks under the guidance of Estabrook & Company, the hospital's investment counsel. This trend accelerated under new counsel, Nathan Bugbee of Boston, retained in 1943, on whose advice all new commitments were made in such securities. The only bonds bought for several years thereafter were those issued by the federal government.

Public Relations and a Fiftieth Anniversary

During its early years the hospital had but scant publicity; in fact, the Trustees tended to avoid public discussion of its affairs. The Prentiss Wing program opened their eyes to the possibilities of favorable newspaper coverage, however, and from then on stories appeared more frequently. The fund raising during the 1940s and the need expressed by Dwight Folsom for more communication simply emphasized the point.

John Radcliffe, influential at the *Times* and a hospital Trustee since 1928, was undoubtedly a factor in encouraging coverage during the 1930s. When the Board decided to formalize the procedure in January 1944 by appointing a Publicity Committee, he was named to chair it, an assignment unfortunately cut short by his sudden death that spring. The busy Bob Thompson, a diligent guardian of hospital affairs, replaced him as spokesman, publicist and archivist.

One chore neither he nor Mr. Radcliffe had, however, was preparation of the annual report. The small circulation compendium of statistics and other hospital information, which had been published yearly since the beginning, became a casualty of the hard times of the period after 1930. It was not issued again until 1936 when it covered the six years 1931 to 1936, and then it was dropped for twelve more years until a new Administrator revived it to cover the year 1948. The hiatus meant loss of a valuable source of statistics and other factual information, but because of its limited circulation, it was hardly missed by the outside world.

In February 1947, anticipating the hospital's fiftieth anniversary, President Carroll Steele appointed a new Public Relations Committee to assist in planning the celebration of that birthday, seen as a golden opportunity to tell the hospital's story. Over two days in June the *Times* devoted several pages to the hospital and related organizations. The highlight was a chronological history compiled by reporter Paul B. Kenyon,[1] who based his work on material contained in the annual reports. There were also articles on the Medical Staff and on Addison Gilbert, with histories of the Women's Auxiliary, the Nursing School and the local Red Cross Chapter. A congratulatory editorial pondered what Gloucester would be like without a hospital and expressed hope for its future.

The Auxiliary took charge of an Open House during which tea was served to all comers in the Longan Room, from which guided tours left to inspect the plant, which the *Times* described as "impressive, spacious and well-

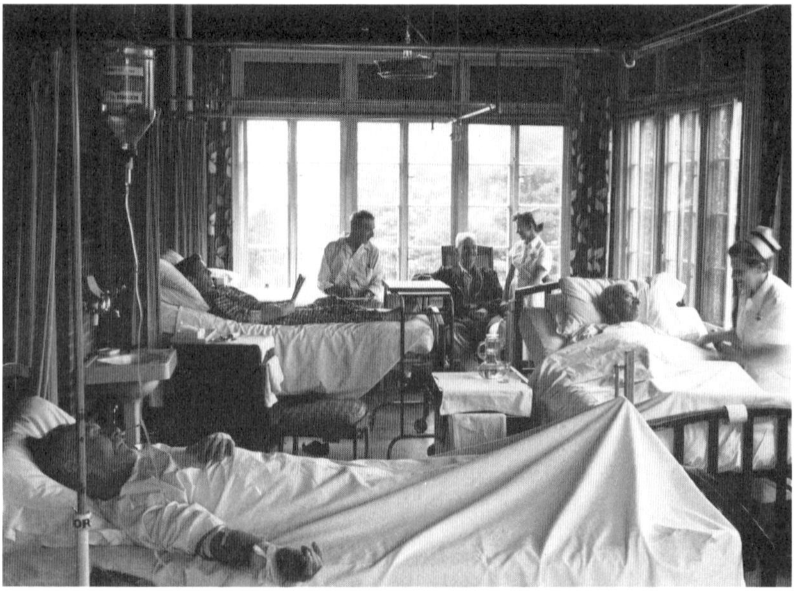

By 1947 the open sun porches at the south end of Prentiss House had all been converted to six-bed wards to provide badly needed space.

equipped." Noted among the visitors was Martin Lofquist, still hale at eighty-seven and reminiscing about "the way it was." Martin also returned for the reunion held a few days later by the Nurses' Alumnae Association, of which he was an honorary member.

During its fiftieth year the hospital admitted 3,296 patients and treated 3,173 outpatients while logging 28,357 patient days. There were 1,484 surgical procedures and 644 babies were born, a record high. It was a busy place employing 107 people and chronically overcrowded, with sixty-four licensed beds plus six more in each of the two Prentiss sun porches that could be pressed into service when needed. It cost $796.16 a day to operate on an average daily income of $619.50, an obvious source of some of its chronic financial difficulties. Its pathology laboratory performed almost 14,000 examinations that year; the X-ray Department took more than 8,500 pictures.

The front entrance had been graced by a porch added in 1936 with a $1,500 gift of the unspent funds of the Ladies Auxiliary to the 1923 Gloucester Day Committee. The Gloucester Day Auxiliary[2] had been part of a large committee headed by Fred W. Tibbetts to organize the 300th Anniversary celebration of the first settlement. The week-long event was a huge success that brought thousands of visitors, but was marred by Mr. Tibbetts' death a short time prior to the celebration. A large bronze tablet recognizing his work and that of the many others involved was placed adjacent to the new porch, where it remained until 1973, when the entrance was completely rebuilt.

The School of Nursing: The Old Order Changeth . . .

The nursing school flourished before and during the war years. In fact dormitory and classroom space was, by 1941, too small to accommodate the school as Miss Jackson, then its Director, envisioned it. She hoped for a total enrollment of forty, ten more than previously, but was finding it difficult to house that number plus nine teaching nurses and other hospital staffers given quarters at the fifty-two-bed residence. Even with extra beds rented at the 222 Washington Street home of Mrs. Molly Post, in July 1941 Superintendent Jackson had to advise the Trustees that without more space she could not admit a new class that fall. It was only the loss of staff nurses that made it possible, indeed advisable, to admit the twelve-student Class of 1944 in February 1941; several further applicants for that class were rejected for lack of space.

Additional housing was found the following June at the home of Mrs. E. Archer Bradley, who was able to take twenty in the large gray gabled residence at the corner of Washington and Baker Streets. The house was already owned by the hospital, which had inherited it subject to her life tenancy in 1935 under her husband's will. It seemed like a good solution when she and her sister consented to act as house mothers at $3.50 per week for each occupant. It was a short-lived arrangement, however, lasting less than three years, until the winter of 1944 when the house's ancient heating plant finally failed. Pending repairs, almost impossible with the war on, the eight students then living there were squeezed into the Nurses' Residence. The crunch was eased when Faulk Brothers offered the old Cunningham residence which the firm owned at 258 Washington Street, much nearer than Mrs. Bradley's. Available at a nominal rent to cover its maintenance, it was too good an offer to refuse, and the house was used until December 1947.

By that time the question of housing was no longer important, for the School of Nursing was fighting for its life. Every effort, including a revised oversight committee, had been made to meet the increasingly stringent requirements imposed by the State Board of Nursing. The end finally came in April 1947 when the Trustees received a report of the most recent inspection by the State Board outlining further demands. The faculty must be upgraded, it said, and its members must be college graduates. Students, while not required to be college graduates, must have had the equivalent of two years of college-level science, and the higher-level curriculum required would be almost equivalent to a four-year college course without the liberal arts.

With this the Trustees sadly reported that the future of the fifty-year-old school was in jeopardy and dependent "upon the willingness and ability of the hospital to meet recommendations." Discussions continued that spring, but it was soon apparent that a three-year, registry-approved school was no longer feasible except at prohibitive cost. The June 17, 1947 Board meeting closed the issue when it voted "to discontinue the admission of students . . . with the proviso that present students be permitted to continue . . . until graduation." Determined not to lose the prestige of having a school, however, it authorized the Superintendent to start planning for a new school. And in August "it was voted to establish a school for nurse-attendants, the name to be Addison Gilbert Hospital School for Nursing Attendants."

Miss Jackson's Director of Nursing, and Director of the old School of Nursing, was Miss Marjory V. Howlett, RN, who had come here from Beverly Hospital in 1944. As School Director she had been deeply involved with the State Registry, and it was only natural that the task of organizing the new program would be assigned to her. Her experience at the successful School for Attendants which had been in operation at Beverly for six years, a pioneering one-year course graduating nursing assistants to be licensed by the state rather than registered, had convinced her that a similar school would succeed here as well.

She had no difficulty convincing the State Board, where she had several friends and contacts, of the need for another hospital-based school that could train high school graduates and fill a great need of hospitals everywhere. So it was that on Florence Nightingale's birthday, May 12, 1948, the Addison Gilbert Hospital School for Nursing Attendants opened with two students; eight more would be added before the year was out. It was to teach a fifteen-month course, and for its first two years it operated in tandem with the remaining students from the old school, which graduated thirteen in September 1948. A year later the last three Registered Nurses joined their 293 predecessors in the right to wear this hospital's distinctive black-ribboned cap.

The new school's curriculum was a simplified version of the old. It included six weeks with the Gloucester District Nurses on home care, and that agency also established a course in public health nursing at the hospital, an affiliation described as one of the first in the nation. The Susan B. Tracy Fund, designated for occupational therapy training or for patients, could not be utilized in the new curriculum, however. In seeking a redesignated purpose, it seemed only proper to use it as nearly as possible in keeping with the donor's wishes, and after considerable study it was reestablished, with the same name, in support of a library for patients. As such it operates today, under the supervision of the Auxiliary, as a Library on Wheels, familiar to patients and staff alike as it makes its rounds of the floors.

The new school would produce what soon came to be called Licensed Practical Nurses for another thirty years.

Matron/Superintendents: . . . Giving Place to New

Ever since Matron Emma Gordon opened the hospital in 1897, she and her nine successors had, with varying degrees of skill and results, directed its day-to-day operations. For fifty years they had contended with an often stubborn, always demanding Medical Staff, had helped the Trustees keep the wheels turning through war and hard times, and above all had tried to make their small hospital a *good* small hospital. For the most part they had succeeded.

But times were changing. Government regulations, higher standards being set by the American College of Surgeons and the American Hospital Association, and the hard facts of the complexity of size all combined to make the business of running a hospital an undertaking that required a professional also trained in hospital management. It had simply gone beyond the ability of someone trained only as a nurse, no matter how capable, to handle.

The impetus for change at the AGH came first from the Medical Staff, whose younger members recognized the need for adjusting to changing times and saw that the older doctors were too often taking advantage of the Superintendent in their effort to avoid that change. The young men wanted someone in charge who could and would stand up to the Staff, able to speak to it as an equal in completing the recovery from the recent struggle with the Trustees. They felt, too, that a male, carrying the then new title of Administrator, could better direct the hospital.

The quest had its formal beginning at the Staff meeting of August 14, 1947, when the Staff Council voted a motion by Dr. Irving "that the Staff Council . . . contact the Trustees with regard to obtaining a specially trained, qualified male administrator for the hospital." Drs. Irving and Babson then took the idea to Board President Steele who joined them in seeking outside advice, most of which can be summarized in the views of Dr. N. W. Faxon of the Massachusetts General Hospital, who told them that any hospital of more than a hundred beds should, if possible, have a male Administrator.

Thus armed, Mr. Steele passed the proposal to the Board, which held a joint meeting with the Staff Council on December 8, 1947 at which the Staff's wishes were discussed. President Steele took responsibility for the search and, after three months of interviews, was able to report on March 16, 1948 that he and the House Committee were ready with a recommendation. Taking immediate action, the Board voted "that Mr. Tucker M. Vye be appointed administrator at an annual salary of $8,500," – $5,500 more than Miss Jackson's highest level.

Meanwhile, she had submitted her resignation in late December to take effect immediately. Although she left under some strain, she received high praise for her eight years of effort. The Trustees, the Medical Staff, the Auxiliary and her nurses all presented gifts, and the Auxiliary further honored her with a large formal tea in the Longan Room. She went on to become Superintendent at Portsmouth (N.H.) Hospital and died, after a long illness, in 1959.

As interim manager the Board appointed the capable and already busy Marjory Howlett. She graciously took one more load on her slim but strong shoulders and did the job well during the six-month changeover. This pleasant, physically small woman, respected and loved by all who knew her, remained here in her two regular positions until October 1955, when she retired to her home in Beverly and the care of her aging mother.

The newly appointed Administrator was a thirty-eight-year-old graduate of the Massachusetts Institute of Technology with postgraduate study in hospital administration at Boston University and the Harvard School of Public Health. Prior to his latest post as Administrator at nearby Winchester Hospital, he had worked his way up to the position of Assistant Administrator at Norfolk County Hospital in Braintree, his place of birth and early schooling. When he took the post at AGH, he and his wife Betty had a year-old daughter. All three were in residence at a rented home in East Gloucester by early June, and soon thereafter established permanent domicile in their own home in Rockport.

Vye's first order of business was attendance at a reception by the Trustees and Medical Staff. His remarks to the optimism-filled gathering, as reported by the *Times*, were perhaps the key to his philosophy. After acknowledging the problems he saw, he said they and those which would certainly follow could be solved if everyone worked in a cooperative spirit of understanding. He asked for open minds and closed with a bit of personal opinion:

> *There are three groups of salesmen who can best sell the hospital: satisfied patients, the Staff and nurses by spreading good will, and the Trustees by stepping on unjustified rumors quickly and decisively. The hardest thing hospitals really have to contend with is the false story. When you hear a rumor about the hospital, call me to get the facts, because it will otherwise spread, and rumors never lose anything in the telling and re-telling.*
>
> *You can be proud of your hospital. It is the cleanest I have ever seen. The nurses are a fine type. We are fortunate in having a woman of Miss Howlett's calibre. Other departments are also running well, and I don't intend to come in here and turn things upside down. I am pleased with the physical plant, the staff and the way things are functioning.*

A new era had begun.

NOTES

[1]Paul B. Kenyon was a long-time *Times* reporter noted for his sensitive insight concerning local affairs. Since the hospital was among his regular reportorial assignments, he was a logical choice to prepare its history.

[2]This was a separate organization, unrelated to the hospital's Women's Auxiliary.

PART III
THE BUILDING YEARS
1948 - 1974

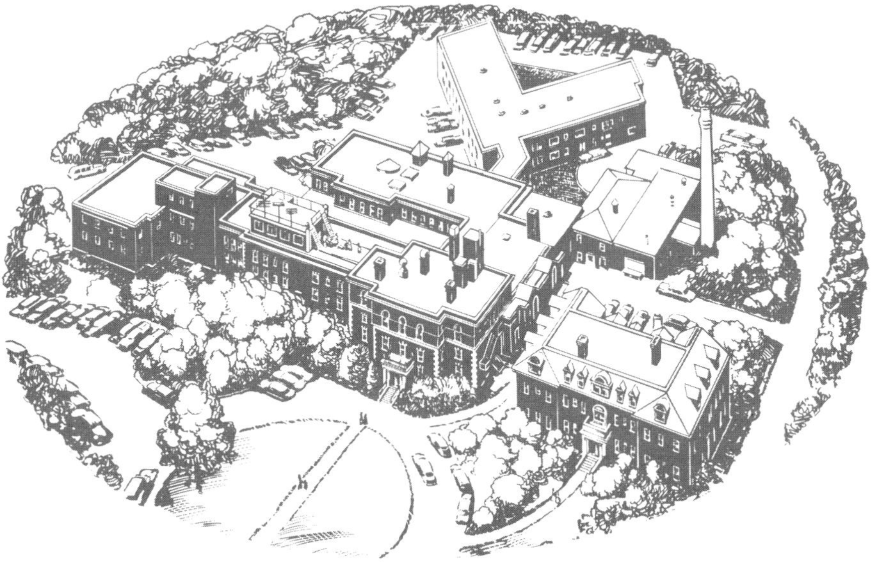

6

Facing Old Problems

The Changing Scene

THE NEW ADMINISTRATOR found himself at a hospital with what he considered a good plant and staff all functioning well. The earlier problems of human relationships between the Board of Trustees and the Medical Staff were history, and they had found it possible as well as advantageous to work in harmony. Now, with the appointment of a trained professional manager, the team was complete. Having passed its fiftieth birthday, the hospital was mature in fact as well as years.

The team would continue in reasonable harmony during a period when hospitals everywhere were coming under increasing pressure from the federal and, to a lesser degree, the state governments. New laws and the consequent regulatory power would become major factors as government impinged ever more deeply on the health care field. All hospitals would soon look back nostalgically to the days when the government's chief weapon was the power to issue licenses and the American College of Surgeons was a hospital's sternest overseer.

Some of the control would take the form of direct intervention, but it would also be assumed more subtly through such programs as the Hospital Survey and Construction Act of 1946 (the Hill-Burton Act) and, later, through Medicare and its companion, Medicaid. These and other laws would give rise to a bureaucracy responsible for their implementation. Devices such as planning councils and commissions governing such issues as determination of need and the setting of rates were also to come at the state level.[1]

Resistance to such control was probably only natural, and, like the doctors earlier, hospital Trustees viewed much of the regulation as interference in their right to handle their own affairs. In simpler days antagonism to such regulation as was proposed was effective in minimizing it, but now, facing a government encouraged by a surging civic conscience and aware of its own power, that resistance must assume a more constructive mien as hospitals and doctors alike faced the fact that a new day was at hand. Loss of independence thus becomes one of three major factors influencing the story of the period ahead.

A second is found in the emergence of health insurance, which eventually would assure that almost everyone would have some form of third-party coverage. Blue Cross and Blue Shield along with a few other private plans were already in place by 1948, and they would be complemented a few years later by two government-sponsored programs, Medicare and Medicaid, one covering the elderly and disabled and the other the financially weak. The ability to pay thus made the services of the hospital available to all, and that led inevitably to the third major influence of the years to come.

Not only could more and more people come to the hospital on a paying basis, but advances in the state of the art also made hospitals the primary location for increasingly sophisticated techniques as good medical practice more and more demanded use of them for testing, diagnosis and treatment. As a result they soon found themselves running out of space and facing the need for larger facilities, an expansion that was encouraged and assisted by government during the 1950s and 1960s. The need for bricks and mortar thus became the third important element influencing the future.

The Governing Body

Tucker Vye liked what he saw on the surface in 1948, but he was also aware of some long-standing deficiencies. In order to correct them he knew he must confront the Board of Trustees with new approaches and new ideas, some of which would be controversial. These were men who had long been accustomed to doing things their way and had never even considered leaving management to an employee they viewed as a nurse who happened to have the title of Superintendent. Vye, recognizing this, also believed them to be men who would respect ability in a leader who could and would take charge once he gained their confidence.

Despite the Board's long role as sole decision maker, Vye perceived its limited first-hand knowledge of the hospital and its daily operation. He also

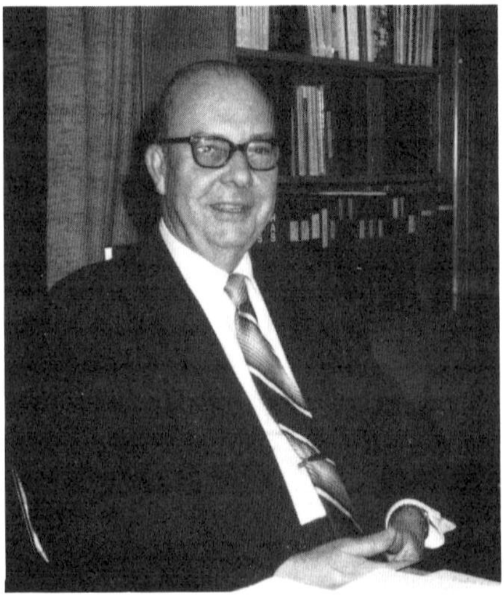

Tucker Vye became administrator in 1947 and instituted many operational changes during his 25-year tenure.

saw what he believed to be a too narrow spectrum from which its members were drawn, a bank-oriented tradition that had endured for more than fifty years and was typified by the fact that rarely had the Board met anywhere but at the Cape Ann Savings Bank. Of its thirty-four members in 1948, twenty-four were either officers or directors of the several banks in town. He was aware, too, that only two were from Rockport, the community in which he had chosen to reside.

Another weakness manifested itself in the almost total lack of interest by the Members of the Corporation who, once elected, were seldom heard from again unless tapped to become Trustees. They were never asked to serve on hospital committees other than those involving fundraising and, unless they became patients, had no reason ever to set foot on the premises. The Annual Meeting, held in the cramped board room at the bank, was certainly no attraction.

The new Administrator lost no time in correcting what to him was part of the problem. He broke precedent at the first meeting of the Board after his arrival by insisting that he could do his job only if he attended all its meetings as a full, though nonvoting, participant. He also recommended that all Board meetings to be held at the hospital, where space was available in the Longan Room, and that to encourage attendance and permit more time for deliberation they take place in the evening instead of the traditional 4 PM. Support of his stand by President Steele convinced the Board, and thus, on June 15, 1948, three customs dating back to 1889 passed from the scene.

The evolution of the Board had its start that day with a proposal for the first revision of the hospital bylaws. Its seriousness of purpose and commitment to a new way of doing things was demonstrated when the Bylaws Committee was appointed with representatives from the Medical Staff, the Auxiliary and the Nurses' Alumnae Association, each of which was invited to nominate a member who would attend all Board meetings "until such revision is accomplished." This took six months, and on December 21 the new bylaws were approved by the Board for adoption at the 1949 Annual Meeting, a first step in bringing the hospital on course in a changing world.

The 1949 bylaws brought several changes respecting hospital governance and management. Rotating three-year terms for Trustees replaced the annual election of the entire Board. Their number was set at twenty-seven with a minimum of eighteen which in evenly divided groups was to comprise the Board from that day on. A provision for Life Trustees made it possible to honor longtime members, retaining their availability while creating openings for new members. The President of the Auxiliary became a full participating member of the Board during her term in that office. A monthly Executive Committee meeting with full power would act in place of the full Board, which thenceforth would meet quarterly.

Other standing committees were Finance, Investment, House & Grounds, Nominating and Public Relations. The Joint Advisory Committee, a combination of the Executive Committee and the Medical Staff Council, made for a formal point of contact between the two bodies and made it possible for Vye in his 1957 report to describe a "close cooperation and understanding . . . between the Trustees and Staff . . . a situation which is tremendously important but unfortunately does not always exist." A detailed description of the Administrator's qualifications and duties included a directive that he attend all Board and standing committee meetings.

The Trustees soon came to appreciate Vye's experience and ability to counsel their deliberations in an atmosphere of mutual confidence and respect. He became their trusted manager as he accomplished what no Superintendent could ever do in maintaining a comfortable and cooperative working relationship among the essential triumvirate of any hospital – governing board, medical staff and management.

The Annual Meeting of 1949, despite being the first held at the hospital and the first to use individually mailed notices, hardly taxed the capacity of the Longan Room. It attracted seventeen Board members and two other Corporators plus Chief of Staff Harold N. Baker, MD; Marjorie Howlett, Director of Nursing and the Training School; and Mrs. Arthur J. Hall, President of the Auxiliary. It duly elected twenty-seven Trustees and designated seven of long service as Life Trustees. Advancing the Administrator's hopes for better participation, it also elected fourteen new Corporators while dropping eight others, among them former Treasurer Horace Smith, who had remained a member despite his 1925 peccancy.

New Annual Meeting dates were tried in an attempt to find a time better suited to the membership: the second Tuesday in February from 1950 to 1952, in March for 1953, back to January from 1954 to 1963, when the last Tuesday in January was made permanent. Attendance at the Annual Meeting began to improve in 1953, when a buffet dinner was served in the Nurses' Dining Room. Of the thirty people present that year, thirteen were non-Trustee Members of the Corporation. By 1956 attendance had expanded to forty-two with twenty-six non-Trustee Corporators, a phenomenon that perhaps proved once again that the way to a man's heart is through his stomach.

Elimination of dinners due to construction from 1957 to 1961 was accompanied by a drop in attendance during that five-year span, but at the 75th Annual Meeting in 1963, with dinner served in a new cafeteria, there were fifty-nine in attendance including forty-six members of the Board and Corporation. At that meeting the presentation of rose bouquets to the presidents of the Auxiliary and Alumnae Association, a custom that had begun in 1958, was duly noted in the record. From 1963 on, except when winter weather sometimes intervened, attendance continued to grow, and in 1972, the seventy-fifth anniversary of the actual opening of the hospital, 66 of the then 156 Corporators showed up. Dinner for the quarterly meetings of the full Board was introduced in 1966 and has remained the practice ever since.

The move to Board and Corporation diversification passed another milestone in 1973, encouraged if not actually instigated by a question raised by the Auxiliary at a Board meeting on October 11, 1971. The record of that meeting notes that "Mrs. Lloyd G. David, Auxiliary President, wondered if women might be considered for nomination to the Board of Trustees in [the] foreseeable future." Her question was answered at the 1973 Annual Meeting when, after almost eighty-five years of male domination, four women, Jane P. Brown, Mollie A. Rodgers, Barbara M. Simpson and Janis D. Stelluto, were elected Members of the Corporation. Mrs. Brown was also elected to the Board at the same meeting, where Mrs. Stelluto and Mrs. Simpson joined her in 1974 and 1975 respectively.

Paying the Piper: Financial Problems

Although Board reorganization was helpful and essential in meeting what Tucker Vye saw as his responsibility, it was by no means his first priority. That was the precarious financial situation he found during his first days on the job. He realized he must immediately overcome the reluctance of the Trustees to "borrow," and later replace, endowment in meeting current expenses during that first critical year. He saw also the old reluctance to raise room rates as the Board clung to its long-held conviction that the people of Cape Ann were paying all they could be expected to, an attitude that must be overcome if the hospital were to be put on a sound financial footing. On the positive side, he was grateful to find in place a developing tradition of public gift support that could be used in solving the perennial money problems.

At his first Board meeting he explained the urgency of becoming current with suppliers who were by then threatening cutoff or the imposition of cash payment on delivery. Arriving at a current payment basis would also, he reminded them, permit discounting of invoices and offer greater flexibility in seeking the best prices. The Finance Committee acted promptly, selling off almost $28,000 in securities to meet all outstanding accounts payable.

The Trustees, to their credit, soon found it less difficult to confront the need for rate increases. That of 1947 was followed by another in 1949 and again in 1951, limited that year by a federally imposed price freeze on industry in general. Fees for ancillary services such as laboratory, X-ray and operating room use were also being regularly adjusted to reflect costs, to take advantage of third-party allowances and to maintain parity with other area hospitals. Room rate increases, once started, continued almost annually, with the Board agonizing over the decision each time. By 1957 the price of a private room had reached $22 per day, semiprivate $18 and ward and children's beds $14.

These fees were justified by escalating costs. There were more employees, many in relatively highly paid technical services needed to meet the expectations of a Medical Staff that by then included several young physicians putting into practice the modern concepts they brought from medical school. And after 1950 government-mandated minimum wages in the less-skilled, lower-paid occupations created a ripple effect that more often than not resulted in the need for increases to those higher on the pay scale.

Goods as well as services also cost more as a postwar inflation became a nationwide problem. Hospitals everywhere were feeling the same pressures, and as long as one didn't charge more than others in the area, Blue Cross, in those lightly regulated days, would pay. Unfortunately it was not always easy for patients not yet covered by insurance, and during the fifties there were still many in that situation.

Collecting from some remained difficult with too many Cape Anners without insurance in the habit of putting hospital and doctors' bills at the bottom of the pile. The Administrator was given a free hand to use such means as he saw fit, including use of collection agencies if necessary, to overcome this problem. He was also authorized in October 1948 to employ an assistant to the Treasurer "in the matter of collections and billing [and] to render regular and more frequent statements."

A local credit agency was retained to follow up the more serious situations, and in 1954 Vye was authorized to give 272 past due accounts totaling $17,000 to the harder-hitting Professional Service Company of Boston in a short-lived trial of this method. Most cases were handled inhouse by the hospital's diligent Treasurer, Robert Thompson, who continued his efforts valiantly despite his many critics. It was said that he was worse than a dog worrying a bone in chasing down delinquents — his discovery of one of the newfangled television aerials or a new car owned by someone who owed the hospital led to many showdowns.

With $140,000 in such uncollected accounts in 1958 it again became necessary to borrow from endowment in a reprise of an old refrain that troubled the Board every time it was required. A new Credit Department, established in 1960 and expected to tighten up a still too liberal credit policy, helped but couldn't cure the problem as accounts payable continued to exceed cash on hand.

Despite all efforts to control operating expenses, deficit balances on the annual financial reports remained the norm, although bright spots were occasionally seen. In 1950, for example, on a $390,000 expense budget with a loss on operations of $39,203 and a "Free and Uncollectible Care" account that totaled $36,175, there was a small overall surplus after other income, mainly gifts and income from endowment, was added in. But operating losses, the excess of expenses over income from running the hospital, continued year after year. For the year 1957, the last before a new wing went into service, these were just over $88,000 on an expense budget of $660,000. Even the first $1 million budget, a milestone reached in 1962, was hardly cause for celebration without the cash to meet it.

Saved by the Gift

Fund raising loomed large in the Administrator's mind in the early days of 1948 as an immediate though partial solution to the hospital's financial difficulties. He and the Board knew the importance of regaining the enthusiastic momentum of earlier campaigns, lost in 1946 and 1947, although he viewed them as somewhat haphazard and overshadowed by the YMCA drives each summer. The District Nurse Association favored continuing the joint health concept in proposing a campaign that year with the Massachusetts Society for the Prevention of Cruelty to Children again a partner.

Vye, preferring that the hospital not dilute its effort, was hesitant about linkage with others but was willing to go along with the Trustees in a joint effort to raise $35,000 voted in July. He did insist, however, on use of professional fund-raising counsel and suggested Hugh M. Spalding of New York, who was engaged to direct a fall campaign starting in early September. With businessman-banker William Moore as General Chairman, a full panoply of workers, special emphasis divisions and massive newspaper publicity, the effort raised $43,054 less $4,328 in campaign expenses. The GDNA and MSPCC received their scheduled shares of $6,500 and $2,200 respectively, and the hospital, having borne the major share of the responsibility, was allotted the balance.

This successful drive convinced the Board that Vye's desire for outside counsel was sound, and annual giving campaigns became an integral part of the hospital's funding. With Spalding as director the Joint Health Campaigns continued through 1955, giving way only to the hospital's need for a capital funding campaign in 1956. By that time these annual drives had become truly Cape Ann efforts, with Rockport entering an eager and outstanding group each year under an agreement that money given by its residents would go solely to the hospital. With such added input the hospital consistently exceeded its expectations, and by 1955, after eight campaigns, it had received a total of just over $250,000 in essential operating funds.

The MSPCC dropped out after the 1953 campaign, the only one during Spalding's time that fell short, failed to make its goal in a year described by Campaign Chairman Frank B. Sullivan as involving "the poorest economic condition which has confronted the city in many years." In general, if there was any flaw in the operation of these efforts it was one of timing, since they were all run in the fall of the year. Hugh Spalding, once he became familiar with the area, recognized the possibilities inherent in a summer campaign; but summer was traditionally "the Y's time," and the Trustees, some of whom also worked on its behalf, were unwilling to compete with it. The best Spalding could do was obtain a list of nonresident taxpayers in 1952 so summer residents could at least be approached by mail.

By 1955 both Spalding and Carroll Steele, the dynamo behind all the drives though Chairman only in 1949, had come to the conclusion that the hospital could do better alone. Mr. Steele, as Finance Committee Chairman, brought his concern to the Board "in forceful but friendly terms" in January 1955 but was directed by its vote to maintain the status quo ante. The question became moot when the annual effort gave way to capital funding the next year.

Other traditional means of support continued, complementing the more formal efforts. The Auxiliary, which in 1947 requested assignment of special projects beyond its regular role as "supplier of linens," took on procurement of equipment, starting small with a $450 bedpan sterilizer in 1948 and working its way up. In 1949 it purchased an electrocardiograph and, for the Maternity Wing, fifteen bassinets and an autoclave. By 1956 the energetic ladies had presented the hospital with a new food conveyor system, a water still, a "preemie" bassinet, bed side-rails and a new laundry press, all while continuing to supply about $3,000 worth of linens each year.

Further equipment and funding needs were also being met by individuals and outside groups. Dr. Pett was always generous in giving equipment for the Pediatric Unit, and others too numerous to list could be counted on if they learned of some special need. The employees of W. G. Brown's Department Store staged "Brown's Showboat" in 1948, which added $1,612.47 to help in that time of trouble. The Long Beach Mother's Group gave the proceeds of its 1953 summer dance to benefit the Children's Ward, and when the upper-crust Roundabout Club dissolved in 1948 it voted, as had the Cape Ann Camera Club the previous year, to give the balance of its treasury to the hospital.

In August 1950 the Trustees recorded a $2,000 gift for a new operating table "from Friends of the Hospital who wished to remain anonymous." This group is believed to have been a consortium of fisheries and Main Street businessmen who regularly gathered for lunch and gossip. Undoubtedly encouraged by Carroll Steele, between 1951 and 1955 they privately gathered funds for further surgical needs, for pediatric equipment, and for air-conditioning in the laboratory and the labor room directly above it. Their desire for anonymity was sincere; the Board never did learn who they were, or, if it did, never recorded their names.

Through it all the Nurses' Alumnae Association maintained its active support. An oxygen tent in 1950, bed side-rails in 1954 and several over-bed tables in 1955 were but a part of this loyal group's mission of assistance to its hospital.

A further source of gift support came into being in October 1951, when the Trustees noted a gift of $165 "in lieu of funeral flowers . . . from 29 donors." These were local friends of a long-time Annisquam summer resident, Sally Damon Littlefield, whose obituary here and at her winter home in Connecticut made the suggestion: "Please omit flowers. Those so wishing may make a contribution to Norwalk General Hospital, Norwalk, Connecticut." Her Gloucester friends, in preferring to honor her memory where she had summered for many years, saw Addison Gilbert Hospital as equally appropriate and thus introduced a new practice to Cape Ann where, in keeping with widespread custom, flowers had always been the means of honoring a deceased friend. During the early fifties an occasional death notice included the phrase "please omit flowers," but the suggestion of memorials to a charity, locally at least, does not seem to have been mentioned prior to Mrs. Littlefield's death.

Intrigued by the possibilities suggested by these gifts, the Trustees decided "to encourage gifts of money to the hospital instead of the purchase of funeral flowers [with] the money used [for the] purchase of needed articles of equipment." Frederick M. Bundy, the keen-minded, old Yankee head of Gorton's and the hospital's President at the time, suggested the name Friendship Fund, and it became, remaining to this day, a means of honoring friends or recognizing special events while also supporting the hospital's ongoing need for medical equipment.

Bequests, usually to endowment, were becoming a more important source of funds. Possibly stimulated by the considerable publicity given the hospital's financial problems and by the excitement of the fund campaigns, more and more people began to remember the hospital in this way. From a total of $52,000 recorded in the thirteen years from 1934 to 1947, bequests rose to a total of almost $1 million received from seventy-seven benefactors between 1948 to 1974. These ranged from the relatively small to what, at least to this small hospital, seemed very large. Those of Helen H. Beal, Henry R. Reed and Louise Sturtevant alone totaled $341,135, and many others were in five figures. Large or small, these additions to invested endowment added thousands of dollars to the all-important nonoperating income of the hospital. Added to those received since and yet to come, they will continue to produce income and perpetuate their donors' names.

The hospital also became a Main Street landlord as the result of a bequest by Frank M. Shurtleff, the proprietor of a news and stationery store at 114 Main Street, then as now popularly called The Waiting Station. He owned the block of two buildings there named for their former owners, Tappan and Patillo, and containing several stores and offices. Among his tenants in the Tappan Building were two hospital Trustees, insurance man Carroll Steele and druggist Frank B. Sullivan.

The Board learned shortly after Mr. Shurtleff's death in April 1950 that he had left the Tappan Building to the hospital and the Patillo Building to the YMCA. Conscious of the unusual responsibility involved in the ownership of a business block, President Bundy appointed a special committee chaired by Mr. Sullivan to administer it.

Problems soon cropped up. The Chamber of Commerce, a second floor tenant, wanted renovations to its rooms. Toilets needed replacement, the stairwells and corridors required plaster and paint and, worst of all, the roof leaked badly. Another tenant, Nichols Candy Company, wanted to sublet to TicToc Doughnut Shop, which meant higher insurance costs to cover the added fire hazard. Sullivan's Drug Store needed work, but Trustee Sullivan was unwilling to request it. Trustee-tenant Steele needed more space but did not feel he could ask for it at the expense of other tenants. The single stairway to the second floors of the two buildings made for problems between their new owners.

Rents, although maintained at fair market value, never returned more than $5,000 annually, which barely covered expenses. All in all, it did not seem a wise long-term holding. The committee, facing repairs and heavy maintenance expenses and sensing the inappropriateness of the hospital as landlord, decided early the next year to place it on the market. The building was carried on the books at $64,000; the asking price was set at $75,000. After six years of holding out for that price, the Board gave up. Sealed bids, subject to refusal, brought three offers, and in August 1957, the high bidder, Martin Levy, relieved the hospital of its role as landlord for $62,510.

With the expansion of what by the mid-1960s was becoming a reasonably impressive endowment, special skills in managing it were needed, and the Board, cognizant of its fiduciary responsibilities, recognized this. The Investment Committee continued to rely on the counsel of Nathan Bugbee and his faith in good common stocks. That committee, which during most of the period included bankers Temple A. Bradley, "Fritz" Bundy and J. Hollis Griffin plus Treasurer Thompson, welcomed a good second opinion, though occasionally disagreeing with their advisor's recommendations. Mr. Bugbee was replaced in 1969 by the Wellesley firm of David L. Babson & Company, which bore the name of its founder, a Gloucester native and the son of the deceased veterinarian and Trustee Dr. Elmer W. Babson.

Under the Babson influence the committee altered its policy slightly in setting standards for the invested funds. The Endowment Fund was to emphasize income while the General Fund, from which capital could be drawn more readily, would concentrate on growth. And all, said the prudent committee, should be done with the safety of principal firmly in mind. Emphasis remained on industrial common stocks which constituted about 50 percent of the portfolio through most of the period, the balance being placed in utilities as well as industrial and government bonds. Aside from a few years during the fifties when sales to raise cash again became necessary, purchases and sales were made only to improve the mix and increase income and growth. By 1973 and with all "borrowed" endowment restored, total invested funds had grown to $1,398,299, based on cost value, from the $360,956 reported in 1948.

NOTES

[1]It seems neither necessary nor appropriate to examine the detail of the evolution of these laws and regulations, which were to grow more complex and far-reaching with the passage of time. Where necessary to the story we may briefly describe some of them, but we believe the detail is best left for more scholarly exploration. It will be helpful, however, to keep their existence in mind for a better understanding of what was happening locally.

7

On Things Medical

THE REORGANIZATION of the Medical Staff in 1946 essentially ended what might be called "the troubles." It now operated under new bylaws, and its Chief of Staff, a new title replacing the former designation of President, was Dr. Harold N. Baker of Rockport. Elected at the Staff's Annual Meeting in December 1946, Dr. Baker was a quiet, middle-of-the-road leader of the type required during a period of readjustment. He served, somewhat reluctantly, until 1950. The division into clinical departments, each with its own Chief of Service, was in place, and within the Staff and between it and the Board of Trustees there was a new sense of harmony.

Tucker Vye, along with most of the medical-hospital fraternity in eastern Massachusetts, had been aware of the earlier disorganization at AGH and thought hard about coming into a situation that he wasn't sure had been fully resolved. However, he was reassured after meeting with Dr. Baker, Dr. Babson and other influential Staff members that all was well, and, as a full participant in the monthly Staff meetings, he soon gained its respect as he had that of the Trustees. The improving relationship was further enhanced in 1949 when, by invitation of the Trustees, a Staff member was appointed to attend Board meetings. And in 1951 a new Chief of Staff, Dr. John J. Egan, Jr., described in his first annual report an "increased degree of mutual understanding and cooperation [with] a clearly discernible 'esprit de corps'."

With word getting around that Cape Ann had become a good place to practice, the postwar crop of young medical school graduates could be attracted here. The 1950s thus became a time of Medical Staff building, with well-trained men and women bringing new methods and ideas to a Staff that was, to be candid, aging. The first of the young postwar physicians was Dr. Lawrence Ross in 1945, followed by Drs. C. Bruce Brown and Ever Curtis in 1948 and by Drs. Robert N. Lundberg (1951), John S. Gale (1953) and Hamer Lacey (1956). Others would follow, but these bright young additions were a clear sign that a new day had dawned.

Medical Records

Although its major problems of the past fifty years were then history, some troublesome issues persisted, the worst, administratively at least, being the maintenance of medical records. Mrs. Blanchet's constant efforts worked some of the time, but pockets of resistance remained that could not be ignored. Well-completed records were expected by an increasingly strict accreditation program, and Tucker Vye did not wish his hospital to be criticized by the inspectors on this or any other remediable point.

Dictating equipment was installed in 1953 at handy locations to speed the process for the doctors and for the transcribers in the Records Office. The Staff Council also took a hand in cajoling, demanding and threatening those whose records were most often neglected. The combination of efforts kept matters in hand for a few years, with seldom more than one or two members behind more than the two weeks allowed by Staff rules.

By 1957, however, several were again falling behind, and two years later the situation had deteriorated so far that Blue Cross was holding up reimbursement because of insufficient documentation of cases. Only the pressure of an approaching survey by the Joint Commission on Accreditation of Hospitals (JCAH), formed by the American Hospital Association to replace the ACS in critiquing hospital performance, corrected the situation — temporarily. By 1961 it had regressed with 179 incompletes at year end, and two years later, persuasion having failed, a frustrated Dr. Lacey warned his colleagues that he, then Chairman of the Staff Medical Records Committee, would not hesitate to invoke a never-before-enforced rule withdrawing the hospital privileges of those whose records were seriously behind.

This threat brought but short-lived improvement. Only the periodic JCAH surveys seemed to carry enough weight to bring transitory compliance by the handful of Staff members who were habitually delinquent. A new government program, Medicare, added further pressure for better documentation after 1965, but a year later Dr. Lacey could only describe the situation as "appalling." Finally, on November 27, 1968, five Staff members were advised of their suspension from "all hospital privileges other than those pertaining to record writing until records are completed." This stringent penalty, which forced the sanctioned member to turn treatment of his hospitalized patients over to a colleague, was a last resort. Such suspension was invoked several more times during the next year, improving matters to the point where, in September 1971, the Staff Council was able to report all records current.

The cure was again short-lived. A year later a new Records Committee found almost 500 incompletes and threatened fines in addition to suspension of privilege. Nine different doctors found themselves on the "banned" list at least once over the next three years. It is important to recognize this as a problem mostly confined to a very small number of Staff members, and most of the others were rarely more than minimally behind. Nonetheless the few serious offenders made Mrs. Blanchet's life interesting, to say the least.

Human nature being what it is, there may be no sure cure for this chronic problem, in which the AGH is by no means alone. In the year following Mrs. Blanchet's 1976 retirement, a new department director had slightly more success, as record-keeping delinquencies ebbed and flowed depending on internal pressure and increasingly strict requirements by the JCAH. Although suspension of privileges is seldom necessary, medical records maintenance remains a blot on an otherwise outstanding Medical Staff performance.

The Emergency Room

The Accident Room, long located adjacent to the original operating rooms and moved in 1958 to larger, better-equipped quarters beneath Prentiss House, became known during the 1960s as the Emergency Room. By either name its coverage remained a nagging problem, especially irksome to the Medical Staff, whose members resisted being on call for emergencies or, later, being required to have a member always present at the hospital during the day.

A 1929 revision of the "Rules and Regulations of the Medical Staff" had formalized Accident Room coverage in stating that "emergency cases, where no preference as to physician is expressed, shall be assigned to members of the Staff in rotation as far as possible." There was no provision for enforcement, however, and it was not always easy for the nurse in charge to get a doctor to come in. When she reached one, she was sometimes quizzed as to the nature of the case. If it sounded interesting and there was insurance or other means of payment, the doctor might or might not take the case. It was an embarassing situation for the nurse to be on the telephone, often with the patient or family listening, while she made several such calls. Neither was it good public relations for the hospital along Main Street, where such stories spread quickly.

A more structured "officer-of-the-day" system installed after World War II helped to some degree, but like its predecessor rule, it lacked any real power of enforcement. Assignment as O.D. was resisted; Mrs. Blanchet, whose unhappy duty it was to remind doctors of their scheduled coverage, was ordered in November 1957 to "tell them and then hang up," a method that surely didn't improve dispositions on either side. Worse were the occasions when the O.D. failed to provide coverage for himself when unable to take a scheduled duty day, an issue that led to written complaint from Mrs. Blanchet to the Staff in July 1967.

Summer coverage was especially difficult, with an influx of summer residents and tourists adding to the Accident Room load. Employment of an intern, assigned here by Salem Hospital on a two-month rotating basis in 1957, helped some during all seasons, but that extra help ended in 1960 when the American Medical Association, citing insufficient supervision and opportunity for experience at small hospitals, ruled against the practice.

Thus, when a forty-eight-year-old native of Samoa named Bert Williams, in this country for further medical education, applied for summer work in 1960, it was almost the answer to a prayer. Described as a medical practitioner, Williams had been educated at a British medical school in Fiji and had subsequently served as a medical assistant at a U.S. Navy hospital in Samoa during and after World War II and later as a public health officer. He was well recommended, and, after an interview, the Staff Council did not hesitate to employ him. His work that summer gained him the confidence of the Staff, and according to the record he "seemed to be extremely capable and well-liked."

At the end of the summer, although he had to return to school in Boston, he further endeared himself by remaining available for weekend duty "except for morning church" and by offering to return the next summer. After "Doctor" Williams, as everyone by then called him, returned home to Samoa in 1962 an agreement was worked out for weekend coverage by surgical residents from Boston City Hospital. This arrangement, in operation until 1967 and shifting to residents from Chelsea Naval Hospital and New England Medical Center in 1968, worked reasonably well in coverage of busy summer weekends, but it could not solve the basic problem during the week or at other seasons.

A more dangerous situation was evolving by 1971 when the legal aspects were considered. At issue was the very real possibility of a specialist, a pediatrician for example, being O.D. if an adult with complex medical problems was brought in. The conscientious physician, knowing he was not trained for that situation, could only stabilize the patient and hope that the internist could be located quickly and, if anything went wrong meantime, that his malpractice insurance was sufficient. Long discussions held that year were beneficial not only in getting better cooperation and participation but also in assigning specialists to supplementary lists for call as needed.

Small hospitals everywhere faced the same dilemma. Few could afford full-time Emergency Room coverage or interns, and the O.D./on-call system caused delays, misunderstandings and resentment for many years. The situation began to change only after the Massachusetts Legislature acted in 1974. The impetus for change that year had its beginnings in a 1963 report by the Massachusetts Trauma Committee of the ACS, chaired by the AGH's Dr. Babson. The study, which entailed a statewide survey of facilities and the treatment and care of accident victims, revealed among other things that this institution was no better or worse than most of the Commonwealth's small hospitals.

The 1974 legislation decreed rigid requirements for Emergency Room coverage. A "routine" E.R., the operation of which permitted a hospital to post the now familiar blue H signs on the highway, required the twenty-four-hour in-house presence of a physician trained if possible in emergency medicine. The AGH Staff had already met most of its requirements in agreeing in 1973 to have the O.D. sleep inhouse, paid by the hospital for the extra duty. With the new law requiring full-time coverage by someone other than an O.D., another problem was put to rest.

Specialization and Group Practice

This period also marked the rise of specialization and the passing of the old-time family doctor. The American College of Surgeons had been granting certification to surgeons since the 1930s, and this had been recognized here in the bylaws of 1946, which required those applying for major surgical privileges to meet ACS standards. The new rules also meant that a surgeon must confine himself to that specialty, a departure that was difficult for the older members of the Staff to accept. Dr. Mooring especially resented the new order. Older Staff members recall with chuckles his reaction when Dr. Babson advised a Staff meeting that, as a Board-certified surgeon, he could no longer handle obstetrics or other medical practice. Hearing this, Dr. Mooring called out, "And I suppose, Doctor, that means you will no longer be able to order an enema?" To which the usually quiet Dr. Cleaves wryly responded, "Why, Dr. Mooring, do you need one?"

Other specialty boards followed the surgeons, first in obstetrics and internal medicine and, a few years later, in pediatrics with Board certification the cherished, and necessary, goal of all. Adherence to these high standards has meant that the hospital has been able to attract and hold good physicians, with new specialties being added regularly. By 1974 the AGH had specialists in orthopedics, ophthalmology, urology and ear-nose-throat; today, it has nineteen primary specialties, including one called Family Practice, which surely would sound familiar to Drs. Cleaves and Mooring and other old-timers.

The organization of a Dental Service was an offshoot of the trend toward specialization. Selected dentists had been appointed to the Medical Staff since 1919 and, since 1946, had been members of its Consulting Staff, a post filled only by Dr. George Taylor from 1919 and by Irving H. Pomeroy, DMD. In 1954 the Medical Staff and Trustees, recognizing that many others had no hospital affiliation, appointed thirteen Cape Ann dentists as the Dental Service with Dr. Taylor, senior among them, as Chief of Service.

With its own rules and bylaws, the Dental Service became a separate body under the authority of the Board of Trustees and subject to loose supervision by the Medical Staff, as required by the JCAH. Its members could treat their patients in the hospital although admission could be authorized only by a physician after medical evaluation. The dentists sometimes chafed under such restrictions, including that under which only a physician could order medication, an issue that became more significant in 1971 when Alan J. Kace, DMD opened a Cape Ann practice. Dr. Kace brought a new level of dental surgery which required greater diversity of medication and with it the conviction that he was qualified to perform independent of a medical overseer. Medical Staff resistance to any relaxation of its rules was overcome in 1984 when Dr. Kace and Morton A. Levin, DDS were appointed to the Medical Staff with Active Staff status.

Another phenomenon of the times was the development of group practice by physicians in the same specialty. Impossible in the days of jealously guarded "ownership" of patients and still unthinkable to many older doctors, it was another concept brought in by the younger doctors, who had seen it work in privately owned clinics since the Mayo brothers first introduced the idea in the waning years of the nineteenth century. The clinic concept spread during the first half of the twentieth century, probably because it was a practical way to handle financial and other business aspects of practice and later, among the pragmatic younger doctors, because it was a means of lightening the burdens of working alone, of being the slave, as it were, to a job with no time off. It was especially attractive to those whose practice was emergency oriented: internists, obstetricians, pediatricians and surgeons.

The first such partnership here was that of Drs. Babson and Lundberg, who established an office together when the latter came home to practice in 1951. Their quarters in Dr. Babson's Prospect Street residence were soon to prove inadequate, a problem they had in common with many others who, finding commercial office space scarce and often unsuitable, had offices in converted residences, often at considerable distance from the hospital. This was particularly impractical for the surgeons who, with the obstetricians, were most likely to be summoned on short notice.

With other colleagues also expressing interest in group work and better facilities, discussion intra-Staff and with the AGH Trustees was opened in late 1959 as to the possibilities of a medical office building on the hospital grounds. The Trustees, preoccupied with planning for a new wing, delayed serious consideration of the matter until 1962, when they asked Ritchie Associates, the hospital's architectural firm, to prepare sketches for a building to cost between $65,000 and $70,000. Such a building would, the architects pointed out, mean wood construction and thus probably not be permitted. In addition it was almost impossible to get the prospective tenants to agree on space requirements and layout, and, said the planners, standardization was essential to low-cost construction.

It was thus inevitable that when Dr. Lawrence Ross presented Ritchie's draft plans for a proposed building in February 1963, the estimated cost of $95,000 was found to require prohibitively high rents. That, plus the fact that the hospital's auditors had explained the complications of a nonprofit, nontaxed institution owning and managing a commercial enterprise, resulted in a mutual loss of interest.

With that, those most interested, the surgical, obstetrical and pediatric groups, formed a realty trust partnership. Through it they acquired property at 302 Washington Street next door to the hospital on which, in 1964, they opened the Medical Office Building, which today houses the original groups plus others as tenants. A similarly financed building owned by a dental partnership followed a few years later at 321 Washington, also near the hospital.

Meanwhile another group practice had been established by Walter E. O'Donnell, MD, who had been attracted to Cape Ann in 1960 from the Sloan-Kettering Institute for Cancer Research in New York. Attuned to a more sophisticated practice, Dr. O'Donnell began to chafe at what he perceived as small-town medicine lacking modern facilities and concepts and without a broad base of medical specialties. He was also aware of many patients served less than well as their family doctors retired or entered restrictive specialties. His vision of modern practice and a growing patient load together with what he viewed as indifference to his ideas among his fellow Staff members at the hospital soon led him to begin recruiting for colleagues who would share his dream.

He was joined in 1963 by Robert L. Jedrey, MD, a Lanesville native fresh from a residency in internal medicine. They moved into Dr. O'Donnell's newly constructed office building on the corner of Bass Avenue and Thatcher Road which, complete with a small laboratory, could accommodate an expanded practice. Together they commenced the search for a third internist.

It was not an easy task. These were times of a general shortage of doctors, and competition for those available was keen. The best and brightest of the young specialists expected modern facilities and equipment with consultation within easy distances, assets that were to some degree lacking in the small community hospitals of the 1960s. Persistent search eventually brought Peter S. New, MD to Cape Ann in 1967 to join the two pioneers, and by 1969, with the group then totaling five, the Bass Avenue office was becoming crowded.

It soon became evident that the busy practice would require more space if it was to expand further, and that summer planning was begun for a new facility to be located at Gloucester's new industrial park off Blackburn Circle. Although the group had hoped to locate adjacent to the hospital, the Medical Office Building in which they had been invited to participate five years earlier no longer had space available, and there was no other site in the near vicinity. The industrial park, then sparsely settled, welcomed the prestige offered by a medical office complex, which when it opened as Cape Ann Medical Center (CAMC) on July 3, 1971, housed eight physicians.

With a larger laboratory and a small radiology unit directed by Dr. O'Donnell's sister, Ann R. O'Donnell, MD, the original concept of a group practice providing one-stop service in a modern single-story building became reality. At the same time, however, differences between the Medical Center group and the hospital as well as many of its Medical Staff were becoming obvious. There were several issues.

The CAMC, with its lab and X-ray units, was at first open and staffed from 9 A.M. to 5 P.M. weekdays and until noon on Saturdays. The hospital, on the other hand, was ready twenty-four hours every day of the week with technicians on call during the off-hours, a schedule that relied on optimum utilization of its equipment. Radiology was especially affected as the CAMC unit, established independently only after discussions with hospital radiologists failed to produce an acceptable arrangement for a cooperative operation, cut deeply into the hospital's work, which dropped from 50,000 films in 1971 to 41,000 in 1972.

Another facet of the problem stemmed from the situation in the hospital's Emergency Room, where coverage relied on the unsatisfactory O.D. system. The CAMC, which by mid-1971 had an internist on duty eighty-four hours a week including Sundays, was in many ways offering more adequate coverage than the hospital, where, as we have seen, the O.D. could be one of several specialists unversed in the medical needs of a case. The public relations problems in the Emergency Room, already severe, were hardly improved by the need to explain why, if the patient wished treatment by a CAMC member, he must go there if the doctor in question didn't happen to be in the hospital at the time. This problem would be resolved with the eventual full-time coverage of the Emergency Room, under which a qualified emergency medicine specialist was available at all times. At the time, however, what seemed like irreconcilable differences of opinion prevented integration of coverage hours on a scheduled basis, despite efforts on both sides to arrange it.

These and other issues only exacerbated the tense relationship between the hospital-oriented physicians and their Medical Staff colleagues at the center. Many of the former were concerned that the CAMC group did not seem to be hospital-minded, using it only as a place for admission of cases that could not be managed at the center. The Medical Center physicians, on the other hand, prided themselves on being ahead of the times in operating such an ambulatory care facility with ready access to beds at the nearby hospital when needed.

These differences should not have been allowed to escalate. The Medical Center was an advanced idea introduced to an unreceptive, conservative medical community. Its basic concept is today widely accepted as offering day-to-day medical care efficiently and less expensively on an ambulatory, outpatient basis. Of more significance to the community, over the years the CAMC had attracted a fine group of physicians, some for but short stays but all well trained and practicing high-quality medicine. Its current eight members are augmented by fifteen consultant specialists, and Cape Ann has unquestionably benefited from having such physicians as Drs. Choate, Fiero, Mann, Smith and Wolfe who, with others as tenants at the center, now practice with the three founders. All members of the hospital's Medical Staff, which they serve in many official capacities, they might not have come had there not been a separate facility offering the opportunity for group practice supplemented by an outstanding consultant staff.

Because of this the problems of the past, now largely solved, can be put aside and the old antagonisms forgotten and relegated to history.

The Ancillary Services

The laboratory, which continued to function in its original crowded rooms beneath the old Maternity Wing, finally gained the space it needed in 1958, as the result of a building program completed that year (see Chapter 8). Laid out under the supervision of Dr. Nickerson, it could then add new equipment and enlarge its staff.

Hematology work took a significant step forward, for example, with the acquisition of one of the new Coulter Counters, automated for speedier determination of hematocrit, hemoglobin and blood cell counts. The lab's ability to perform more work inhouse was further improved by a new device for the electrophoretic separation of serum proteins. Late in the 1960s, its work was again advanced with installation of a gamma ray well counter for use in the determination of thyroid function by radioimmunoassay.

These new terms and new equipment were surely little understood by the rest of the hospital staff and even less by its patients, but with them the laboratory was entering the computer age, which arrived in June 1972 with the installation of a leased Hycel Mark X. This bulky multichannel chemistry analyzer, capable of performing in minutes a volume of tests that required several hours by hand, was perhaps the culmination of Dr. Nickerson's thirty years of dedication to the creation of a laboratory rivaling that at his "home" hospital in Salem.

By 1972, however, the lab was again becoming overcrowded, with a dozen full-time technicians and far more equipment again making for uncomfortable and inefficient working conditions. Its workload had reached the point where Dr. Nickerson felt he was unable to give it the time required even with the assistance of a third pathologist from his Salem staff. It was time, he said, for the AGH to have its own full-time pathologist. The matter came to a head with his death in 1973 and became critical as a retrenchment plan begun the next year at Salem Hospital reduced its cooperative arrangements with smaller hospitals. As a result, the Staff Council voted on February 23, 1974 to recommend "the hiring of Dr. William J. Cornetta [who] will be available by August 1, 1974." With Dr. Cornetta's arrival that summer, the laboratory came into its own.

The X-ray Department of 1948 still shared space with the lab and remained under the supervision of Dr. Wilson, who continued coming part time from Salem. He was finding it difficult to give the time required, however, and, unlike the affable Dr. Nickerson, he was not popular with the Medical Staff. That body recommended his dismissal in March 1949, suggesting as replacements Raymond A. Dillon, MD and his partner, L. Alexander Vance, MD, with Dr. Wilson retained on the Consulting Staff. The

Trustees concurred, and in April 1949 Vance-Dillon Associates joined the growing hospital family.

The personable pair fitted in nicely. Dr. Dillon, according to Executive Committee records of July 1954, "brought in X-ray equipment from his own office and had rebuilt the small machine . . . involving expenditure of a considerable amount of his own funds." He later gave other equipment, including a sound film projector, and participated enthusiastically in the functioning of the hospital.

Their partnership was joined in 1950 by Edward P. Wells, MD, and became North Shore Radiological Associates. Dr. Wells, the first of several partners the new group recruited from Mary Hitchcock Hospital in Hanover, N.H., soon found himself assigned to the Addison Gilbert, coming here daily for three or four hours with Dr. Dillon or Dr. Vance. In 1957, as he describes it, "we decided to have me come . . . routinely instead of Dr. Dillon, and gradually I seemed to become a fixture at this place." He became such a fixture that he soon was assigned here full time and in 1975 was honored by the Medical Staff in being elected its Chief of Staff. Dr. Wells retired in 1984 and, like Dr. Dillon in 1976, was appointed to the Honorary Staff.

Space remained a problem only partially solved by a 1958 move to newly created space adjacent to the new laboratory (see Chapter 8), where the two basic machines could be more adequately accommodated. The Nurses' Dining Room, at that time located across from the kitchen, became a film storage area, its original china cabinets used for supplies and record storage. Dr. Wells, however, was always frustrated by the need to compromise his desire for more equipment with the lack of space in which to put it, as well as a decided lack of privacy and comfort for patients. The first xeroradiograph on the North Shore, for example, was placed in a small inner office, and a nuclear body scanner funded for $40,000 by the Women's Auxiliary in 1974 was installed some distance from the rest of the department. Portable equipment augmented the heavy fixed machines which, under Dr. Wells, were replaced several times as the state of the art improved.

The workload also increased — from just over 10,000 films in 1950, it had quadrupled to 43,000 by 1967. By the time the count reached 56,000 in 1979 Ed Wells could take satisfaction in the knowledge that his dream of more space would shortly be fulfilled by another building program, even though he would no longer be around to enjoy it. He and his colleagues at North Shore Radiological could take justifiable pride in their management of a fine department under less-than-optimum conditions.

Dispensing of pharmaceuticals was also among the advances of the period. Gone was the practice of dipping into the doctor's bag or having Fred

Barker's drugstore mix a compound on prescription. Gone too was the day when the safekeeping of medicines was a function of the Superintendent and her nurses. As new and more complex medications were developed, the old way was no longer sufficient. The nursing service continued to control and dispense them until the early 1960s, but a change was inevitable. The Medical Staff, concerned over the "duplication and multiplicity of drugs," recognized the problem in early 1958, when it appointed a Drug Committee to oversee the purchase of drug supplies. The committee's mission was enlarged a year later in "the hope that a hospital formulary [could] be established to simplify the confusion and excessive waste of many new drugs."

A more pressing need for change surfaced on May 26, 1964 when the Administrator reported to the Board that "recent court decisions [suggest the need] for a hospital pharmacist [since] hospitals are not exempt in case of administration of wrong medications, and nurses are not allowed to repackage drugs for use on the floors." He was given authority to employ "a competent pharmacist" part time to manage, with nurse assistance, the small pharmacy that was located on the ground floor of a new maternity wing (see Chapter 8).

The department grew, and five years later it was necessary to bring a full-time pharmacist to the hospital staff. Rosemary F. Bigelow, Registered Pharmacist, was appointed to the post, which she held with distinction for many years, managing a department of great importance in the operation of the hospital that, out of the public view, works unrecognized. As recorded in the *Annual Report* of 1969, Mrs. Bigelow's impact was felt immediately in the development of more coordinated drug information and improved pharmaceutical service.

Today the pharmacy employs five pharmacists housed in well-equipped, computerized quarters completed in 1983. There it not only dispenses standard unit dose medications but compounds many sophisticated intravenous solutions including antibiotics, chemotherapies for cancer treatment, and total parenteral nutrition. It also offers medication counseling to patients and participates in the hospital's cardiac and pulmonary rehabilitation programs.

The State of the Art

The period following 1948 was to become known as the space age, and the many medical advances during it would reflect the high technical sophistication which made space exploration possible. Diagnosis, while remaining very much a hands-on skill, would benefit from the electronic wonders which seemed to come along so rapidly that early obsolescence became a factor in the costs of keeping pace with it all. The new equipment was expensive and sometimes of only marginal utilization, and smaller hospitals had to think long and hard before giving in to the wishes of their medical staffs and a shared desire for the latest technology.

Despite care, the urge to "keep up with the Joneses" sometimes led them to acquire equipment they didn't really need. Costs could only rise under a lax policy and, as they did so, so did the attention of a cost-conscious government which was, after 1965, helping to underwrite health care through Medicare and Medicaid. This in turn led to more regulation and the creation of more watchdog agencies. Outside oversight of planning as an element of cost control would follow later.

Surgery joined diagnosis in making advances. The skills learned during World War II were further developed as the large teaching hospitals, and later even small community hospitals, performed work undreamed of when Dr. Babson opened his practice. Open heart surgery, while not common until a few years later, had its start in Europe. Organ transplants were being done by the early 1960s — first the kidney, then the liver and finally, as the 1970s progressed, the heart and lungs.

None of these was attempted here, but the development of joint replacement techniques at the large urban hospitals during the sixties offered opportunities for the smaller institutions. That technique came to the AGH as the period was ending with the appointment of Mordecai E. Berkowitz, MD, an orthopedic surgeon who proceeded to give the mobility and comfort of new hip and other joints to many formerly hopeless Cape Ann sufferers. Eye surgery came to this small hospital at about the same time as ophthalmologist David W. Sauer, MD, transformed cataract surgery from a three-week ordeal to what is now often a day surgery procedure.

The local surgeons began performing major urological procedures, pelvic surgery, and lung, abdominal and cancer surgery along with the surgical treatment of thoracic, thyroid and major neck problems during the 1950s. They were using intramedullary nails in fracture cases during the 1960s, before the technique was commonly accepted by most other hospitals in the state. They introduced the metal prosthesis in replacement of the intracapsular femoral head during the same decade, at that time a forerunner of the joint replacement yet to come.

The art of anesthesia had suffered a setback with the departure of Miss Blandford in 1942. There was no regular service again until 1950, when the department was reorganized under Dr. Lawrence Ross. Dr. Ross, doing obstetrics and other elements of family practice when he joined the Staff in 1945, had had intensive training and experience in anesthesia as an intern at Rhode Island Hospital and was interested in returning to that field while he built his obstetrical practice. The Staff was happy to elect him Chief of Anesthesia, a post he held until 1960, when he came to the realization that he must choose between one specialty or the other. His colleagues, in accepting his decision to devote himself to obstetrics, voted their thanks for "the fine anesthesia service the hospital has had."

Dr. Ross' decision left a void that had to be filled. The interim appointment of John C. Roberts, MD, now an ophthalmologist in Hawaii, did so for two years before Lloyd G. David, MD, a well-trained specialist from Lowell, was recruited. Although willing to devote full time to anesthesiology, Dr. David also realized that the growing workload was too much for one person to handle alone. Thus, when Dr. John Bloomburgh, a veteran member of the Staff, returned from a year's leave of absence as resident in anesthesia at New England Medical Center, they became a team. They were joined by H. Elizabeth Cherry, MD in 1972, and others joined her as departmental associates for varying lengths of stay after Dr. Bloombergh's retirement in 1973. Dr. David served, usually with no more than one assistant plus a nurse anesthetist, until his own retirement in 1983.

Medical practice was, like surgery, also advancing with cardiology, neurology and radiology all gaining benefits from the space age. The Secretary's annual report to the Medical Staff in 1971 recorded "an increasing number of difficult medical problems . . . being treated here. There have been several abdominal aortic aneurisms [and a partial] hepatectomy. . . . Increasing use of sophisticated equipment in the coronary care unit resulted in more complex cardiac problems being treated here [and] therefore obviate transfer to the major medical centers."

Among the more significant developments of the period was improvement in the treatment and management of coronary cases. It was no longer accepted that the victim of a heart attack, if he made it to the hospital in the first place, would simply be put to bed in an oxygen tent for total bed rest. New diagnostic capabilities were making it possible to detect and more effectively evaluate early symptoms and, in many cases, prevent a cardiac attack.

The hospital had acquired its own electrocardiograph, funded by the Auxiliary, in 1949 and had been given a bedside monitor by the Massachusetts Heart Association in 1951. It also had the standard oxygen hoods of the day, but, except for the application of care and bed rest on a regular nursing floor, that was about the extent of coronary treatment prior to the sixties. Extra care was available from private nurses until their increasing cost and a trend away from in-hospital private care led Tucker Vye to advise the Trustees in late 1960 that the hospital must soon consider installation of a special nursing

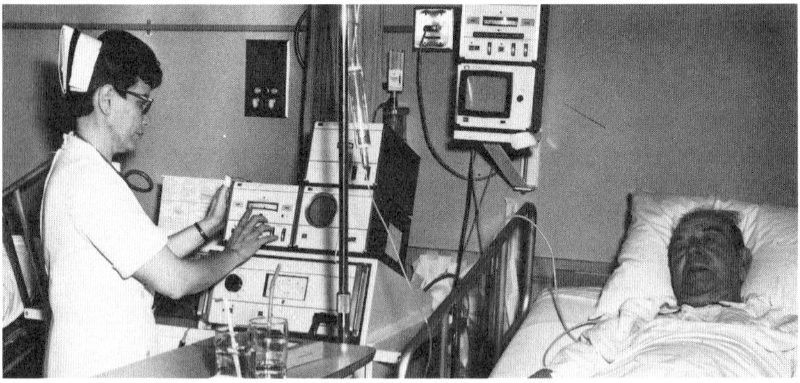

RN Virginia Webber administers to a patient in the first coronary care unit installed in 1969 in a four-bed room in South Wing.

unit for cardiac and other cases requiring intensive care.

Dr. Gale and the other internists kept the idea alive and under study. His report to the Staff Council in January 1967 followed a survey exploring the need for and feasibility of what he described as a coronary care unit and was the first positive step toward its realization. He explained the cost, about $8,000, of installing such a unit and advised that staffing it would require "a disproportionately large number of highly trained persons." Gale was asked to study the matter further and in October reported back with a recommendation for a two-bed unit on the second floor of the South Wing, then in its ninth year of operation (see Chapter 8). His report indicated that five physicians were interested in a rotating coverage plan to provide constant medical supervision. On October 17, 1967 Administrator Vye presented the Gale plan to the Trustees, but, already faced with more patients than space, they were forced to compromise by authorizing special training and acquisition of a mobile unit as a temporary measure until space became available.

A "crash cart" with monitor, defibrillator and other equipment and supplies was given by the Auxiliary, and nurses Virginia Webber and Alicia Dench were sent to Salem Hospital for a six-week course in the care of coronary patients. They and others like them across the nation were about to break new ground in their profession, as their special training made it possible to entrust the initial emergency and longer-range care to these nurses. Until the needed space could be found and an in-place unit installed, they, the crash cart and Dr. Gale's physician team covered the heart cases anywhere in the hospital.

The general patient load had lightened a year later, permitting the conversion of a four-bed room on South II in January 1969. From that time on Cape Ann patients who got to the hospital promptly could count on effective care, and the cardiac mortality rate decreased. The in-place unit proved its value early and received accolades in a full-page story in the May 4 Boston *Herald Traveler,* headlined "*HEART ATTACK!*" The story detailed the onset of the reporter's coronary occlusion while on a visit to Gloucester.

I was very, very lucky. It was not - as I kept insisting it must be - Hong Kong flu. It was a heart attack, and within 45 minutes I was in a hospital under treatment. That part of my luck was due to fast action by my family, an accurate diagnosis by a young physician who had never seen me before and tender loving care from a pair of burly policemen. The other and more important part of my luck was that all this happened in Gloucester where I ended up at the Addison Gilbert Hospital. Addison Gilbert is not exactly a big, urban medical center . . . but it does have a Coronary Care Unit, electronically equipped and staffed by nurses especially trained.

The story went on to detail the treatment and endorse the need for such units in all hospitals, citing estimates that "some 2,000 other heart attack victims die every year in Massachusetts hospitals for lack of such equipment." The new unit was indeed kept busy, and the next year, after 247 admissions in 1969, it was necessary to add eight beds for intermediate care, the recovery period, in order to keep the closely monitored two-bed unit always available for emergencies and the early stages of treatment. That first small unit, primitive by today's standards, prepared the way for the advanced Coronary Care Unit (CCU) to come three years later with construction of another new wing. From it also came the formation of "code teams," units of selected nurses and technicians assigned on each shift to drop whatever they were doing at the time and respond to cardiac emergencies within the hospital or meet such cases on arrival at the Emergency Room.

Better training for ambulance attendants was also an important factor, and this, later augmented by radio communication, shares credit for the subsequent decrease in mortalities from cardiac failure as well as accidents. By 1960 each Cape Ann community was operating its own municipally supported ambulance service, although, lacking any real training beyond first aid, the crews were little more than chauffeurs. Aware of this, in 1966 the Medical Staff had sponsored the first of several one-day courses in cardiopulmonary resuscitation (CPR) for the Gloucester and Rockport Fire and Police departments. The program, being voluntary and attended during off-duty time, was only marginally successful until it was reorganized on a mandatory, on-duty basis in 1972.

With reorganization, the first thirteen-week course for Emergency Medical Technicians (EMTs) was offered in March 1974 under Alexander N. Gunn II, MD, of the hospital's surgical staff. During eighty-five hours of training, which included far more than first aid and CPR, the Gloucester fire fighters and police and Rockport and Essex volunteers were exposed to a course that set a standard for a series of similar courses that followed. Realistic disaster drills, refresher training and much actual experience has continued to assure skilled transportation as a significant factor in emergency treatment at the AGH.

Other Health Problems and Clinics

Among the epidemic illnesses remaining dangerous into the 1950s was poliomyelitis, commonly known as infantile paralysis or polio. It was much feared as a crippler of children and postadolescents, and at a time when other infectious diseases were largely under control it remained a major threat. During the decade from 1945 to 1955 there were some 360,000 cases in the United States, 20,000 of which resulted in death.

The disease hit Cape Ann with periodic heavy onslaughts in the same way it was seen nationally. After a fifteen-case year in Gloucester in 1927 only fourteen cases were recorded over the next twenty years until 1945, when eleven cases were diagnosed and reported. Only eight cases occurred here after 1945 until, in 1955, another epidemic resulted in ten more being afflicted before a new vaccine developed by Dr. Jonas Salk and tested under supervision of the University of Michigan became available.

The Gloucester Board of Health, then chaired by Dr. Lundberg, obtained sufficient vaccine that year to immunize all first- and second-grade schoolchildren, and during the next two years it conducted mass immunization drives to reach the remaining groups at risk. Clinics established at the hospital through 1962 reached any missed earlier and were also able to offer the newer Sabin oral vaccine. As a result of such breakthroughs polio here and around the world soon joined the list of "has-been" diseases.

A scourge of a different sort replaced polio a few years later, one for which there was no vaccine and no sure cure. In many ways it was worse than the diseases that preceded it, since the only cure rested within the individual victim. Drug abuse, a product of the counterculture restlessness of the 1960s, was becoming a major problem in Gloucester by 1970. In August that year, urged by psychiatrist Philip D. Cutter, MD and Dr. New, the Medical Staff approved the idea of a joint effort by the hospital and NUVA, a drug counseling organization, involving the use of methadone as a possible treatment.

Proponents of the methadone method argued that, as a substitute for heroin, it would be a low-cost means of removing the addictive attraction of that drug and eventually permit the user to cease its use completely. Others saw it as helpful but doubted its long-term effectiveness, since methadone was itself considered addictive. In any case, a methadone dispensary was opened at the hospital in late 1970 to administer the substitute under Outpatient Department (OPD) supervision with counseling offered by NUVA.

The clinic, which received Federal Drug Administration approval in early 1973, soon became involved in further controversy. Problems developed within the OPD through misunderstandings by addicts as to the clinic's schedule and function. The Medical Staff and Trustees questioned its effectiveness and feasibility as well as its sometimes embarrassing disruption of normal OPD operation. With rarely more than twelve participants at any one time, its $20—30,000 annual expense was also of concern. Arguments pro and con were a source of friction within and outside the hospital until mid-1975 when, with the clinic down to four clients, the Medical Staff was advised that those remaining would become private patients and that, in effect, the clinic would cease to operate.

The methadone method was then, and continues to be, open to question as to its value. It was a meritorious concept that withered after 1975 and is only now being reconsidered by NUVA with the hospital as a possible partner. New regulations for dispensing methadone and more effective counseling carry the hope for a partial solution to a problem of vital concern nationwide.

Another short-lived clinic, also a product of its times, was that devoted to family planning. The Family Planning Clinic operated under the North Shore Family Planning Council with funding assistance from the Department of Health, Education and Welfare. Expected to supplement one already established at Beverly Hospital, it opened with considerable publicity in July 1972. It was to be available one day a week for a four-hour period under a Family Planning Council nurse with counseling available also from the three AGH obstetricians, each of whom was to be in attendance every third week.

According to its proponents it was designed to serve low-income singles and families and "would not limit its scope simply to birth control . . . but would deal with all related problems when they come up." It was confidently expected to enroll ten clients a week and thus counsel approximately 500 young women a year. Three months later it was still far from that goal, citing a lack of community interest in its services. Cut back to two sessions monthly and in danger of losing HEW funding, the Family Planning Clinic was closed in 1976 with its remaining fifty clients referred to its more popular companion at Beverly.

A clinic of far greater significance arrived on the scene in 1968. The care of the mentally ill had by long tradition been a public function largely left to the individual states to deal with as they saw fit. What they saw as fit was too often institutional care of patients, out of sight and away from their homes and families, "warehoused" in large, centralized facilities. A few privately owned treatment centers also served, although their function was usually limited to alcoholism and psychiatric counsel. One of this type, Villa Atlanta, was owned and directed by Dr. Bernard A. Williams on Shore Road in Magnolia from 1965 to 1974, when it closed in the face of increasingly restrictive regulations.

The traditional approach remained the rule into the 1950s, when it began to give way to the development of a generally more liberal philosophy. With the promotion of community participation in this and other matters by the short-lived Kennedy administration, and encouraged by the possibilities offered by newly developed medication, many patients were deemed treatable in responsible community-centered facilities. Elderly patients, sometimes victims only of senility, could be brought closer to home and freed from the stigma of mental hospital confinement by transfer to nursing homes. Others with varying degrees of mental disability could also leave the isolation of often distant hospitals and, with local centers overseeing their treatment on an outpatient basis, return to a more normal life and place in society.

The new approach, with state encouragement, materialized on Cape Ann in early 1968 when Mr. Vye was authorized by the Trustees to work with representatives of the North Shore Mental Health Association in finding space for an outpatient facility at the hospital. The vacant third floor of the original 1897 wing was made available and, with concurrence by the Medical Staff, a clinic opened there that summer as an outpost of the North Shore Child Guidance Clinic under joint sponsorship of the Gloucester School Department. Within a year the School Department concluded that the clinic should expand its services to other age groups, and the Staff Council, responding to the eloquence of Dr. New, voted its support.

The program began to gain momentum in 1969, when the Mental Health Association and the state's Department of Public Health allocated three full-time, state-funded staffers to the clinic. Dr. Philip D. Cutter, a psychiatrist who had summered on Cape Ann as a young man and was eager to return there from Wiesbaden, West Germany, where he was Director of the USAFE Child Guidance Center, joined the Medical Staff in late 1969 and was appointed Clinical Director. He was shortly joined on the small clinic staff by a clinical psychologist and a psychiatric social worker.

By 1972 its staff included three social workers, a psychologist, a psychiatric nurse and two secretaries, and the clinic was well able to expand its services to include adult treatment. With expansion its designation changed to the Cape Ann Children and Family Center. A second psychiatrist, Allan B. Rosansky, MD, joined the clinic staff in 1973 when Dr. Cutter was appointed Program Director for the area that included Beverly, Essex, Gloucester, Hamilton, Manchester, Rockport, Topsfield and Wenham, all of which were served by the Cape Ann clinic.

Local sponsorship and funding assistance soon made possible the formation of a separate corporate entity, Greater Cape Ann Human Services, Inc. (GCAHS), called "G-Kiss" by its staff, to operate the clinic. Thus separated from the North Shore Mental Health Association, GCAHS continued to maintain its affiliation with the state Department of Public Health. By 1978, with an average caseload of 350 patients a year and facing a growing problem of drug abuse in addition to its other work, the clinic was rapidly outgrowing the limited space within the hospital.

In 1979 it was renamed the Mental Health Center of Greater Cape Ann, a term more descriptive of its expanded mission, and during the next year its need for larger quarters, by then critical, was met. With the support of a Block Development Grant from the City of Gloucester, the second and third floors of the former nurses' residence were renovated and converted to a modern mental health outpatient center. With that move the Mental Health Center and its staff of eighteen was firmly established as an important member of Cape Ann's health care community. Its programs included a twenty-four-hour emergency service, a psychiatric day treatment program, two residential facilities for mentally retarded children and adolescents, and a community education program plus satellite offices in Beverly, Essex and Hamilton.

8

Expansion: South and Babson Wings

IT WAS OBVIOUS by 1948 that the hospital was severely under-bedded. With an average daily patient load of seventy-five or more in a hospital with eighty-four beds, almost a fifth of them in the single-purpose, restricted Maternity Wing, there was little flexibility. When there were more than sixty-five acute-care cases beds had to be placed wherever space could be found, and this meant putting patients in the corridors.

Such overcrowding was not confined to the Addison Gilbert; all across the nation other hospitals were feeling the same pinch. Increased insurance coverage and better medical technology made a hospital admission the norm during serious illness or for surgery. The young physicians added during the fifties were more hospital oriented, fresh from residencies in the teaching-center hospitals, where they had access to diagnostic tools and facilities they couldn't hope to match in their own offices. They were not hesitant about admitting their patients for the more effective treatment and diagnostic testing even then available within the hospital here.

Some of the demand thus created had been taken care of in the former open sun porches on the south end of Prentiss House, which had been glassed in some years earlier. Although popular with patients because of their airiness, these rooms could accommodate only five on each of the two floors. They were also what today are called "unlicensed beds," not counted in the formal tally but winked at by the state authorities in those less-regulated times. Not so acceptable, especially to the Gloucester Fire Department or to those who were placed in them, were beds in the corridors. The firefighters saw them as traffic-inhibiting hazards while the patients, shielded by portable screens, suffered the loss of any semblance of privacy.

Although crowded conditions had been noted as far back as 1940, when the Superintendent blamed it on large numbers of patients eligible for home or resthome care but kept at the hospital "for the convenience of the doctor," it was not until the war ended in 1945 that the Trustees could consider the matter constructively. A survey begun that year by Curtin & Riley, hospital architects, was described at a joint dinner meeting of the Board and Medical Staff in May 1946. The participants found it interesting, but problems over billings by the architects led to argument rather than progress, and when the dispute was finally settled in 1950, five years had been lost without relieving the worsening bed shortage.

In October 1950 architect James Ritchie was retained on a five-year contract to prepare "a long-range plan" which, after exhaustive study of the hospital and the area it served, was presented to the Board on August 20, 1954. The Ritchie Plan outlined an ambitious program, and the report accompanying it was critical of almost every aspect of the physical plant, which was deemed, probably to nobody's surprise, totally inadequate for the job it was called on to do. The plan proposed a single-story wing attached south of Prentiss House to contain nineteen beds, with a new operating suite on its ground floor. Another single-story wing was to extend west from the 1925 Maternity Wing, which it would replace; the wood-framed 1925 wing would be converted to nonpatient use. The ground floor of the new maternity wing would contain a cafeteria and maintenance/storage space. The lab and X-ray would each get new quarters by roofing over the open area between Prentiss House and the old Maternity Wing.

The original operating room area would be converted to office space into which the Administrator and Business Office could move, finally, from the crowded first floor of the original building. That area, the architects suggested, could, be used for coffee and gift shops and a waiting lounge. The doctors would gain a new lounge and a libary in space to be created by attaching the separate laundry building at the end of the old operating room ell. The project could be done in successive steps and, including an optional second floor on the proposed south wing, was estimated to cost $1,052,568.

A Million Dollar Fund-Raising Goal

The prospect of a million-dollar project made for a year of agonizing indecision, during which corridor beds became frequent to the point where patients regularly registered complaints at being charged room rates while enduring the discomfort of corridor living. It was not until December 4, 1955, at a well-attended joint meeting of the Trustees, the Medical Staff, the Dental Staff, representatives of the Auxiliary and the Nurses' Alumnae Association plus delegates from the architects and Will, Folsom & Smith, fund-raising counsel, that the die was cast. The physicians and dentists reported unanimity for the proposal, the Auxiliary and the Alumnae promised to help, and with that evidence of support Trustee William F. Moore made the motion to hold a fund-raising campaign for $1 million to get the job done. With unanimous support from the twenty-one Trustees present, the real work was about to begin.

The Plant Improvement Committee, a combination of the Executive, Finance and House & Grounds Committees, was renamed the Campaign Committee under the chairmanship of Carroll Steele. Already recognized as a dynamic leader of such efforts in many years of summer YMCA drives and, more recently, the Joint Health Campaigns, always an optimist, he was eager to get this one started. In this largest ever effort on Cape Ann he was joined by William S. Webber, Jr., who became the hospital's President at the 1956 Annual Meeting.

By April 1956 campaign headquarters had been activated in a Duncan Street storefront loaned by Charles T. (Cap) Heberle and his Gloucester Coal and Lumber Company. Furnished and equipped by Gloucester Safe Deposit & Trust Company, it became the hospital's downtown base under "Pete" Wilson of the Will, Folsom & Smith firm. Prospect lists were drawn up over a spring and summer of work, during which hardly a day passed without some sort of hospital story in the newspaper.

The Board also devised a questionnaire in which it sought public input – the hospital's place in the community and opinion as to the need for a costly expansion were among the subjects covered. The results revealed overwhelming support for the institution and its proposed program, with a gratifyingly large number, 80 percent, of the respondents indicating approval of the rates then being charged. It gave the Board confidence that a campaign was likely to be successful.

The first gift officially credited had arrived immediately following announcement of the December decision to proceed, when Sam Gordon of Gloucester Supply Company sent in the funds he usually spent on Christmas gifts to his good customers. The Ford Foundation, with fortuitous timing, announced a $500 million grant to be divided among hospitals nationwide, based on recommendations made to it by the American Hospital Association. Among 128 Massachusetts hospitals, the AGH share was set at $45,500, and this unrestricted gift was placed in the infant Building Fund.

Other gifts, made during the spring and early summer of 1956, seemed to justify the Board's confidence.

The Trustees backed slightly away from the original idea of raising the entire million dollars locally, deciding instead to obtain 75 percent via gifts with the balance from a grant under the Hill-Burton Act. This program, adopted in the postwar haste to create more hospital beds, operated under supervision of the individual states, which determined need based on a rather loose beds-per-thousand population formula with emphasis on grants to low-income states. Any hospital awarded such a grant was expected to raise at least two-thirds of the construction funds and to demonstrate financial stability. Another provision, unenforced for many years, required "a reasonable volume of hospital services to persons unable to pay." This proviso came back some three decades later to haunt many hospitals that lacked the AGH tradition of free care when, in an excess of cost consciousness, the federal government decided to require pro rata free care from any hospital that had ever received Hill-Burton funding.

The Addison Gilbert joined the frantic Hill-Burton chase in August 1956 with its application for $250,000. It made a good case for itself, and the Massachusetts Department of Public Health gave prompt approval. It was then that Dr. A. Daniel Rubenstein, for many years the Department's Director, became something of a godfather to this and other hospitals across the state. The relationship formed then would serve to open many doors and ease many situations for Tucker Vye, who carefully nurtured Dr. Rubenstein's friendship.

The community campaign was organized and ready to go in June. Early large gifts, essential to any such effort, started to come in, and, after a barrage of stories in the *Times* detailing large memorial gifts and identifying the campaign leadership, the drive "went public" in September. The special gifts campaign had raised $573,261.88 in gifts and pledges, and three weeks later at the final report meeting on September 24 the drive had recorded 3,231 gifts and pledges totaling $806,927.

It was the largest amount ever raised on Cape Ann until then, and it was truly a Cape-wide effort. Gloucester residents and businesses logged $616,716 and Rockport $114,935. The Medical and Dental Staffs pledged $66,150 and hospital employees gave $9,126. The sources were diverse: an anonymous ten $10 bills to Dr. Babson with a hand-lettered note, "This is toward your new surgical unit"; a Rockport "Fireman's Frolic"; summer residents; three paintings by Anthony Thieme, among other gifts of art. The *Times* summed it up in an editorial: "In the end it was the response of the people that counted. 'Wonderful people,' as Carroll Steele said, 'the people of Cape Ann.'"

The euphoria felt by the Trustees at the close of the campaign soon gave way to reality. By the following spring it had become obvious that the cost estimates of 1954 were now much too low, and the original program must be cut back. When the first phase, the new south wing, estimated in 1954 at $650,000, was bid in June 1957 at $816,545, the Building Committee (the former Plant Improvement/Campaign Committee) knew it must seek alternatives.

Cuts and alterations were made and subcontracts were re-bid, but meanwhile bids on equipment and furnishings also were coming in higher than expected. The final result was a projected cost of $856,000 for construction of and furnishing a single new wing with a second floor added and roofing in the space for the lab and X-ray, and that was it. Gone were the new Maternity Wing and the renovated areas so optimistically described in the campaign brochure and for which specific gifts had been designated. The decision made, the deeply curtailed construction project was begun July 5, 1957 when General Contractor Russell M. Curtis of Gloucester broke ground.

The September 1956 euphoria dimmed even further when, by August, it was becoming apparent that pledge collections were lagging. Troubled by rumors of higher costs and postponement of the balance of the program to which many gifts had been allocated, pledge makers were having second thoughts. Appeals in a newly inaugurated hospital *Newsletter* and in the *Times* helped some, but by December, when collections had been scheduled to be almost complete, only 70 percent had been paid. An additional Hill-Burton grant of $50,000 helped as did a grant of $20,000 by the Godfrey Hyams Trust of Boston, but overall it was a classic hand-to-mouth situation.

Meanwhile construction was proceeding. By November the lab/X-ray area had been roofed in, to be followed on January 9, 1958 by the roof of the main wing. The latter led to a race between Faulk Brothers and the onslaught of a long arctic freeze that made it necessary to pour the concrete slab under a heated tentlike covering. Subcontractor Faulk won the race by doing the whole job in six hours.

Back in the boardroom authorization was given the architects to proceed with plans for renovation of the old Maternity Wing to bring it up to 1958 requirements. Plans were also made to renovate the boiler plant and install new boilers at once, a previously postponed step now necessary to meet the additional steam requirements of the new wing.

March and April were spent in contemplation of $475,000 still due on construction payments with only $350,000 remaining in the Building Fund and the next Hill-Burton installment not due until July. Although uncollected pledges stood at $200,000, a vote in late April to proceed with the deferred work "at the earliest possible date" manifested the Board's determination to keep the faith. It seems to have helped, as by late November the unpaid pledge total was down to $106,000.

That autumn, with construction and furnishings almost complete, the project was judged ready for the necessary formal inspection by Hill-Burton authorities. This was done in November by a delegation led by Dr. Rubenstein and guided by the Administrator and two specially designated Trustees, as required by the terms of the grant. But even more exciting was the public Open House held on December 6 when some 1,500 people guided by hostesses from the Auxiliary trooped through the facility which, not yet named, was called simply the New Wing. Later dubbed South Wing by common usage, it did not receive a formal designation until the Annual Meeting of 1978 when a plaque was dedicated naming it Webber House in honor of Bill Webber, its enthusiastic protagonist in 1955, who had retired in 1974 after eighteen years as President.

The new wing received its first patients two days before Christmas, when an emergency admission brought in Kathleen McGillivary, age five. Later that day five more children were moved to the new Pediatrics Unit from the former Children's Ward on the original building's third floor. The opening of the second floor was delayed by staffing problems and minor completion work, but on January 13, 1959, with a hospital census of 102 again bulging the walls, the first adult patients were moved in. With that, the Administrator had a total of 117 beds including maternity and pediatrics and could at last relax on the issue of corridor beds.

The new surgical suite, spacious and sophisticated compared with that in continuous use since 1897, was opened in February. With the closing of the old operating area, the adjacent Accident Room also moved to a new Outpatient Clinic in renovated space under Prentiss House. The laboratory had moved to its spacious new quarters a few days earlier, radiology gradually expanded into its new space, and the first phase of the job was complete. Prentiss House, of course, lost both its popular sun porches when the new wing was attached to its southern end.

Further Funding and Expansion

With the South Wing project completed, the Trustees had to consider the fact that two years of capital funding had left the cupboard bare of gifts to help with operations. The painful truth was that income from patient fees and endowment without the support of annual giving simply was not enough, and in consequence during 1957 it had once again become necessary to borrow from endowment principal.

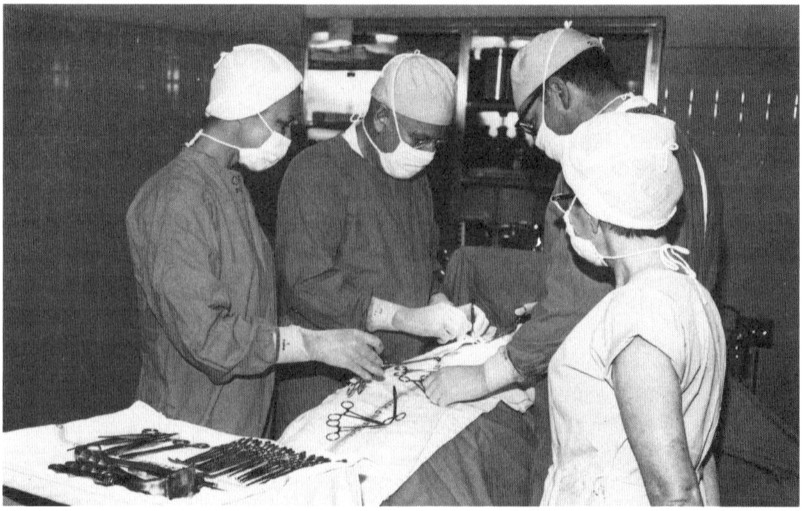

Surgery moved to a new suite in 1958 with completion of South Wing. Doctors Babson (left) and Lundberg, shown here with Head OR Nurse Virginia (Bellie) Bergeron and OR Nurse Claire O'Brien (left) were doing almost all AGH surgery in 1969 when this photo was taken.

The Gloucester District Nurse Association was also feeling the pinch, having done only minimal fund raising in 1956 in expectation that the Joint Health Campaign would be revived in 1957. Without endowment, that agency depended even more than the hospital on annual giving, and it was a serious blow when a joint meeting between representatives of the two groups in November 1956 resulted in cancellation of plans for a drive in 1957. All the hospital delegates could promise was to give the GDNA such assistance and advice as it might require.

Both organizations felt relieved when, in September 1957, the hospital Board voted to hold a "sustaining campaign" in the summer or fall of 1958, one purpose of which was to make a start toward replacing borrowed endowment funds. Unable to retain Hugh Spalding who was on assignment elsewhere, the Finance Committee selected Denton Associates of Holyoke to direct the revived effort for a fixed fee plus expenses. The Gloucester goal was set at $48,000 plus a further $7,800 from Rockport. The GDNA was to get $5,500 from the Gloucester gifts with everything after expenses to come to the hospital.

It was not a successful effort. No one was happy with the precampaign publicity or the campaign material. The GDNA wanted a house-to-house effort as before and felt that the limited number of prospects for solicitation was far too low. Although more prospects were added, the campaign grossed only $38,500, $7,325 of which came from Rockport. That failure ended the affiliation with Denton as well as fourteen years of joint effort with the District Nurses. The latter's preference for smaller gifts through house-to-house visits plus a general uneasiness with a divided effort loomed large among the factors ending the relationship.

Will, Folsom & Smith returned as counsel for a 1959 sustaining drive for $49,700. Things went well that fall in raising just over $50,000 before expenses, convincing the Trustees that the hospital was indeed better off raising funds independently. By then, moreover, it was time to fulfill the promise made in April 1958 to build the Maternity Wing, and the 1959 success made it easier to contemplate another capital campaign.

Early thinking suggested simply proceeding with the wing as proposed in the 1954 Ritchie Plan which, with conversion of the former surgical area to office space and further work on the boiler plant plus all furnishings and equipment, was estimated at $522,795. Since Hill-Burton had already funded that program to its limit, nothing could be expected from that source, and, although $100,000 in late gifts and uncollected pledges was still left from the 1956 Building Fund, that and the limited amount considered feasible through public funding was realistically seen as far from enough. That realization led the Trustees to consider venturing into a previously untried method.

A proposal in May 1958 on their behalf by Cape Ann Savings Bank to Provident Savings Bank of Boston for mutual participation in a $450,000 mortgage loan brought a chilling refusal by the latter and the Board's reluctant conclusion that if that bank wouldn't do it, no one would. Simple rebuilding of the old Maternity Wing seemed the only possibility until Dr. Rubenstein suggested in November that a totally new plan would possibly warrant further Hill-Burton support, perhaps as high as $300,000; but only if construction was started by the end of June 1959.

Faced with that very big *if*, Ritchie moved fast to come in a month later with a totally different concept for the new wing which would comply with Hill-Burton requirements by avoiding any direct connection with the old Maternity Wing. There was even consideration of tearing it down altogether if doing so would assure the availability of those funds, a drastic step and happily not required so it could remain in use for patients during construction of the new wing. This phase could also include alteration of the old surgical wing and lobby and would permit converting the boilers from coal to oil. Complete, the program was estimated at $627,251, of which Hill-Burton would cover 40 percent. The balance, about $375,000, would have to be found elsewhere.

The hastily drawn Ritchie plans called for a two-floor, L-shaped wing extending westward via a short passageway from the old surgical wing. Its ground floor was to house a cafeteria, a combined conference room and doctors' dining room, the pharmacy and a central sterile supply room. The main floor would have nine rooms for seventeen beds and two nurseries with labor and delivery rooms plus doctors' and nurses' lounges in its ell. Years later the peculiarly shaped wing would become an architectural puzzle in its effect on future planning, but it looked good in December 1958 when it received final approval.

A month later Dr. Rubenstein confirmed a $250,000 Hill-Burton grant. A mortgage began to appear more feasible, and in April a four-bank consortium, which included Cape Ann Savings Bank and Granite Savings Bank (Rockport), granted a $325,000 loan, using the entire hospital plant as collateral. With $575,000 thus assured plus about $80,000 available from the 1956 Building Fund, the $555,425 low bid made the project a reality. Planning was begun for a "completion campaign" during the summer of 1960.

O. D. Purington & Company, the low bidder from Providence, started work following ground-breaking ceremonies on June 17, 1959. Construction, slated for completion in the fall of 1960, moved along on schedule despite a steel strike and some untimely bad weather, and the wing was ready for a tour by campaigners on September 6. The formal, public Open House was held a month later, and, with the funding campaign by then almost complete, the facility, known simply as the New Maternity Wing, opened for use a few days later.

With its opening another significant milestone had been reached, and the old wing, with 13,589 newborns to its credit since its own opening just thirty-five years earlier, could be closed. Ellen (Mother) Coull, RN, its feisty head, moved her crew over, and the first baby, nine-pound Michael Sullivan, was born there October 12. The Trustees had already moved their meetings from the Longan Room to the new ground floor Conference Room on September 20, the employees' cafeteria opened on November 1, and the Medical Staff held its first meeting in the new Medical Library upstairs on November 10.

The new cafeteria marked the end of the Nurses' Dining Room, which had for years occupied the space opposite the kitchen. It had always been restricted for use only by nurse and ranking staff employees who enjoyed reserved seating, linen napkins with personalized rings, and the luxury of tablecloths and waitresses. Tucker Vye had found this somewhat elitist and had done away with the table covers and waitresses soon after his arrival. The special privileges ended entirely with the opening of the new cafeteria, which seated all employees on an equal basis.

Fund raising for the wing had begun in earnest in June. Carroll Steele continued as General Chairman of a campaign with a goal of $605,000, of which $100,000 was earmarked to cover the amount that would normally have been raised in 1960 and 1961 annual drives. The Gloucester National Bank, having recently moved to new banking rooms further down Main Street, loaned its old quarters on Post Office Square[1] as campaign headquarters. The organizational work, again under Will, Folsom & Smith, was completed expeditiously, and the effort was launched at a dinner meeting on June 29, 1960.

Special gifts work that spring had already produced $169,100, including a $15,000 pledge by the Auxiliary, and this plus further major gifts were duly publicized in the *Times*. A fall public campaign with almost 300 workers raised $71,693 for an overall total of $512,699. Although sufficient to cover construction, this amount failed to replace the needed operating money, but despite not reaching its goal, the campaign was called a success at an all-out Victory Dinner in the high school cafeteria on September 22, 1960. A special feature of that affair was the presentation to Carroll Steele of a bird's-eye view watercolor of the hospital in recognition of "his inspiring leadership in the community effort which produced for the people of Cape Ann the expanded Addison Gilbert Hospital."

Rockport, under Trustees William J. Dean and Robert Simpson plus Barbara Marshall (later to become Mrs. Robert Simpson), had raised a record $112,095, a feat that was recognized shortly thereafter with the unveiling of a plaque in the labor/delivery ell of the new wing "in honor of the Town of Rockport and its citizens." They had indeed labored and delivered, but the record does not suggest that that was what the Trustees or the Sandy Bayers had in mind in selecting that particular unit for the plaque's location.

Insight into that choice, however, may be gained from a skit presented by the Rockport division's workers at the earlier 1956 campaign opening dinner during which they sang:

Why can't I be born in old Rockport,
Then a native of Rockport I'll be,
For there soon will be no native Rockporters
In just a few years, don't you see.

With the dedication of the delivery room area to the town, a bit of Rockport was symbolically established at the hospital so that, born there, future children of Rockport parents could claim Sandy Bay nativity.

The final phase remaining from the 1954 Ritchie Plan was then begun. A local contracting firm, Cooney & Feldman, was low bidder and got the project under way in early January 1961. The work progressed on schedule with no problems beyond the ususal upsets to routine caused by construction clutter, noise and displacement of staff. When the job was completed a few months later, the old Maternity Wing and surgical floor had become office space, the almost-sixty-five-year-old wooden stairway in the 1897 building had been replaced by one of steel, and a single nursing unit had been created combining Prentiss House II with the second floor of the old building, long known as Ward II.

The latter step joined what many saw as a very special floor of private rooms to an old ward. No distinction remained between the two, and paying patients were to be housed in either section of the unit. Although they didn't mind that, since the fireplaced rooms in the old building had a certain ambience, they did object to hearing the old section spoken of as Ward II. Aware of this, the unit's new Head Nurse, Muriel Walker, suggested designating that part of her unit as North II, and, with the passage of time, the entire original building came to be known as North Wing.

The Auxiliary pledge to the 1956 campaign had been designated for the Coffee Shop, and, with the Washington Street lobby no longer housing offices, that dream was about to come true. The Gift Shop, to the left just inside the front door, opened October 3, 1961. The Coffee Shop, located adjacent to the Gift Shop, was ready and opened with considerable flutter December 4. An open lobby with a counter for the main switchboard and reception desk on its inboard wall occupied the entire space on the side toward the Nurses' Residence. The Administrator and the business office staff moved to their new offices in the old operating rooms with the Nursing Service and Admissions Office across the corridor overlooking the new roof of the laboratory.

The program begun five years before was finally complete, and with it the hospital's plant, for insurance purposes, took on new value at $2,500,000. Its value in terms of community service could not be similarly measured, although one yardstick might be the fact that in the twelve months since its opening the previous October, 619 new citizens had already been born in the new wing.

"We are looking forward to the comparative peace and quiet of normal hospital operation after these years of contractors working in the most important areas of the hospital," Tucker Vye said in his report for 1961. President Bill Webber said it differently: "Historians of the local area may someday comment on the vitality of our communities of Rockport and Gloucester which have contributed approximately $1,350,000 for the development of their modern community hospital."

The construction may have been completed, but the hospital still faced its $325,000 mortgage. The balance of funds raised in 1960 helped, but by April 1962 the obligation was only down to $193,402 and holding. Repayment from that point loomed as a long, slow process, and the Trustees were understandably concerned when they assembled for a hastily called special meeting on July 30.

Carroll Steele lost no time in dissipating the concern with the announcement that he had spent two hours the previous day with Roger W. Babson, and, as a result of that conversation and others between Mr. Babson and his cousin, Dr. Warren Babson, earlier, he had a letter to share. Addressed simply to "Mr. Carroll K. Steele," it said:

If the directors of the Addison Gilbert Hospital will erect a bronze plaque by a vote which cannot be withdrawn or changed, naming the entire second floor of the new wing "THE ISABEL BABSON OBSTETRICAL FLOOR," I will give the hospital Two Hundred Thousand Dollars ($200,000) – One half this fall, and the other half in January of 1963, with no further "strings" thereby.

P.S. It should be understood by the directors that my interest in the Isabel Babson Memorial at 69 Main Street will continue. No "strings" can be attached to this, although every doctor is free to criticize it, irrespective of this gift.

Discussion was brief, and the vote to accept with "grateful thanks" was unanimous. The new wing had a name, and repayment of the mortgage was assured.

Roger Ward Babson

Roger Ward Babson can be variously described as eccentric, brilliant, self-made, visionary or vain. Born in Gloucester in 1875, he was a direct descendant of Isabel Babson and the son of Nathaniel, a Trustee of the hospital from 1900 until his death in 1927. Babson College in Wellesley, founded by Roger in 1919, is perhaps his best known monument, but this multimillionaire financier left many others.

Gloucester's Babson Reservoir and Sanctuary attests to his conservationist leanings. The Isabel Babson Memorial and Library, established at 69 Main Street on land occupied three hundred years earlier by his ancester Isabel, keeps alive his belief that the right type of reading by a pregnant mother would influence her child; he described it as "the power of positive thought." His Middle Street birthplace is the home of his Open Church and Gravity

Research Foundation and perpetuates his conviction that if gravity could somehow be overcome, many of the world's problems would be solved.

He once owned Milk Island off Rockport, using it to provide an outdoor experience for deprived Boston children. Many of Dogtown Common's boulders bear carved inscriptions which he commissioned as testimony to his moral beliefs. His belief in himself led to his Prohibition Party candidacy for President of the United States in 1940, although only about 58,000 voters shared that faith.

The postscript to his letter refers to a controversial 1961 proposal for the Isabel Babson Pre-natal Clinic, Inc. to operate out of the 69 Main Street building. The hospital's Medical Staff recorded itself as opposed to this supposed intrusion into its territory, and the Trustees, concerned over its effect on the hospital, asked Dr. Rubenstein for his intervention. That influential doctor was able to persuade Mr. Babson of the responsibility of the Massachusetts Department of Public Health if it were indeed a clinic and lying-in center. The proposal was withdrawn and the idea reconceived as the Isabel Babson Memorial Library Foundation. The medical opposition to it obviously still rankled in 1962.

The passage of time has long since healed any rift existing then. Mothers-to-be and others find the Babson Library a source of information and answers to their childbearing and child-rearing questions, and the hospital and its Medical Staff have joined it in sponsoring prenatal classes. In 1979 the hospital's Board was invited to nominate three of its members to serve on the Babson Foundation Board. The Foundation's well-managed endowment funds have also been the source of generous gifts designated for maternal care equipment such as the hospital's busy ultrasound. Through such continuing gifts Roger Babson's interest in his native community lives on.

His personal gifts to the hospital often reflected his individuality. The first, in 1938, was for a railing on the granite steps at the front of the old building so that others would not slip and fall as he once had. Another, influenced by his interest in maternity care and the promotion of thrifty habits, took the form of a $1,000 Treasury bond in 1963 to make possible a $25 savings deposit for the first baby born at the hospital each year. The child was to be designated "Master Gloucester," which was interpreted for many years to mean its award only to a son of Gloucester parents, a practice that changed during the seventies so that now Cape Ann's first boy and first girl each benefit regardless of home community.

His most unusual gift, however, was the so-called Babson Venture Fund, first proposed by him in 1957. As established two years later, a gift of $12,500 was to be invested only in DeBeers Consolidated Mines, Ltd., with all dividends to be reinvested therein. The stock, under the strict terms of the gift contract, was to be held intact until December 31, 1996 when, he believed, it would be worth at least $400,000. Always subject to wide price swings, it has twice exceeded that figure, in 1980 and again in 1983. The variations in value plus a developing disaffection for South African investment led the Trustees to vote in April 1982 to investigate the possibility of the deed of gift being "altered or changed so as to permit investments consistent with market conditions." On being advised that the Probate Court would be very unlikely to permit this in view of the firm and precisely expressed wishes of the donor, they abandoned the proposal. Only time will tell what its value will be when the Investment Committee of 1997 has the opportunity to determine its use beyond that point.

Eccentric though he may have been, Roger Babson will always be remembered as a most timely benefactor at the AGH. Payments on his 1962 pledge, sometimes accompanied by a wry comment, came faithfully although on his own, somewhat altered, schedule. One, for $34,000, was predated by three months but bore the promise of more "which I will take my time for as money comes in." Another requested the hospital to open a $5,000 account, presumably with its own funds, at Gloucester National Bank, which had been founded by his ancestors, "in honor of Isabel Babson." His final payment on the pledge arrived in March 1963, and in September of that year the mortgage was discharged and all remaining Building Fund money was transferred to the hospital's General Fund.

NOTES

[1]The junction of Pleasant and Duncan streets with Main Street, known by old-timers as Post Office Square from the days when the stately old stone postal building dominated the area.

9

Living with a Growing Hospital

WITH HOSPITALS across the nation facing financial difficulties and dependent on patients, some of whom still were without insurance, a new approach to making health care available to all was inevitable. Attempts toward this end had been made over the years, always with strong opposition by the medical establishment, which labeled them socialized medicine or worse.

Medicare-Medicaid

Finally, in July 1965, with assistance from the by-that-time compliant American Medical Association whose own proposal for an Eldercare Plan contained many of the elements of the bill, Congress passed the act creating Medicare for the elderly and Medicaid for the poor. Quickly signed into law by President Lyndon Johnson as part of his Great Society program, it became effective a year later.

Under it were three essential elements: hospital insurance under Social Security, which became Part A of Medicare; partially subsidized, voluntary insurance, which became Part B; and the federally assisted, state-administered program to assure medical care for the poor, which became Medicaid. Of the two, Medicare was the more easily accepted by hospitals and physicians, with federally mandated standards and, most important to the doctors, permitting charges above what the program reimbursed. Medicaid, on the other hand, left responsibility with each state to decide how extensive its program would be, thus becoming dependent on the individual state's ability or willingness to pay for its people's care.

The hospitals had a year in which to prepare before the act became effective. A major concern to many was an anticipated heavy influx of patients coupled with vastly more paperwork than small hospitals were accustomed to. The first was not seen as a problem at the Addison Gilbert. As Tucker Vye explained in the *Times*: "When I came to Gloucester I was emphatically informed that [this hospital] accepted patients whether they were able to pay or not; that policy has been strictly observed. We have amply cared for our elderly people . . . [and] I do not expect any influx of patients after July 1." He did, however, stress his concern for the administrative problems and the lack of nursing homes to assume the care of patients who, no longer requiring hospitalization, would lose their Medicare eligibility. At least three additional staff members would also be required: a Patient Service Coordinator to ease elderly discharges, a Medicare clerk, and a secretary for the new Utilization Review Committee, which would oversee length of stay and discharge.

Vye was only partially correct in his estimate as to census, but he was on target as to the administrative problems and the effect of too few nursing-home beds. Meeting Medicare reporting and compliance requirements demanded a better accounting system and closer attention to costs. This would result in a more efficient operation after the first few years of adjustment, but the shift from the relatively unregulated old days was not easy. In addition, the problem of older patients unable to find nursing-home beds was to become chronic and will remain so until more such beds can be provided in the Cape Ann area.

Most important of all, the Medicare-Medicaid program eased a major concern of the elderly and the less affluent in assuring them, their hospitals and their physicians that their care would be paid for, if not in full then at least on a basis that would presumably keep all of them solvent. It would inevitably lead to greater federal and state regulatory power over almost all aspects of hospital operation, a development that would become more evident as the 1970s unfolded. It also was to change the health care industry by stimulating the move to investor-owned hospitals, nursing homes and clinics, the formation of health maintenance organizations (HMOs) and the development of home care services.

An immediate effect of Medicare-Medicaid at the AGH was elimination of the Ward Service, which had been a problem for the hospital and its Medical Staff since 1897. With reimbursement available to cover the majority of patients, there was no further need to maintain the wards which for years had provided free beds and free doctors' care. Now all patients were on equal footing, free of the old stigma of being "on the Ward."

With the advent of Medicare-Medicaid, it was the rare family that did not have some form of hospital-medical insurance coverage. Blue Cross-Blue Shield, as administrative manager for the Medicare program, expanded with the additional duties, and the fact of its participation encouraged further enrollment by the general public, to the point where wholly self-pay patients are now rare. Since more of its patients' care was being reimbursed, the hospital's financial problems also eased, and in 1968 and 1969 its operating statements showed more income than expense. Cash flow, however, remained a problem because of slow payments, now not *by* patients but *for* them.

The cause of this was twofold. Blue Cross was part of the problem, as after 1960 it began to permit hospitals to draw funds from it by writing drafts against charges that would then be periodically audited and adjusted. The adjustments seemed always to result in discounts, often well below actual costs, which each hospital must then return.

But the major responsibility for the cash flow problems lay with the federal and state governments, which were frustratingly slow in making payments. As early as October 1966 Vye reported to the Trustees that Medicare, by then covering 35 percent of the patients in the hospital, was forty days behind in its payments, perhaps understandable during the start-up and adjustment period. After it adopted the Blue Cross system of estimated payments with year-end adjustments that problem eased, but, as with Blue Cross, its discounts usually meant yearly refunds by the hospital.

The worst offender was Medicaid. Underfunded and poorly administered by the state, its affairs seemed always to be in what can only be described as a mess, with delays in reimbursement payments causing problems for everyone involved: hospitals, physicians, nursing homes and pharmacies. Hospitals, with the largest billings and relying on steady income to meet payrolls and suppliers' bills, were very hard hit, with many being forced to borrow.

By 1971 the unpaid Medicaid backlog here averaged $125,000 with payments running up to six months behind. Reminiscent of a time believed long since past, at the end of May that year there was only $107.07 cash on hand. By late 1972 the state owed the hospital $225,000 with the situation further complicated by a dispute between the state rate setters and Blue Cross, which delayed payments from that source. The combination of backlogs soon brought the Trustees to the Cape Ann Bank & Trust Company for a $200,000 line of credit. By March 1972, with $100,000 owed Medicare after billing adjustments and $250,000 due from Medicaid, it was necessary once again to sell securities from unrestricted endowment funds. Fiscal 1973 ended with

Medicaid payments overdue by $306,000 and no solution in sight.

Adding insult to injury was the need to purchase some $5,000 worth of National Cash Register (NCR) computer equipment and tapes solely to gain some degree of compatibility with the state's computers in hope of receiving faster payment. The whole situation was nicely summed up by Tucker Vye in the *Annual Report* of 1972:

> *The Commonwealth is unable to find out from the Department of Public Welfare either the total amount due its vendors or even who the vendors are. It seems almost unbelievable that [it] is forcing hospitals and other health suppliers to borrow money to continue their work in serving the public. Everyone involved in the government seems very sympathetic to our plight, but . . . no one has been able to do anything to resolve [it]. . . . The financial picture is not bright.*

Vye's earlier optimism to the contrary, the new law also brought more patients. The Staff Council noted on October 1966 that corridor beds were again in use and urged restraint on the Staff in admitting only the most acute cases. The new Utilization Review Committee placed part of the blame on the administratively necessary days (AND) situation whereby the hospital was obliged to keep patients, mostly elderly, who no longer required the hospital level of care but could not be cared for at home and could not find a vacant nursing-home bed. In 1967 Vye advised the Trustees that the situation was "very serious," with 636 patients having used corridor beds during the previous twelve months and only seventy-nine days that year when the corridors did not double as patient rooms.

Nursing Homes: Partners in Health Care

Nursing homes gained an important role in health care during this period. In their earliest form they had been simple homes for the indigent aged, typified on Cape Ann by the Gilbert Home established under Addison Gilbert's will in 1890 and, to give its seldom-used proper name, the Huntress Home for Old Ladies of Native Birth, then located at 110 Prospect Street. As hospital treatment shifted from long-term stays to confinement only during the acute stages of illness, other facilities opened. These were usually small, privately owned homes for convalescence without true nursing care. There were seven, listed as "Rest Homes," in Gloucester in 1951.

The significant development of this field dates from 1956, when amendments to the Social Security Act offered federal assistance for support of the elderly in nursing homes. It made care available to those previously unable to afford it and allowed those who could not be properly cared for at home to survive in reasonable security. From then on the small rest homes began to give way to the skilled care facilities we know today.

In 1957 there were still twelve of the smaller variety listed in Gloucester. Appearing among them for the first time was one called Cape Ann Nursing Home, located just down the street from the hospital on the old Curtis Greenhouse site. Also listed for the first time that year was the Hospitaller Order of St. John of God at 210 Western Avenue, operated by the Archdiocese of Boston. Rockport had Den Mar Nursing Home, which had begun as a rest home about 1948.

The number of rest homes diminished significantly with stricter government supervision, which followed the establishment of Medicare-Medicaid. The consequent need for better-trained staffs was partially met by a federal/state grant program under which selected hospitals offered six-week courses of instruction for nursing-home aides, an activity in which hospitals were willing participants since it would ease the demand for the too few nurses available. The AGH offered two such courses during 1965 with forty participants, who were then qualified to join nursing-home staffs.

By 1986 there were five facilities listed as Nursing Homes or Rest Homes on Cape Ann. The Gilbert Home had become an attorney's office, the Huntress Home existed in name only as a shelter for the homeless on Emerson Avenue, and the Hospitaller Order had closed some years before. The two leading local homes, Cape Ann (which became Greycliff at Cape Ann in 1982) and Den Mar, have followed a national trend to professional management, which has brought many such establishments under the control of investor-owned chains. A chronic shortage of beds is also leading many hospitals to build and operate them, and perhaps future historians will be able to number Addison Gilbert among them.

The People of the AGH

With the increase in patient load and the need for more sophisticated equipment came an increase in the size and composition of the hospital staff. Such changes meant higher payroll and benefit costs in every department, a trend that was slow to be recognized by those who held to the tradition that hospital work was a privilege of service to be compensated less by money than by good feelings. Change came slowly, but by the close of the 1960s hospital people would be in step with the rest of the working world in expecting and receiving a fair share of that world's rewards.

As the period opened the Administrator's staff listed nine department heads. These had increased to twenty-four by 1973, almost as many as the total number of employees in 1897. Each department was also something of its own fiefdom with its head establishing wage policy, hours, vacation and sick-leave standards for his or her share of the more than 300 employees. It had become a chaotic situation, which the Board tried to remedy in 1970 with the appointment of a Personnel and Wage Committee. When this proved ineffective without professional staff assistance, the first Personnel Director (today called Director of Human Resources) was appointed the next year. With completion of a personnel policies manual two years later, the old, loosely constructed system was gone. In its place was a tighter, more manageable organization free of most of the jealousies and misunderstandings engendered by as many different policies as there were department heads to set them.

In 1948, when Tucker Vye came to "a spic and span hospital if I ever saw one – you couldn't find dirt anywhere," the housekeeping was still being performed by the nurses with the help of "floor maids" and one man, Frank Gagliano, who had done minor maintenance and the heavy floor polishing since the early 1920s. On his retirement in 1957 the first designated "houseman" was appointed as a working foreman with responsibilities as orderly and maintenance assistant. By 1969 the department had grown to the point where it seemed feasible to contract its management out, and the Servicemaster Corporation took over in an arrangement that lasted until 1975, when in-house control was restored.

Maintenance work underwent a similar evolution. Originally among the duties of the boiler-room crew, it assumed separate status when Edward O. Griffin, the hospital's long-time, constantly paged "Mr. Fix-it," joined the staff in 1950. By 1959, when Ed Griffin was given a full-time assistant, the department had doubled in size, and in 1972, with several more people and skills added, it got its first Director, Joseph Huntley. Joe had come first in 1956 as Clerk of the Works on South Wing, returning for Babson Wing and, in 1969, for yet another construction project. He was thoroughly familiar with the hospital plant, and it was an easy transition to a post he held until his retirement in 1975. By that time the Maintenance Department was sufficiently broad-based to render the hospital capable of performing much of its own general repair and renovation work utilizing the skills of a ten-man staff.

The kitchen got its first supervisor in 1948 when Hilda Andrews, with whom Tucker Vye had worked at Winchester, was appointed Dietitian, with additional duties as Administrator's Assistant. Her program for modernization of service and higher food standards culminated in 1965 when she persuaded the Trustees that a dollar per patient day could be saved by contracting the food service out.[1] The subsequent arrangement with Crotty Brothers, hospital and airlines caterers, continued until 1975, following almost total rebuilding of the kitchen complete with new stoves and refrigeration. The kitchen, incidentally, is the only department still operating where it was when Vye came here, having been moved to its present location in 1933 after the boiler house was built.

The Business Office of 1948 had already gone far beyond the day when the Matron and a clerk-bookkeeper kept the accounts in a handwritten ledger, but changes had been slow until 1937, when Robert F. Thompson was appointed Assistant Treasurer to handle purchasing and collections. By 1948 the conscientious Thompson had become a Trustee, Treasurer and general financial manager and was well able to become the new Administrator's chief advisor. The two worked well together until Mr. Thompson's sudden death in December 1967 left a void, which was further complicated a few days later with the death of Bob Thompson's long-time secretary and general office assistant, Miss Hazel Johnson.

By 1956 the hospital had reached the point where hand posting could not handle the complexities of accounting to third-party payors, and the purchase that year of a National Cash Register bookkeeping machine brought it at least to the fringes of the still infant computer age. This machine and its mate, added a few years later, served until 1968, when what the Trustees described as "electronic bookkeeping machines" made the clanking monsters obsolete and ripe for replacement by a new NCR 500 computer. The new machine did not eliminate people, however, and by 1973 the Business Office Staff numbered thirty, directed by a Comptroller and his assistant, an Office Manager, and a Patients' Accounts Supervisor.

The largest and most visible department in any hospital is its nursing service. Their numbers and the essential nature of their function give the nurses considerable weight in setting pay and other standards not only for themselves but, almost by osmosis, for all other employees. The stampede to add hospital beds during the fifties and sixties that made competition for their services acute also increased their influence. The combination of circumstances gave them a new sense of strength, and they took advantage of it.

The shortage began to show at the AGH in 1950, when the nursing staff still numbered only thirty, including supervisors. An increase of $10 per month and the assistance of a recruiting agency eased the situation somewhat, but only temporarily. Another $10 a month plus $35 "maintenance pay" for nurses not living at the Nurses' Residence, plus reduction in hours from forty-eight to forty a week, was hardly more attractive a year later.

Encouraged by the growing militance of their state associations, nurses everywhere were winning similar increases on an almost annual basis. Locally these ranged from $10 to as much as $30 per month, with two in 1965 totaling $39. Each RN increase usually meant an additional smaller one for the growing group of Licensed Practical Nurses (LPNs) who, by 1968, were themselves strong enough to ask and receive 80 percent of whatever level the RNs gained.

The increases kept the hospital competitive but failed to eliminate the nurse shortage, which soon became chronic and a regular topic for mention in Nursing Service annual reports. Although many hospitals were occasionally forced to close floors, that move was never necessary or even possible here and could be avoided by greater use of the LPNs who, on graduation, chose to stay on at their school's hospital. And surely the opportunity to live and work on Cape Ann also helped.

Among the side effects of the shortage was the gradual phasing out of private-duty nursing. Essential in the past when nursing staffs were smaller, private-duty nurses were available for special individual care at the hospital as well as at home. As employees of the patient they served only that person, always ready and in extreme cases sleeping on a cot in the same room. Their presence freed staff nurses to care for the other floor and ward patients, who sometimes were more acutely ill than those employing their own nurses.

By 1956 the fees charged by nurses in the private registry had reached $15 per eight-hour shift, and even the affluent had difficulty accepting the extra expense. Ten years later further increases had made special nursing almost a thing of the past as its practitioners moved on to meet the demands of industrial nursing or to work in doctor's offices. They are rarely seen today, and home care is more often given by visiting nurses.

Nurses were also gaining an increasing sense of profession as, relieved of some of the more routine tasks by the LPNs, the ward or nurses' aides added in 1958, and a growing Housekeeping Department, they began to take on work once done only by physcians. By 1953 qualified nurses, the first here being Edith B. Lord, RN, were allowed to administer intravenous solutions. Twenty years later Medical Staff policy had broadened to permit strictly qualified nurses to do endotracheal intubation "if a physician is not immediately available" and to start and administer blood transfusions in the E.R. and on the floors. In-service training had become standard practice, and every nurse was expected to maintain skills and learn new methods by participating in hospital and outside programs as well as by attendance at clinical sessions of the Medical Staff.

This growing professionalism was also manifest in the care and treatment of patients. No longer totally subservient to the doctors' commands, nurses were becoming participating members of a team, preparing and executing detailed nursing plans covering every aspect of the patient's hospital stay from admission through rehabilitation and treatment to discharge. This upgrading of the nurses's role was universal, but it may well have been expedited here by the appointment of a new Director of Nurses in 1969.

Pauline A. Metras, RN, was one of a new level of nurses with advanced degrees. When she came here each nursing floor was an almost independent entity controlled by its Head Nurse, who assigned shifts and time off, set policy, and only grudgingly allowed "her" nurses to substitute on other units. Miss Metras was quick to perceive that without a centralized, coordinated policy it would be impossible to administer the large staff effectively, and she set out to correct the situation. She knew that what she had to do would not be popular and at one point suggested that she would not survive two years in her position.

She was often outspoken and controversial, at odds with many on the Medical Staff and the nursing staff itself, especially the LPNs, whom she refused to recognize as professionals. But she knew what was needed and she did it, introducing the concepts of modern nursing and nursing management and gaining the respect, if not the affection, of many who earlier decried her methods. The changes she wrought and the concepts she introduced during her brief tenure (true to her prediction, she stayed only until 1971) remained in place and were enlarged upon by her successors, Irene M. Gavin, RN and Rebecca C. Brown, RN, BS, appointed following Mrs. Gavin's retirement in 1978.

Although the nurses were a major factor in the hospital's salary budget, other employees also had to be considered. Traditionally the executive and technical staffs had been given increases individually, though sometimes only if requested, while the blue collar staff was all too often overlooked by the money-conscious Trustees. Significant change in this way of doing things did not appear until a relaxation of the postwar wage-price freezes after 1948.

Small cost of living adjustments in 1948 and 1949 were followed by a general 5 percent increase in 1950. An increase in the minimum wage to 65¢ per hour brought the payroll to what then seemed an astronomical level, at 59.6 percent of the hospital's budget. That was only the beginning as, pressured by rising inflation, the minimum was raised almost every year with more and more work categories being influenced by it. The ripple effect was increasingly felt as lower-paid employees approached those who had previously been at a relatively higher rate, and in 1958 the increase to a $1 minimum had a direct effect on even technical and clerical staff members. The situation was further complicated when the forty-hour work week was mandated for hospital employees, a ruling that included provisions for extra overtime pay for work beyond forty hours.

With the minimum at $1.25 in 1963 the Administrator expressed his concern that $14,135 was thus added to the annual payroll, a figure that appeared miniscule four years later when he reported to the Board a ripple-induced increase of $158,400 for the year and urged authorization to retain a job analyst in an effort to control further staff growth and consequent payroll increases. The reimposition of federal wage-price controls slowed the rise for a short time after 1970, but despite all efforts, the growth of the people factor had brought payroll plus benefits to 65.7 percent of the budget by 1974, with nursing accounting for just over 30 percent.

As hospitals approached parity with commerce in pay levels so too was there an evolution toward some of the other benefits. Health and welfare programs covering employees and their families for illness were becoming popular through group or other insurance plans, and the AGH had formed a Blue Cross group in 1941 to supplement the hospital admission privilege then in effect. The availability of improved Blue Cross coverage removed the need for such free care after 1961 except for the few still spurning group participation, opting instead to take the 40 percent discount applied to their hospital bills. By 1966, with the hospital assuming a large part of the premium cost and with Master Medical coverage in effect, it was the rare employee who did not join the group plan.

Social Security coverage was also slow in coming to nonprofit institutions. Although hospitals could participate on an optional basis, the program was already fifteen years old when the AGH Board authorized its implementation here for all employees if two-thirds of them wished it. A canvas of the staff in November 1950 resulted in an 85 percent acceptance, and the hospital joined the vast majority of American institutions in adding FICA payments to its benefits budget.

Social Security was, however, not much help for many older employees with little vested in it. Too many of them retired only to join the welfare relief rolls, and that troubled Tucker Vye. The Trustees, anxious to hold down expenses and avoid rate increases, were reluctant to consider even the minimal retirement plan being offered by the Massachusetts Hospital Association in 1952. In those days when relatively small local businesses were still the rule in Gloucester, Board thinking did not include what its members saw as a luxury even for their own employees, and, despite his often expressed fear for the public image of the hospital with many of its retirees on welfare, Vye was unsuccessful in changing their position.

He finally persuaded the Board to face the issue in May 1965, and a committee to "report with recommendations" was authorized. This reported back a year later with a plan devised by the American Hospital Association which, including Social Security, would provide 50 percent of a full-time employee's highest five years of salary at a cost estimated at $28,000 annually. Six months of further deliberation led to a vote on December 15, 1966 adopting a plan along those lines, with the First National Bank of Boston as trustee. A final vote the following March funded the plan and appointed a Retirement Committee with Boston actuaries, Warner Watson, Inc., as advisors. It became effective October 1, 1967 — better late than never.

Under its terms the hospital bore the entire cost. Payments on retirement varied with salary level and length of service, and in the two examples cited in the descriptive booklet given all employees that summer, "Your Retirement Income Plan," benefits ranged from $1,200 to $1,908.75 a year plus the individual's Social Security payments. It could be taken in various ways, including payment to an employee's surviving beneficiary, and it covered early retirement due to disability. It was not a large-income program, but it was certainly an improvement over welfare.

The fifties and sixties were also a time when labor unions, encouraged by the Taft-Hartley Act, were growing in strength and militancy. Hospital people had not yet been brought under the collective bargaining umbrella, however, and although they could organize, their affiliation thus meant little. By the early 1960s this was becoming a sore point, especially for nurses, who were the best organized of all health care workers. Their state groups, of which the Massachusetts Nursing Association was typical, joined with others to correct what they considered an unfair discrimination. Their goal was achieved in 1967 with legislation giving the Massachusetts Labor Relations Commission jurisdiction over nurses, and with it the right of collective bargaining.

The new law covered only nurses. Other hospital workers, lacking similar clout, would have to wait a few more years. Nurses, especially in the large urban hospitals, began to avail themselves of the opportunity, with most of them designating the MNA as their collective bargaining agent. In the smaller hospitals the trend to regular and relatively generous wage increases along with increasing benefits minimized the effectiveness of organization, and for the most part the status quo was maintained, at least among RNs.

LPNs, among them those at the AGH, saw the situation differently. They were a fairly large group here by the late 1960s, comprising half the full-time nursing staff and with a sizable group also of part-timers. Their pay remained some 20 percent lower than that of the RNs, but the real issue lay in a sense of discrimination against them by Director Metras. The LPNs, some of whom capably served as charge nurses in a pinch, resented being considered little more than nurses' aides.

This resentment led to action, and at a special meeting on December 19, 1969 the Trustees received notice from the state Labor Relations Commission of a petition for an election to certify the Massachusetts LPN Association as collective bargaining agent for the local group. The Board, recognizing the need for expert counsel, retained the services of the MHA Labor Relations program. The election that spring favored the LPNA by a 3 to 1 margin, and on August 4, 1970 the first negotiated contract was accepted by the Trustees.

It was described by the MHA negotiator as "honorable, middle of the road and workable," and, indeed, both parties lived with it in reasonable comfort through its first few years. With coverage of wages and conditions such as vacation, sick leave and other benefits, it approximated the policies already in effect for all employees but added a formal grievance procedure and a no-strike clause. One-year renewals through 1974 were reached usually with little more than normal across-the-table bickering although general wage adjustments for all employees were made necessary by a substantial wage increase in 1973.

The Schools

Miss Howlett's first class at the new School for Nursing Attendants graduated six of its eight students in October 1949 after a difficult year during which she closed out one school and opened another with too few students (see Chapter 5). Recruiting in those first few years remained a problem despite the assistance of a part-time staffer whose assignment was to "call on schools in neighboring cities at a charge of $5 and travelling expenses for each visit."

It was 1953 before the school's continued existence could be assured. By then, in response to a new state regulation, its name had been changed to the Addison Gilbert Hospital School for Practical Nurses. Its aim, according to the attractive catalogue issued that year, was "to present to the student a well organized program of study in the art of nursing, that she may learn to give skilled nursing care to the patient in the hospital under the supervision of the professional nurse and to the mild or chronically ill patient in the home under the supervision of the physician."

The course of study covered fifteen months and cost $60 for four uniforms plus $7 for textbooks. Each student received a stipend of $15 monthly after the first three months and was enrolled in the hospital's medical-benefit pro-

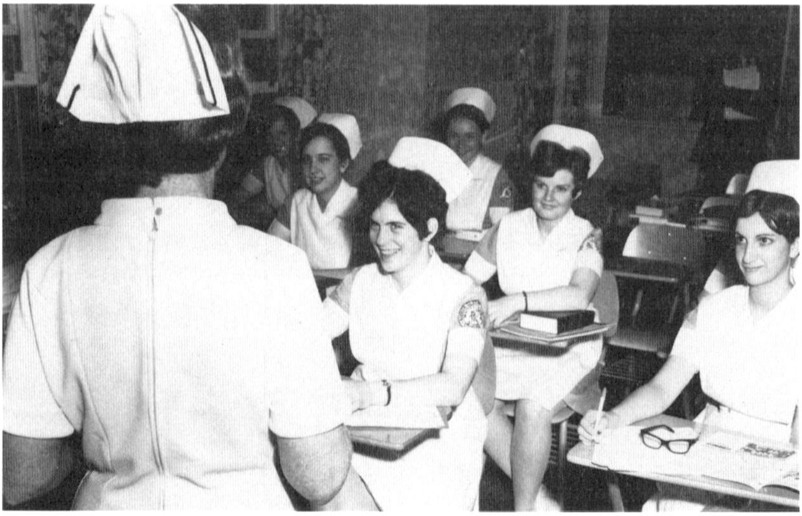

The AGH School for Practical Nurses replaced the school for RNs in 1949. Between then and 1978 when more rigorous requirements forced its closing it graduated 412 nurses.

gram. In addition to classroom instruction students were expected to learn by working on the floors, an assignment that included two months of night duty "to help the student gain an insight of the individual patient's needs during the night," which some construed as a way to add coverage during a traditionally unpopular work shift.

The school received general oversight from a committee appointed by the Trustees. This was broad-based with ten members – a Trustee, a doctor, a public health nurse, the high school principal and two residents of the community, one knowledgeable of nursing and the other "interested in community affairs" – and ex officio, the Administrator, the School Director and the presidents of the Auxiliary and Nurses' Alumnae Association. As a standing committee of the Board, its members were appointed each year.

Fifteen students enrolled for the class entering in September 1953, and this record class became something of a bellwether for those which followed. It was the first to be "capped," a ceremony that endured throughout the school's existence. It was this class which formed the LPN Alumnae Association a year later, and it was that organization which added the distinction of blue bands on the graduates' caps. By the school's 10th anniversary year, with a new high of fourteen graduates in its Class of 1958, it had awarded diplomas to ninety-seven young women and two young men, Brother John and Brother Gerald of the Hospitaller Order of St. John of God.

Success appeared even more assured with eighteen enrollees in 1959 and with applications running fifty or more each year. Jean Deming, RN had been named its first full-time Director, enabling Miss Howlett to devote all her energy to direction of the nursing service. The curriculum was expanded by adding a week of work experience in the newly opened pediatric offices of Dr. Hamer Lacey to give students a better understanding of children's problems. Between 1959 and 1964 it graduated seventy-eight more nurses, many of whom stayed on to augment the chronically short-handed AGH staff. For the publicity-conscious hospital, its commencement exercises at the West Parish School during the 1950s and 1960s were always good for a story and a picture or two in the newspaper.

A significant change took place in the fall of 1964 when H. Claire Chaffee, RN, BS was appointed to replace Miss Deming. Mrs. Chaffee brought a new dimension to the school, along with much nursing and teaching experience. Hers was a hands-on administration that involved her deeply and enthusiastically in every aspect of the school's life. Diligent study and good behavior by "her girls" was of great personal concern, and her enthusiasm transformed ceremonial occasions — opening day, capping and graduation — into great events.

Despite increasing its $300 tuition of 1966 to $500 by 1973, the school grew in strength and prestige under her guidance. Her first change was to upgrade the curriculum to meet the standards of the Massachusetts Board of Registry of Nurses. The course of study was further enhanced in January 1968 when the Trustees voted to affiliate with the Associate Nurse Degree Program of the relatively new North Shore Community College for some of the work. A change to a twelve-month course in 1971 meant that, except for periods of floor training, far more time was required for classroom instruction, with almost none left for floor duty.

Applications went from 130 in 1966 to 223 in 1973, and classes were filled to capacity, with twenty to twenty-four students enrolled each year. Commencements, held at Fuller School after 1971, were well attended by families and friends of the fifteen to twenty who made it through each year. The AGH school, one of some forty in Massachusetts in 1970, was doing well.

But it was not to last. By 1976 the shortage of nurses had become an oversupply, and with hospitals almost universally experiencing severe financial pain, most were reviewing their schools as a possibly avoidable drain on funds. The first hint of change at AGH was the August 1977 decision to close the dormitory. Only four of the twenty-two students that year had elected to live there after the Board, recognizing that many students were married or desired the freedom of independent living, made dormitory residence optional.

Three months later, on October 18, 1977, a more drastic decision was made, one Board member dissenting, to terminate the school after the eight-member Class of 1978 graduated. The AGH was then one of only three hospitals in Massachusetts still operating a practical-nurse training program, and, with tuition still $500 but operating expenses some five times that per student, training people for whom there might not be employment was simply not practical. As with Registered Nurse training thirty years earlier, the LPNs' schooling was being better done at the college level with such courses readily available at the nearby North Shore Community College. All in all, despite a lingering sentiment against the move, closing, was the only possible decision.

During its existence the LPN School had graduated 412 students, 234 of them during Claire Chaffee's tenure as Director. Among them were many Cape Ann residents and several young men. Many had joined the hospital's nursing staff, and several had gone on to gain the RN degree. But in the summer of 1978 a tradition of eighty years in which the hospital can take justifiable pride came to a close.

The smaller school for X-ray technicians had its genesis in an exchange arrangement with Winchester Hospital initiated in 1949. The plan was for students to train for three months at each hospital, a course giving them experience on a wider range of equipment than either could offer alone. The idea was a good one, but problems with transportation and living arrangements made it impractical to continue after the first trial year.

The school idea was revived in 1957 to meet a growing need for skilled technicians when Dr. Wells and Dr. Vance organized a one-year course to operate entirely within the hospital. Under their guidance and directed by Chief Technician Helen Page, it soon earned accreditation by the American Registry of X-ray Technicians, a step that allowed it to award the Registered Technician degree to its first three graduates. Among these was Mrs. Billie Jensen of Gloucester, who then joined the AGH department and, two years later, herself became the school's Director in addition to her other duties as a working technician.

In 1961, many hospitals having established their own courses, the AMA and the American College of Radiologists (ACR) realized the need for stricter criteria. Their new standards mandated a two-year course with four hours of classroom instruction weekly at an accredited college during the second year, a requirement met here by affiliation with Northeastern University in Boston. Although the small department at AGH could accommodate only three students, it met all standards and was regularly accredited after each biennial survey by the ACR.

The small school operated quietly and largely unknown, except for its annual graduation story and picture in the *Times*. But small though it was, operating under what the Administrator's report for 1965 called Mrs. Jensen's "continued enthusiasm and teaching skills," it performed its mission well. The outside college affiliation was transferred to North Shore Community College in 1969, permitting an increase in the number of classroom hours, and its well-trained graduates were eagerly sought by this and other hospitals.

It did, however, suffer from a lack of diverse equipment in the still cramped Radiology Department, and as the ACR requirements became stricter, it was becoming difficult for any small hospital school to meet accreditation standards. A few years later the AGH would house a highly modern well-equipped department, but that expectation was no help in December 1975 when, with no other alternative, the Board voted to close the school. Its final class graduated in June 1976, adding three more Registered Radiological Technicians to the almost sixty young men and women who had learned their profession here.

Deficit Operations, Giving and Public Relations

Expansion of the entire national hospital system remained government policy throughout the 1960s. Improving but costly technology, higher wages and the burden of capital expenditure faced by all hospitals were being further complicated by the economic inflation that had followed World War II and continued to worsen. Since as expenses increase so must income, hospitals, no different from any other business in that respect, could fill the gap only by charging more for their product. But such increases by hospitals everywhere soon began to attract a closer scrutiny of health care costs by government regulators.

At AGH the two new wings offered an opportunity for slightly higher room rates. When South Wing opened in 1958 its beds were set $2 higher than their equivalents in what was being called "Old Hospital." The rate trend begun earlier continued with increases put in place each year, first $1 or $2 per bed, then, after 1966, going up $5 every year. By 1969, when the Trustees recorded praise for the Administrator in maintaining rates "still much lower than surrounding hospitals," a bed in South Wing cost $53 to $57, with other units scaling down from there.

Such rates were still too low in August 1970 when the Board was told that wage and benefit increases would add $300,000 a year to the expense budget and inflate costs per patient day by at least $10. An agony session at the meeting the next month resulted in the largest increase to that time at $15

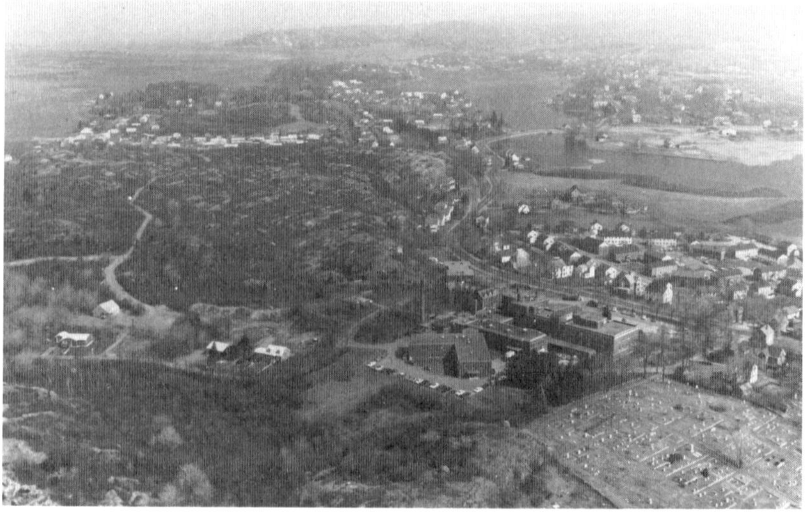

Aerial view of AGH in the 1960s looking north across Riverdale and Wheeler's Point to Annisquam and Ipswich Bay.

per bed, and by October 1973, with a third new wing open, bed rates ranged from $77 for a multibed room in Pediatrics to $94 for a private room in the newest wing. The Trustees could presumably draw consolation from the fact that AGH was not among those area hospitals forced to roll back 1972 increases that exceeded the federal wage-price freeze then in effect, but they also were becoming aware of the increasing vigilance of the newly established Massachusetts Rate Setting Commission. They could only wonder where it would all end, and when.

The other road to meeting deficits called for a return to annual gift seeking once the Babson Wing campaign was closed, now, however, with a different approach. It had become evident during the last annual drive in 1959, and particularly after the 1960—61 capital effort, that everyone had had enough of the organizing, the visiting and the other paraphernalia of the old-style campaign method.

Will, Folsom & Smith's new AGH contact, Ed Call, had proposed in September 1961 a combination of personal solicitation coupled with a continuing follow-up by mail. He also pointed out that larger hospitals were formalizing their gift-seeking programs by establishing development offices, suggesting that even a small institution could profit by such an addition. The idea appealed to the Board which appointed one of its members,

Lawrence J. Hart, the first salaried Director of Development.

Larry Hart had been manager of the Gloucester Chamber of Commerce and was then serving as Executive Director of the Gloucester Fisheries Association. He had the advantage of being well known in the business community, although he had no fund-raising experience except as a Trustee who pitched in with the others when needed. Brought in first to clean up the outstanding pledges from the 1960 campaign, he used the time also to organize his office, and was ready when the Board decided early the next year to try the new approach.

The responsibility was placed on the Trustees to call on selected prospects, with others to be approached in a direct mail appeal. All were to be asked to make a current gift and to indicate future continuing support in a "Statement of Intent," so that once the first year's work was complete all donors could be followed up annually by mail by the new department. The 1963 goal of $84,327 matched the anticipated operating deficit; Will, Folsom & Smith sent Ed Call to guide the first-year trial; Carroll Steele again took the chairmanship and the effort got under way.

Twenty Trustees plus ten other Corporators did the visiting. The two-person Development Office, assisted by twenty-three volunteers from the Gloucester Girl Scouts, handled the mailing of 10,000 letters. When it was over President Webber could say in his annual report that "the results of the first year's experiment which raised over $70,000 gave the Trustees encouragement to continue the program for ensuing years."

Continue it they did, relying entirely on mail each year thereafter, except for special efforts and capital campaigns. Concern over asking for help with deficit funding when operations began to show black instead of red ink led to use of annual giving for equipment acquisition, and whatever the purpose, the people of Cape Ann continued to respond generously in support of their hospital. In 1968, the last year before another capital campaign, a high of almost $85,000 was reached, and during the later 1970s results over $100,000 a year were not uncommon. The mail only, year-round method had proved its value and everyone was pleased. After all, the Development Office was doing all the work.

The Trustees had also developed an increased sense of the value of maintaining good relationships with the people of the communities in the hospital's service area. Fund-raising activities had perhaps been most influential in this public communication, and the Board had come to recognize also the need to stay in touch between campaigns. The little things that happened were in many ways just as newsworthy as the big events and could be used in the cultivation of public or community relations.

It helped that Cape Ann had but one daily newspaper. It surely helped also that the paper's editor, Roy L. Parsons, had been a member of the hospital's Board from 1946 through 1954 and that, after his retirement therefrom to become a paid hospital consultant, he had been invited to continue to attend and report on Board meetings. After his death in September 1969, the practice was carried on by Paul B. Kenyon, who replaced him as editor. This strange but effective relationship continued until 1971, when it ended by mutual consent of the parties.

Publicity was initially sought as far back as 1906. The quest for it was not active except for special events, however, until 1954 when Mr. Vye proposed "weekly publicity in the *Times* to be written by a professional and edited by himself." Allotted $500 to spend on the idea, he approached editor Parsons, whose service as Trustee had made him knowledgeable concerning hospital affairs. The resulting series opened in February 1956, coinciding with the start of the Building Fund campaign, and ran in fifteen long articles during the next three months.

Planned, according to the editor's note accompanying the first story, "so that readers may become more fully acquainted with the Addison Gilbert Hospital, the series will tell the hospital's story [and] will tour departments and present the men and women responsible for the hospital's development." The idea was revived for a further Parsons series which ran sporadically from 1959 to 1962, by which time planned series were no longer needed as almost any happening, large or small, at the hospital was good for a story.

From New Year and Leap Year babies to the annual "Christmas at the Hospital" story, the coverage was constant. A guest "Lookout" column[2] by Henry Bollman, ceramicist, film producer, musician, writer and summer visitor converted to Cape Ann residency, appeared annually from 1953 until his death in 1962. The Bollman "Lookouts" always had something in praise of the hospital he came to know well as a patient, and they somehow always coincided with whatever fund drive was under way at the time. Even such mundane occurrences as National Hospital Day each year prompted a *Times* story or editorial, and any Auxiliary activity was covered complete with photographs.

Other than through the newspaper, however, there was almost no printed PR from the hospital until 1957. The *Annual Report* had been revived in 1948 after a lapse of a dozen years, but with its limited circulation it was valuable chiefly as a record of major events and statistics. It and fund-raising pamphlets were the only in-house publications during the first sixty years.

The Administrator was anxious to have an informative publication from the hospital on a regular basis, and Roy Parsons' expertise was again sought to help meet this desire. The result was the first *Newsletter*, which began as a modest 7-by-9-inch four-page general mailing piece for distribution to a list based on the donor and prospect list from the 1956 campaign. The first issue, dated January 1957, was followed by two more that year, each containing a plea by Carroll Steele to laggard pledge payers along with news of hospital events and people.

Vol. II, No. 1 in February 1958 graduated to the more standard 8½-by-11-inch format followed thereafter, which permitted more news and pictures. The next year saw a more sprightly masthead, and three years later the December 1962 issue blossomed forth on colored paper. An expanding mailing list, created in an effort to maintain a firm base of gift support, sent each issue to what the combined Development and Public Relations Department hoped were 5,000 readers.

Paul Kenyon took over as advisor following Roy Parsons' death and assisted through Vol. XIV, No. 1, Spring 1971, an issue that carried the news of Larry Hart's death. Without Larry the impetus for further publication was gone, and that issue, also bearing a photo of another new wing in process of construction, was the last of the series until 1973, when *Newsletter* was revived as a completely in-house project.

The Auxiliary

The growth period of the 1950s and 1960s had a comparable effect on the Auxiliary as, encouraged by the Administrator's appreciative interest, its members brought new vigor to their efforts. By 1956 its membership base had expanded from the small, cliquish group Vye discerned on his arrival to include women from all over Cape Ann. Equally important to its development, the increased emphasis on fund raising and equipment procurement was giving it a renewed sense of purpose and transforming its earlier social club image to one of businesslike activity.

The projects it assumed took money — and money its members raised! They held auctions and rummage sales. They sponsored lectures and held theatre parties at the flourishing Bass Rocks Theatre. The tradition of annual dinner dances and the Easter Monday Bridge was born during those years. In 1954 and 1955 they outdid themselves in staging their own extravaganza, a local talent musical which they felicitously called "Cape Anntics." As it entered its own new era, the Auxiliary was becoming very effective in fulfilling its stated purpose.

Its pledge of $15,000 to the 1956 Building Fund had been designated for the Coffee Shop planned for the elevator side of the entry corridor to Prentiss House. Swallowing their disappointment at losing it in the change of plans, the women completed their pledge in 1959, and, with $1,000 remaining in their treasury, they promptly made a first payment on a new $15,000 commitment to the Babson Wing Program. Again they selected the Coffee Shop, this time slated for the front lobby area. This second pledge was completed with the presentation of a final check for $5,000 by a jubilant Auxiliary President Kay (Mrs. Carroll K.) Steele during the hospital's 1962 Annual Meeting.

Other projects followed in rapid succession. The Longan Room and the Date Room in the Nurses' Residence required $4,000 in 1964 for renovation. Upgrading the thirty-year-old Prentiss House rooms needed some $11,000 between 1964 and 1966, and between 1965 and 1969 they also gave a portable X-ray, a film processor and the cardiac crash cart, all totaling another $24,000. And in 1969, with another Building Fund underway, they accepted the challenge of a pledge for $100,000.

During all this the ladies continued to supply most of the hospital's linen requirements. This combined purchases with labor, since the task also included cutting and sewing the "johnnies" and other items. It had been a long-standing obligation that they took seriously — so seriously, in fact, that Theresa (Mrs. Harold) Maddocks always took material to Florida each winter and brought back a good supply of finished johnnies in the spring. As with so many other traditions, unfortunately, this labor of love succumbed to practicality in 1966 under a Medicare-induced accounting change that made it inadvisable for the hospital to accept linen or other such in-kind gifts. Lovingly offered labor was replaced by a more mundane cash gift of $2,000 annually for purchase of factory-finished linen goods.

Increased funding activity required more than just the social events of the past, and that need brought a more pragmatic approach. Sensing the appeal of television, for example, the women proposed supplying sets to patients, and in 1954 the Trustees authorized them to install 25¢ per hour coin-operated sets in private rooms. This first small business, with sets supplied until 1961 on a loan basis by Trustee Arnold Morton, brought in $500 to $1,000 each year. After Wells TV Service took over the operation in 1961, when all rooms were equipped, the Auxiliary continued to manage it, averaging some $1,500 from it annually by 1973.

The Gift Shop, one of the jewels in the Auxiliary's collection of money-makers, also had its start in the early 1950s. It began small when in February 1954 Mrs. Elmer W. Babson gave the first Hostess Cart in memory of her husband. Pushed to all nursing units each afternoon by High School Girls' Club volunteers, this proved so successful with its supply of candies, stationery and small comfort items that three months later a fixed display

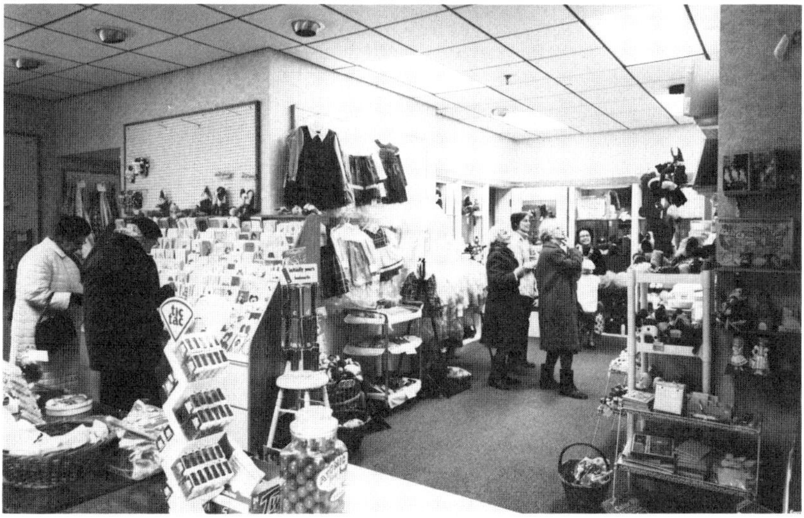

The Gift Shop, operated since 1954 by Auxiliary volunteers, grew steadily and by 1977 occupied new space in the Washington Street lobby. Long-time manager Vi Souza is in the background at the extreme right. The long-dreamed-of Coffee Shop which opened in 1961 was equally successful.

case was installed in the front lobby. As the Auxiliary President reported that year, "the enterprise was dignified with the name Gift Shop in May" and was staffed by members, with the juniors continuing to push the cart.

The 1960 renovations provided a real shop to replace the lobby display case and inspired a level of activity resulting in a steady growth of profits. The new shop was an immediate success under its first volunteer manager Eleanor (Mrs. Robert J.) Harris. It required a larger corps of workers, some of whom, teachers or office or store employees by day, came evenings to help out. When Mrs. Harris became Auxiliary President in 1966, two years prior to her untimely death, her place was taken by Vivian Souza, whose firm hand and determined resolve managed the shop for the next nineteen years.

"Vi" Souza brought the shop into the five-figure annual profit range during her first four years, and before she retired in 1986 had turned in just over $230,000 in small increments proudly presented at each annual meeting of the Auxiliary. Under this diminutive and feisty lady the Gift Shop became a place to go for a wide range of merchandise, which expanded even more after the shop's move to larger quarters across the lobby in 1977.

The long-dreamed-of Coffee Shop opened just before Christmas in 1961. Like the Gift Shop, it relied on a large corps of willing volunteers during its day and evening hours and, again through the efforts of Kay Steele and the Business and Professional Women's Club, its evening hours were staffed by "working gals," as Mrs. Steele called them. In its first full year it turned in $2,000 adding more each year until ten years later it was netting $10,000 and more annually.

It soon found it necessary to employ a manager to prepare the muffins and daily luncheon specials which, along with "the best and cheapest cup of coffee in town," made it a favorite gathering place for hospital employees, visitors and not a few Main Street businessmen. And, as with the Gift Shop and all other moneymaking projects, all its profits were dedicated for use in funding its hospital support.

A wide variety of special events continued to augment funds to assist the hospital. The first Tour of Homes was conducted in 1958, a Fashion Show first sponsored in 1961 became a regular and popular event, and the annual Dinner Dance was always good for a Bill Cahill story in the *Times*, complete with a page of pictures. The Christmas in October fair was established in 1962, first as an adjunct to the Gift Shop but over the years expanding as a successful two-day crafts and ethnic foods bazaar netting over $8,000 in its best years. The imaginative ladies viewed any project with the prospect of raising money as grist for their mill, and most of the ventures had long runs. Some, such as Christmas cards in 1967 or the cookbook of 1973, were one-time efforts.

Not all its activities were designed to raise money. The Patients' Library, funded by the Susan B. Tracy Fund with the donor's approval, was opened in 1951. Counseled during its first years by Sawyer Library personnel, it proved a popular feature among hospital staff as well as patients, who could select from a wide variety of reading material brought to their bedsides on a wheeled book rack by Auxiliary volunteers three times a week. Today, with fewer patients and shorter stays, its rounds are reduced to no more than one a week, and its many books are seldom read.

The Anniversary Quilt project was a fundless venture of another sort, inspired by the 1973 celebration of Gloucester's 350th Anniversary and the Auxiliary's desire to participate therein. Under President Janis D. (Mrs. Michael) Stelluto and project director Bea Allen Dyer, thirty-five women, none of whom had ever made a quilt but were blessed with artistic imaginations, each volunteered to design and execute her own twelve-inch square depicting a Gloucester/Cape Ann scene or historic event. Six months of labor brought forth a full-sized quilting masterpiece, an artistic triumph and not for sale despite generous offers made each time it was displayed. After its anniversary year of public exhibit it came home to the hospital to be hung, framed and with each square identified, in the Washington Street lobby.

The many adult volunteers who comprised the heart and soul of the Auxiliary were augmented by a smaller group of Junior Volunteers of high-school age. Their program had its start in 1954 when thirty-four members of the Gloucester High School Girls Club signed up to serve one day each week as hospital aides. First identified by cherry-colored smocks, the juniors soon adopted the red-and-white striped uniform from which comes the cognomen "Candy Stripers."

The junior group soon grew to more than fifty, and its brightly uniformed, enthusiastically youthful members have been welcome additions among patients and staff alike ever since. Although perhaps not as popular an activity among young people today, many girls and boys gained their first exposure to voluntary service as they performed various chores — delivering mail and flowers; playing with and amusing pediatric patients; feeding, reading to or simply offering companionship to other patients; and sometimes pushing the book cart as they once did the gift wagon. As with their adult counterparts, the chief reward is in the knowledge that they're helping where they are needed.

There is, however, some tangible reward for both groups. Since 1978 a scholarship has been awarded by the Auxiliary each year to an outstanding Candy Striper, and the custom of Volunteer Recognition Teas actually began as a way of thanking juniors in 1957. The teas, continued each year since, were expanded in 1961 under the presidency of Marjorie O. Ross to recognize adult members, and remain an annual event featuring the presentation of pins based on hours served. The number of those hours over the years given by volunteers is enormous and, like the love with which they are offered, beyond count.

Kay Steele described it well in her recapitulation of the Auxiliary's history. "In summing up the contribution of the Women's Auxiliary it is clearly evident that behind every successful man there stands a woman — in this case, a great many women."

Miscellany: The Little Things Also Count

Perhaps not so little in the opinion of the Administrator and the staff members who had to prepare for them were the hospital accreditation surveys. Although always worth a brief mention in the newspaper, except for the fact that the community was again assured that its hospital was performing its mission properly, they held significance chiefly for the Administrator, the Trustees, the Medical Staff and the heads of the various departments. Their approach always loomed large and everyone prepared for them carefully, anticipating them with considerable anxiety and breathing a sigh of relief when they were over.

First carried out here in 1933, when the American College of Surgeons added hospitals of fewer than a hundred beds to its list, the early surveys were pointed primarily at Medical Staffs. Then as now, they were voluntary in the sense that a hospital can operate without undergoing them, but hospital leaders are also acutely aware of the value of the phrase "accredited by" in the eyes of licensing and other authorities. It is the rare hospital that doesn't offer itself for these periodic scrutinies.

By 1949 when the ACS added what it called the Fundamental Principles and a point-scoring system to its criteria for approval, the entire hospital was under examination. About 4,000 of the nation's hospitals were being surveyed each year, with 70 percent scoring above the 70 points required for full approval and 10 percent with 60 to 69 points being provisionally approved and due for a follow-up survey the next year. A score below 60 indicated something seriously wrong with that hospital. On that basis things can be said to have been satisfactory at the AGH from 1933 through 1952 since, with the single exception of a provisional approval because of the Medical Staff problems of 1938, the hospital never received less than full accreditation.

In 1953 the survey responsibility was taken over by the Joint Commission on Accreditation of Hospitals (JCAH), established cooperatively by the ACS, the American Medical Association and the American Hospital Association. Administered by the AHA, its survey teams — a physician, a hospital administrator and, after 1972, a nurse — were stricter and more searching than even the ACS had been. Nothing was too insignificant for their probing eyes as administrators, trustees, medical staffs, nurses, recordkeepers at all levels. All the ancillary services — literally everything except fund raising and public relations — came under intense study during two tension-filled days. Significantly, under JCAH in 1954 only 2,920 of the nation's 7,500 hospitals gained fully approved ranking.

Between 1954 and 1973 the AGH was surveyed ten times, always successfully and four times for the maximum three-year approval. One-year accreditation was given twice, once in 1968, when the Medical Staff came under criticism for inadequate documentation of its subcommittee work, and again in 1969 because of poor Trustee attendance at Board meetings, lack of annual peer review before Medical Staff reappointments, and a lack of sprinklers in the North Wing, all items which had been suggested previously and all of which were promptly corrected. By 1970, with two years then the maximum accredited term, conditions again merited full approval, a happy conclusion repeated in 1972 and, except for one more one-year approval in 1976, continuing since.

Apprehensive though he may be during the process, any hospital administrator is grateful for it, finding it a good example of the belief that the best expert is an outside expert. Trustees may sometimes have reservations when their administrator advises something, but presented by an outsider, the advice magically becomes acceptable. This is particularly true where JCAH is concerned, since the mere threat of loss of standing casts a dark shadow.

Medical staffs feel its sting in a similar fashion. As Tucker Vye has described it: "[The doctors] didn't want to sit there and have a doctor from the Midwest say, 'Well, you boys are kind of behind the times here – we always thought the East was tops in medical care, but I find this, this and this – what is the matter with you fellows?'" And no matter who the team is talking to, it is always the things needing correction that are stressed. Only rarely is commendation offered for the things that are right, but, after all, doing things right is only what is expected – so why mention it?

Much more in the public consciousness are the things it sees every day. An example of this can be found in the entrance to the old original building on Washington Street, which until 1983 was the hospital's main entrance. There was the lobby with the switchboard/reception desk and, after 1960, the Gift and Coffee shops. With its outside granite steps, however, it had always been a problem, especially in winter when ice and snow created an extra hazard.

Construction of a vestibule and, later, Roger Babson's banisters had helped, but as long as the steps were outdoors the problem would be there. Plans for a portico shelter proposed in 1966 were shelved because of lack of funds, and the matter lay dormant until, in August 1971, Trustee C. Richard Clark suggested that $16,500 remaining from a series of grants by the Sarah G. McCarthy Foundation might be used for such a project. When Mr. Clark, who was also a trustee of the several family foundations established by John A. McCarthy, a Peabody resident with a summer place off Concord Street, advised that $25,000 more from the Foundation would be available, it was easy to vote to commission yet another set of plans from Ritchie Associates.

The foundation announced a second $25,000 grant in March the following year, and by June Ritchie's plans were ready to go to bid. When all bids proved too high the Foundation came forward again with $15,000 more, and the plans were redrawn to reduce the cost. Then, with a bid of just over $70,000 by Feldman Construction Company of Rockport, the job was feasible and the portico was built.

The only condition attached to the grants called for dedicating the new entrance to the memory of Mr. McCarthy's sisters, Sarah, Annie and Frances. The plaque so designating it was placed in an attractive ground level lobby opening onto a classic portico for the convenience of automobile passengers. Inside, carpeted stairs replaced the old granite steps, with two massive planters, a pair of leather-covered sofas, and nicely draped windows completing the decor. Although a few years later the main entrance shifted to the rear of the hospital, at least, after more than seventy-five years, "those damned steps" were finally gone.

Another gift project, the Hammond Deck atop Prentiss House, was facing obsolescence. When the third floor, housing the children's and adult wards, went out of service with the opening of South Wing, the deck lost much of its utility. The roof beneath it was almost twenty-five years old and beginning to show signs of disrepair – actually "severe rot," as reported by the House and Grounds Committee in 1959. Although repaired during the Babson Wing construction, it was never made really tight and continued to be a problem.

The Board's reluctance to abandon the deck ended abruptly on the morning of May 11, 1964 when sparks from the boiler house chimney ignited the deck planking, burning through it and into the roof tar before the fire was noticed. The hospital staff, well drilled for fire emergencies, had it under control when the Fire Department arrived to finish the job and praise the employees for the calm manner in which they had handled the first real fire since one in the laundry in 1928. The fire spelled the demise of the deck, which was not replaced after the main roof was rebuilt. The deckhouse itself remained in place but was used only for storage until its general disrepair and disuse resulted in its total removal some twenty years later.

It is essential that hospitals be assured of a constant supply of electric power. The first auxiliary generator was installed here in 1942, but, too small, it was replaced by a 10KW unit in 1948. Four years later this also was judged too small, and the gasoline-powered giant that replaced it demonstrated the value of preparation in 1954 when twin hurricanes, Carol and Edna, forced it to fifteen hours of continuous operation.

A shift to natural gas fueling came in 1958 when twin generators producing 200KW were installed at a cost of about $20,000. These proved their worth in every power outage and, in the summer of 1964, operated steadily for almost three days when lightning destroyed the hospital's underground feeder cable. Even the great Northeast blackout in November 1965 did not darken the hospital nor did a series of severe winter storms in 1968 and 1969. These generators and their successors have kept the hospital a bright oasis during crises that have left the rest of the community in cold and darkness.

Communication within the hospital, calling the nurse or locating a needed doctor, is also among the less obvious things essential to efficiency. Electric call bells were first installed in patients' rooms in 1903, a system which served until 1926 when the Maternity Wing was equipped with a flip-tag annunciator system. It was modernized in 1940 and served until replaced in 1958 by the current room-to-nursing-station voice-call system first installed in South Wing. After July 1953, when the first audiopaging equipment was installed, it was never again necessary to locate a wandering doctor by telephone within the hospital.

Another communications addition was put in place in January 1953 when a direct telephone line from Rockport was installed so Sandy Bay's people could, by responding "3232" to their local operator's "number, please," reach their hospital without paying for a toll call. The hospital itself switched to an in-house dial telephone system in 1958, installing its first ninety-line PBX switchboard in the front lobby almost four years before the rest of Cape Ann changed over to the dial telephone.

No history of medicine on Cape Ann would be complete without mention of the great water scare of 1961. This erupted in early September that year with release of a report by the Massachusetts Department of Public Health citing an "undesirably high count of bacteria, characteristic of pollution" in Gloucester's water and warning of the possibility of typhoid, cholera and dysentery. The news spread quickly throughout the city, growing worse with each telling. Dr. Lundberg, Chairman of the Board of Health at the time, counseled calm pending further study and stated that there was "no evidence of bacteria that would make anyone sick." But people were advised to boil drinking and cooking water, just in case.

The *Times* reported the story in great detail. For several days its front page described developments in headlines and stories — "City Supply Polluted," "Problem Closes Schools," "Big Spurt in Sales of Beer, Tonic, Bottled Water," "Rockport Offers Pure Water," "Free Water from Milk Company" (Whiting's Dairy), "Thanks to National Guard" (which trucked water in), "Sea Gulls Get the Blame" — to the exclusion of almost everything else.

Rumor and headlines created a situation close to panic, prompting Dr. Lundberg to criticize the state for not advising city officials when the problem was first noted in late August. The hospital's Medical Staff joined him in excoriating the state for the alarming nature of its report and the ensuing publicity in voting to contact the Grievance Committee of the Massachusetts Medical Society and the State Commissioner of Public Health to voice their concern at the way the matter had been handled.

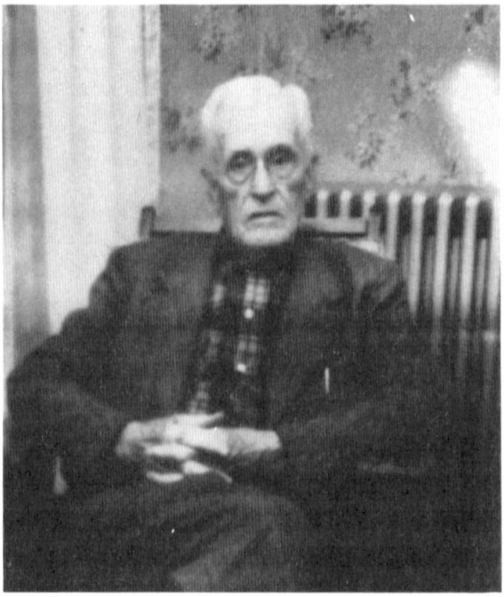

Dr. Scott Mooring detested being photographed. This snapshot, showing an older and more mellow man in retirement about 1960, was permitted an old friend.

The schools reopened September 15. Four days later the *Times* headlined, "Our Water Is Declared Pure By State." The great water scare was over with disagreement among state officials as to its nature and cause, although seagull droppings together with drought-induced low water at Haskell's Pond were offered as a possibility. The bacteria found were determined to have indeed been harmless and not the result of sewage or other manmade pollution. It had been a "tempest in a teapot" from which, nonetheless, came some good. The city embarked on steps to increase its water supply beyond the inadequate Dyke's Meadow reservoir, Haskell's Pond and other scattered sources.

During another dry summer a few years later the hospital itself tried to find a source of water on its grounds. City water had long been blamed for inducing corrosion in boiler and air-conditioning equipment, and the shortage simply emphasized the need for a more dependable supply. Test drillings were made during the summer of 1966, and, although water was found, so was ledge and a nonpermeable sand layer affecting both quality and quantity of the product. The project was abandoned at seventy feet, and the hospital has continued to rely on city water ever since.

The long and distinguished (albeit more than somewhat controversial) medical career of Dr. Scott W. Mooring came to its conclusion with his death on June 9, 1962. Dr. Mooring died at age eighty-four at the hospital he had served since 1905. The Medical Staff, to which he was by then a legend, established a fund in his memory to provide emergency loans to student nurses. A memorial resolution described him as "mentor, friend, confidant and leader to many of the members . . . a man who could not accept compromise [and whose] strong opinions were responsible for many advances." The minutes of the Medical Staff meeting of June 14, 1962 stated that "every member of the Staff . . . felt a true reverence for an outspoken, forthright and capable doctor who will truly long be remembered by this Cape Ann community."

NOTES

[1]Miss Andrews, then holding positions as Purchasing Agent and Assistant Administrator, retired September 1, 1969.

[2]"The Lookout" was for years a daily feature of the *Times* usually prepared by reporter Paul B. Kenyon. It was an editorial page column of Cape Ann tid-bits which delved into the community's life as he saw it with very little escaping his notice or deemed too insignificant for coverage.

10

One More Wing

FOLLOWING TUCKER VYE'S 1967 report on the return of serious overcrowding, the Trustees commissioned Ritchie Associates to conduct another survey of the physical plant. Surveying a problem doesn't make it disappear, however, and while it was in progress matters only got worse. The Gloucester Fire Department was concerned over safety with beds regularly in the corridors and in July 1968 brought its enforcement power to bear by refusing to give its approval for relicensing of the hospital by the state. This crisis, which would have brought Dr. Rubenstein and the State Department of Public Health to the scene, was forestalled when a light census during August coincided with the Fire Department's deciding inspection. With the corridors free of beds on that occasion, the license was approved, but only close cooperation between the Medical Staff and the administration prevented more than occasional use of the corridors for the next two years.

Frequently during 1970 the hospital recorded 100 percent occupancy and was often forced to turn away all but emergencies. Elective surgery postponements were common, and the Utilization Review Committee spent much of its time coping with AND cases. In May 1971 the situation was once again out of hand, with beds frequently in the corridors and some emergency cases forced to make the trip to Beverly Hospital.

The Ritchie survey reached the Board in March 1968, and not surprisingly it pointed out the 97.8 percent occupancy rate among the sixty-seven medical-surgical beds during fiscal 1967, fifteen of which were in the old North Wing and no longer suitable. It recommended adding thirty-six med-surg beds, including a six-bed Intensive-Coronary Care Unit. It also advised providing more space for the Outpatient-Emergency Department; giving the laboratory and X-ray each more space; enlarging the physical therapy unit; moving the kitchen, cafeteria, maintenance, housekeeping and Medical Records; relocating the nursing service to the Nurses' Residence; sheltering the front entrance; and creating a mental health service.

There were no sketches provided with this catch-all scheme nor did the report suggest how to share space with the well-attended LPN School. It can only be assumed that the consulting side of the firm rarely talked with the architectural side, for almost all the relocated departments were to go into the new wing. And thirty regular med-surg beds would be a net gain of only fifteen after North Wing closed. The more pragmatic architects would have to see it much differently.

In any case the recommendations were a start, and in July the Board authorized Ritchie "to prepare complete plans for construction of a new wing." In taking this step it was encouraged by Dr. Rubenstein's suggestion that the AGH was high on the list for Hill-Burton funding and that, because of what he called "the existing emergency," the hospital should arrange to borrow the money to get the program started. With that the Trustees voted to borrow up to $1.5 million and, four months later, to apply for $450,000 of Hill-Burton funds.

Ritchie's estimate that the project as outlined would cost $2.7 million "came as quite a shock," according to the minutes of the Board meeting at which it was presented. The firm was directed to draw plans for a phased program not to exceed $1.6 million for its first step and thus by implication ignore the earlier report's recommendations. Sketch plans somewhat over this figure were ready by January 1969, and, encouraged by warm support at the Annual Meeting, the Board voted to proceed and also plan for a fund drive. A fifteen-year $1,450,000 mortgage at 7.75 percent with nine participating banks was agreed to in April. Capping it all, the indomitable Carroll Steele "in his usual enthusiastic manner stated that he was itching to get started," according to Board Secretary Arthur Murch's record of the meeting.

Carroll Steele appears to have played devil's advocate in his early tactical maneuvering. When the idea of a new wing was first proposed he openly questioned the need for another building program so soon after those of 1956 and 1960. He continued tantalizing his fellow Trustees with doubts and delaying tactics until, by the Annual Meeting of 1969 and the Board meeting later that month, he had them begging for a campaign with promises of all-out support. Having thus convinced his colleagues to convince and commit themselves, he was ready to go.

The campaign goal was set at $1.5 million, and the Medical Staff, having committed itself four months earlier to give 10 percent of whatever goal was set, made an early-bird pledge of $150,000. Carroll accepted the chairmanship, and the campaign was scheduled to open in June, directed once again by Will, Folsom & Smith. Headquarters were established on Main Street's West End near where Isabel Babson had made her home more than 300 years earlier. A special gifts drive to run during the summer would be followed by a public solicitation, all to be based on the proven capital funding concept that about 80 percent of the funds will come from 15 percent of the available prospects. While this went forward the architects would work up plans to permit breaking ground in the spring of 1970.

By September the initial work had brought in $1,063,000 through pledges and outright gifts. The Auxiliary, not to be outdone by the Medical Staff, had pledged $100,000, and other individuals and businesses had also registered their support. The Gorton Corporation early pledged the $73,800 necessary to underwrite the Outpatient Department, and Gloucester Engineering followed with $34,000 for the Emergency Room area. Rockport's Cape Ann Tool Company took five double and two private rooms for a total of $50,400, and the six Cape Ann banks pledged a total of $49,525. Three foundations, those of George and Sybil Fuller, Godfrey Hyams and the McCarthy family, totaled $56,000, and fifty-five other members of Cape Ann's business community gave a further $120,000 among them. The gifts of many individuals, including numerous summer residents, accounted for the balance, and it was on to the public phase of the campaign.

For that some 200 workers, including a group calling itself the Interfaith Team led by Rev. Edmund W. Nutting and Msgr. Daniel Sullivan, obtained 2,120 gifts totaling $189,115. A Victory Dinner on October 9, 1969 celebrated the raising of $1,341,400, and by the time the final report was in there was $1,402,097, a bit short of the goal but a victory nonetheless.

The groundwork for an additional element of excitement at the victory celebration had been laid at a Board meeting in September when an "urgent telephone call" took Mr. Steele from the meeting, which then proceeded to a secret vote. At the dinner President Webber, in his inimitable oracular style, described the vote and announced that the wing would be named for Cape Ann's favorite fund raiser. The standing ovation for what the *Times* described as "a moist-eyed Carroll Steele" was tribute that those who had worked with him over the years knew had been well earned. To his credit were three capital campaigns totaling about $3 million, a dozen or more annual drives which he catalyzed for the hospital, plus several for other community agencies.

The Steele Wing campaign was his last major effort for the community he loved. Carroll King Steele died September 16, 1975 in the wing which, to paraphrase President Webber's words about him in October 1969, would

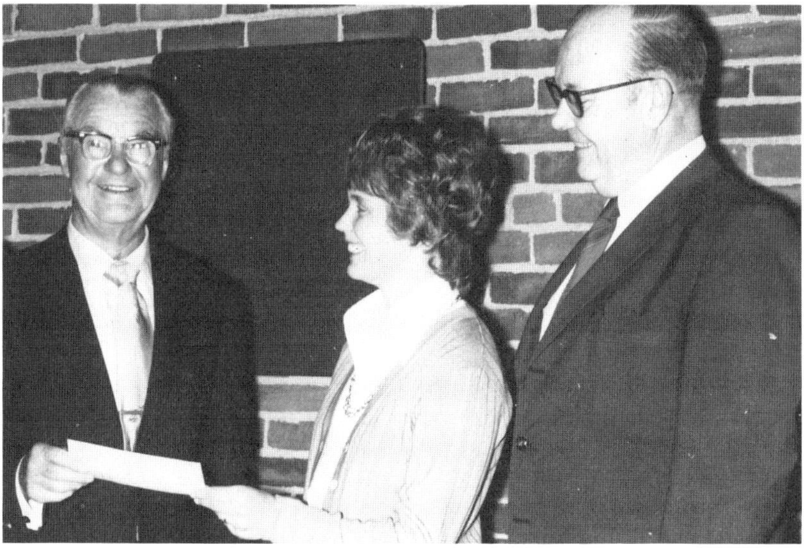

Carroll K. Steele, president from 1947 to 1950, is best remembered as the hospital's enthusiastic leader of all fund-raising activities from the forties into the seventies. Here he happily accepts a check from Auxiliary President Janis D. Stelluto completing the pledge of the Women's Auxiliary to the Steele Wing Fund as Tucker Vye looks on.

remain as a monument to a great and generous man who for fifty years had given of himself and of his own wealth so that his community might be a better place in which to live.

By April 1970 the structural plans had been completed, and, with their acceptance by the state and Hill-Burton authorities, the job was put out for bid. Feldman Construction Company, whose principal, Michael J. Feldman, had resigned as a Trustee so he could bid, was low at $2,408,271 including alternates. Facing the need to move ahead, the Board voted to proceed with a project which, with furnishings, contingencies and all the other extras to be contended with on any major undertaking, would cost an estimated $3,052,100. That total included replacement of the old boilers, which would be too small to handle the load added by the new wing. These and the plumbing subcontract fell within the purview of L. E. Andrews Company, Inc. whose President, Richard L. Andrews, was also a Trustee, a post from which he too resigned to permit him to bid. Low bidder on both jobs, his firm joined the construction team.

Ground was broken May 22, 1970 and, after a hard winter which put the job behind schedule, the building was essentially complete by October 1971. Plans were made to open the thirty-six-bed second floor to patients in January and, after the ground floor with its new Emergency Room and the first floor with thirty more med-surg beds plus a six-bed Coronary Care Unit were ready, to hold a formal dedication and Open House. The first patients moved in on January 26, and a well-attended Open House was held on April 23.

Both events were duly covered by the *Times,* which also devoted twenty-six pages of its weekend supplement to the Open House, telling the story of the hospital and its work and describing the new wing down to the smallest recognition plaque. It was a great day for all, the climax of three years of planning and work; and with it at long last the hospital could return to normal. For the first time in many years it not only had sufficient beds, but, after roofing in the V-shaped area between the 1960 wing and the new one, it also had plenty of storage space.

The uncompleted ground floor, designated "Future Radiology Department," would remain so for another ten years. The laboratory, X-ray, kitchen, cafeteria and all the other candidates for relocation in the early survey remained where they were. Dr. Gale and Nurse Webber left their makeshift unit in South Wing for the highly sophisticated CCU, and the final closing of North Wing[1] for patients was symbolic as well as practical in marking the end of an era.

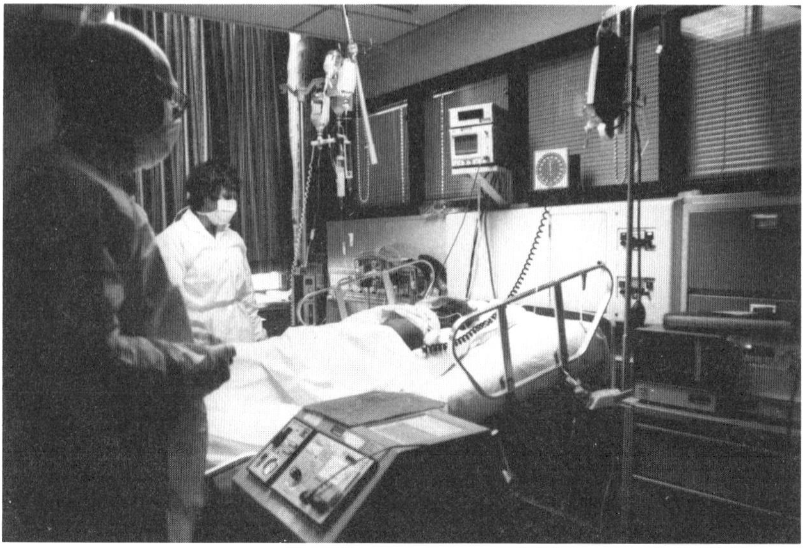

Completion of Steele Wing brought a greatly enhanced capability to coronary and intensive care. The new unit, with all beds in direct view of the nurses' station was equipped to provide ideal care for cardiac, post surgical, and serious accident cases.

The Vye years were coming to a close. The budget exceeded $3 million for a new high in 1971, and with the added burden of interest on the mortgage, further wage-price controls and adjusting to more stringent government regulation of charges and patients' length of stay, the deficits returned, reaching a record high of $418,967 in Vye's last full year. Room rates had been raised to the permissible limit, making it again necessary to invade endowment, an unhappy turn that even a resumption of annual fund-raising could not deter.

The Annual Giving Program had resumed in 1971, with the bulk of the Building Fund pledges then collected. It was promoted as a deficit and mortgage reduction effort, and, despite the gathering clouds of the 1974 recession and fuel shortage, it and other gift income were reaching new highs. A $35,000 grant by the Helen P. & Richard U. Wilson Foundation in January 1974, the first of several it was to make, was designated by the donor to help defray the mortgage.

Thus, as Tucker Vye came to the end of a quarter century as Administrator he saw much that was good and some not so good, but it was time to retire, and on September 25, 1973 he asked to be relieved by April 1974. President Webber appointed a search committee of Trustees Harold Bell, Robert F. Brown and Robert L. French; Chief of Staff Hamer Lacey, MD; Mr. Vye and later Lawrence N. Peterson to replace Mr. Brown following the latter's sudden death that fall. A wide-ranging search for a new Administrator ended in Birmingham, Alabama, where an Assistant Administrator at the Baptist Medical Center was ready to advance his career. On January 29, 1974 Search Committee Chairman Bell announced to the Board that their choice, concurred in by the Medical Staff Council, was Theodore A. Scharfenstein.

Tucker Vye made it final at the Annual Meeting of 1974, which elected him a Member of the Corporation: "It has been a good twenty-five years, and I'm proud of our growth and progress, for we have come a long way together since 1948." A round of farewell parties in March by the Trustees, the Medical Staff, the Auxiliary and the hospital employees, and the stage was set for the new Administrator, who attended his first Board meeting on March 18, 1974. He received a warm welcome on a typical raw New England late-winter day, and, as he said, "I don't even have a winter coat yet."

That was the least of his worries.

NOTES

[1]By 1976 this area had been renovated and was in use as office space.

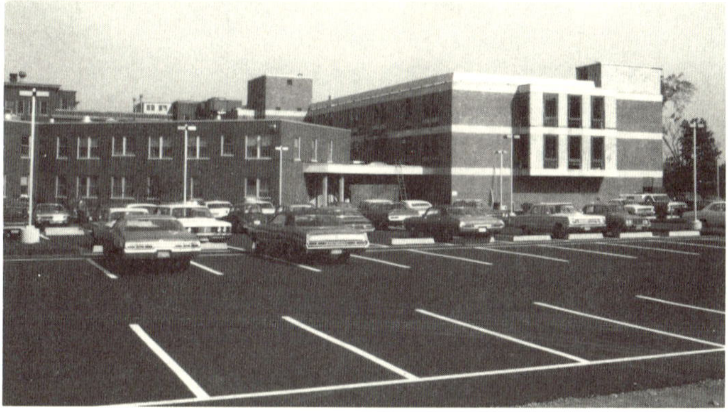

Transition: the newly completed Steele Wing at the right now dominates the scene.

PART IV
CHALLENGE AND CHANGE
1974 - 1983

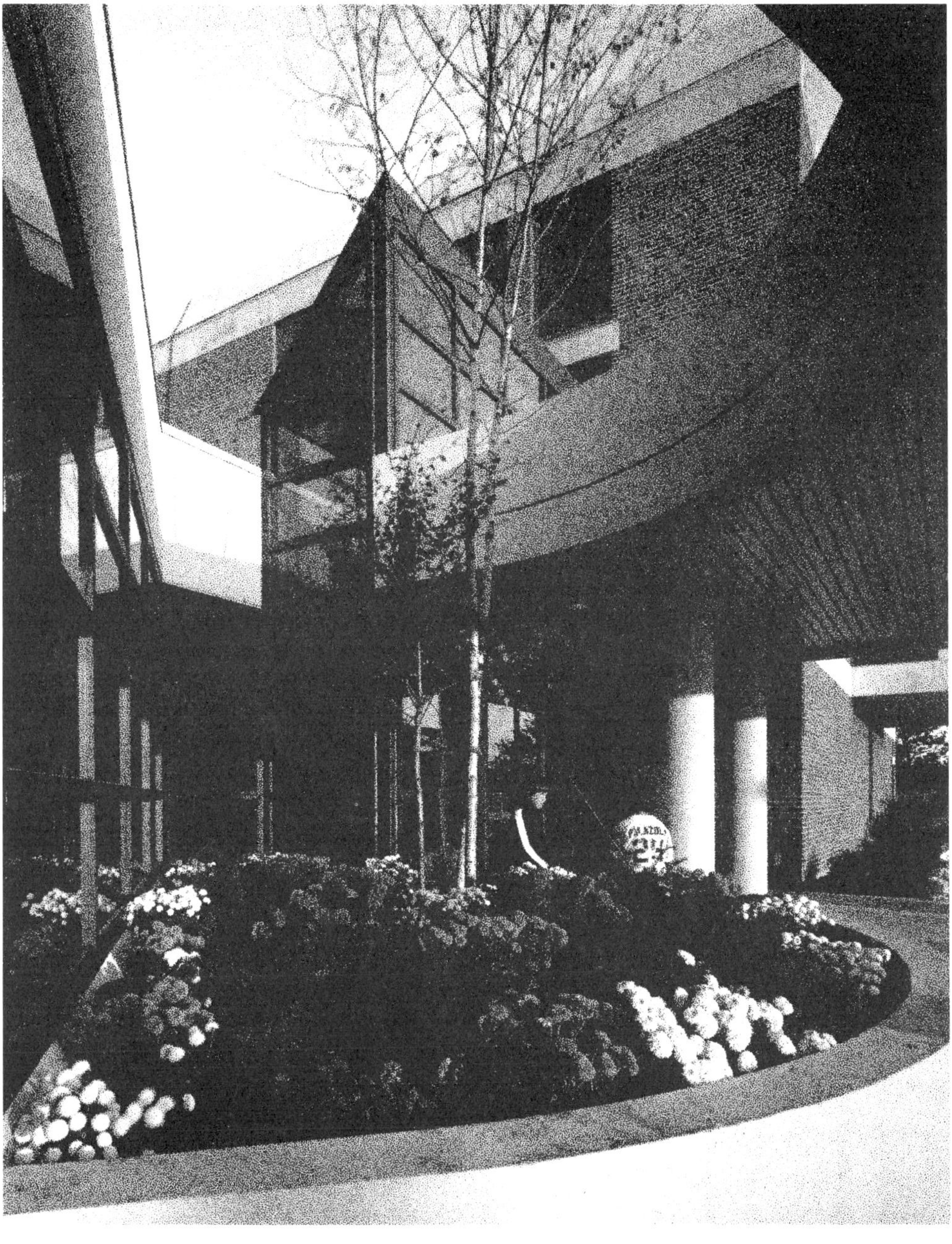

11

Influences of the Period

THE THIRTY-FIVE-YEAR-OLD Scharfenstein, possessor of master's degrees in business and health care administration from George Washington University, took over in April 1974. The new Administrator came to a far different hospital than had his predecessor twenty-five years earlier. It had grown physically and in capability, but it faced in even greater measure those influences, internal and external, which had begun to blossom during the Vye years. In addition to what seemed like chronic financial malaise, the next few years would see still more stringent regulation, third-party intervention, technological growth and competition.

Ted Scharfenstein came to the AGH at a time when its finances were in what Tucker Vye has described as "a desperate situation," his final year having ended with an operating deficit of $418,957 on a budget of about $4.5 million, despite a record-setting 38,824 patient days. But he also inherited a smoothly functioning team combination in its governing body, its Medical Staff and its employees.

"I believe my primary responsibility will be to serve as an expeditor of ideas, concepts and plans [using] the many talents available in the community [which] come together in the hospital . . . the focal point of progress and commitment," he said in an early public statement. Indeed, the involvement and interest of the community in its hospital had been a large factor in his decision to move from a modern urban institution of more than 400 beds to a 142-bed community hospital.

The major outside influences Scharfenstein faced were multiplying far beyond those of the previous twenty-five years and made the "old days," when Hill-Burton, Medicare and federal labor regulations were the chief constraints, look easy. Because these influences bore so heavily on his administration it seems well to examine that changing scene to assist in understanding its effect on the local situation over the period.

Hill-Burton was phasing out as a construction-funding mechanism, but would continue to plague hospitals with stepped-up enforcement of an almost forgotten requirement that its beneficiary hospitals offer free care based on the funding assistance given them over the years. This, while a problem to some hospitals not given to a "whole community" philosophy, had little effect on AGH, where free care had been a fact of life from the beginning. It adopted Hill-Burton's "Open Door" option in 1975, switching to a guarantee of free care amounting to an annual 10 percent of the total funds it had received over the years, only after its more generous "Open Door" option was regulated out of existence in 1979.

More important was government "assistance" in hospital planning which was beginning to be felt more strongly. This had first surfaced here in April 1964 when Mr. Vye reported to the Board that a perceived lack of planning by Massachusetts hospitals in their expansion of plant and acquisition of new equipment was being considered by a special committee of the legislature investigating hospital costs. The committee report suggested formation of regional hospital councils, a step endorsed by the MHA since these would be organized and governed by the hospitals themselves. The MHA guide for their establishment suggested a master plan for each hospital, with groupings to be based on geographic distribution; it would then oversee the whole through its statewide Regional Council.

The AGH Board voted "to favor the philosophy of area-wide regional planning on a voluntary basis," and in late 1964 President Webber was able to report on efforts to get the North Shore hospitals to form such a council "to avoid state control." The North Shore Hospital Council, begun in 1955 by seventeen area hospitals to enable their administrators to meet for sociability and shoptalk, became the basis for a more formally organized group which held its founding meeting on May 19, 1965 with twelve institutions represented.

The resulting North Shore Regional Planning Committee, among the first in Massachusetts, set out at once to address the question of rising costs and to attempt to coordinate such diverse hospital operations as laundry, data processing and medical-technical services. It took as its guide a study by professional hospital consultants that pinpointed areas of feasible and potentially profitable cooperation. Its first chairman was Neil Ayer, President of

Beverly Hospital, and Tucker Vye was appointed a member of its Executive Committee.

It was probably inevitable that self-interest and interhospital jealousies would make true cooperation difficult. A year after its formation the new group had accomplished nothing, although its members each formally reaffirmed support. By late 1967 it had ceased to function, and a new group was forming under increasing threats of state intervention.

The new group materialized in February 1968 as the North Shore Planning Council, again under the guidance of the MHA. The AGH Board authorized President Webber to commit the hospital to the $700 membership assessment if he and Mr. Vye "felt that it was a worthwhile venture." These "dues" were set at $7 per bed the next year and increased to $10 in 1970. In February 1971 Mr. Webber reported his conviction "that this council is apparently on the way to accomplishing its purpose," an opinion concurred in by the Medical Staff, whose representative, Dr. Robert N. Lundberg, reported in late 1972 that "after seven years [it] was becoming increasingly vocal and influential." By that time, although its basis was the council formed in 1968, it had become known as the North Shore Health Planning Council with wider community membership, doctors as well as lay people, and was thus evolving as a more public body.

Such creations lacked authority, however, and could only study and suggest or, at best, bring pressure for change. They had no power to enforce their decisions and were, by their nature, dominated by the hospitals that had formed them in the first place. The long-feared government intervention was coming closer, and by 1973 the United States Congress was leaning toward change in support of the various states' desire for a mechanism governing determination of facilities requirements as well as control of rates and other fees.

The National Health Planning and Resources Department Act of 1974 established regional Health Systems Agencies (HSAs) dominated by consumers instead of providers with oversight of planning within each region. With but limited power to act, however, they could only recommend action to their state regulators or, when appropriate, to the federal oversight agencies. States were required to establish determination-of-need commissions and health-coordinating councils. It put to rest the hope that hospitals, by themselves, could correct the perceived problems; each would now be forced to prove its various needs to a consumer-oriented regional group, which in its turn would report its considered recommendations to the appropriate government agency.

After considerable anguish on the part of the North Shore group over a proposal to include its members in a Greater Boston HSA, the Department of Health, Education and Welfare (HEW) in 1976 granted HSA status to the North Shore Health Planning Council. A Cape Ann Sub-area Council included Beverly, Danvers, Gloucester and Ipswich, each of which had its own hospital.

With this, the hospitals, all members of the reorganized NSHPC, established their own support group as North Shore Hospital Council complete with administrator and physician representatives from fourteen hospitals, an annual assessment, guidance from the MHA, and renewed hopes for the elusive concept of interhospital cooperation. It hoped above all to become a countervailing force in support of the hospitals' stance versus the new agency.

Did the regional planning concept work? Only time will determine its full impact, but certainly its effect had been felt by 1983. Consumers were no longer hesitant to ask questions and discuss the answers. Hospitals were compelled to think longer and plan more constructively before making costly and sometimes duplicating acquisitions or additions. But they were also frequently forced into divisive and costly battles to support what they saw as their own reasonable positions.

An example of this can be seen in the 1977 attempt by the NSHPC/HSA plan to reduce the number of beds in the region. This had its start in the conviction of the planners that the North Shore could reduce costs by eliminating 25 percent or six hundred of the area's hospital beds, even though they could not agree as to how this could be accomplished. The hospitals, for their part, found it difficult to understand the planners' reliance on federal guidelines calling for a set number of beds per thousand people regardless of location, population mix or other unique circumstances.

A public hearing on the matter was scheduled by the area HSA, thus bringing the Hospital Council members to work together with their trustees and medical staffs to support their case before the public. Letters, public forums and copious newspaper publicity preceded the August 18 hearing. From the other side came threats that no more certificated determinations of need would be considered unless a bed reduction was accomplished. A "torrent of opposition," as the *Times* put it, supported by the general public as well as by the finally united hospitals and their staffs, overwhelmed the hearing. Two months later the planners announced withdrawal of the original proposal for further study.

The desired bed reduction came about peacefully the next year under the more natural influence of generally lower occupancy rates. At the AGH "excess" medical-surgical beds were surrendered in favor of a new Psychiatric

Care Unit then in the planning stages, and unnecessary pediatric beds were converted to adult use.

Controversy again erupted in 1978, when the NSHPC attempted to correct what it perceived as a duplication of services by reallocating such services among the region's hospitals. The Hospital Council and a subarea group, Cape Ann Associated Hospitals (Addison Gilbert, Beverly, Cable and Hunt), worked with NSHPC in establishing guidelines and attempting, futilely, to find common ground for reallocation. When it was over, the parties had agreed that, while there was indeed some duplication, it was largely unavoidable given the geographics of the area.

The relationship began to improve after 1979. Area hospitals had accepted the idea that the council concept was a fact of life, and the Council itself had matured and was abating what many had viewed as a "let's get the hospitals" philosophy. Out of it came a more precise planning process within the hospitals, although they continued to resist moves toward regionalization of services, partly because of community self-interest but also out of fear that it would eventually lead to domination of the area by one or two large hospitals. Very probably the rivalries engendered by this fear were a factor a few years later in the growth of intensive marketing of services both in their own and in other hospitals' loosely defined natural service areas.

Other attempts to control health care costs proliferated during this period. The Massachusetts Rate Setting Commission, born of a compromise with Governor Dukakis' demand for a freeze on all hospital charges in 1975, would curb the trend, if not the need, of hospital fee increases. The Determination of Need (DON) process would slow the acquisition and construction of new and possibly duplicative facilities. The latter, requiring extensive documentation of the planning process, would force many hospitals, the AGH among them, to establish costly but essential planning departments.

New state laws, notably Chapters 223 and 372 of the General Laws, imposed further controls after 1982. The former impacted severely on hospital budgets, with AGH projecting $300,000 in reduced income the first year and up to $1 million annually thereafter. Methods to increase volume and significantly reduce costs demanded the hospital planners' time and attention that year and resulted in a nursing staff pattern change as well as the loss of some forty staff positions over the next year. In facing that issue, this and perhaps all hospitals acknowledged the realities of life in the 1980s as, in Ted Scharfenstein's words to the Board concerning Chapter 223, "the hospital must deal with the changing economic environment and do so in an effective and timely fashion."

Chapter 372 had its origin in a bill sponsored by the state Rate Setting Commission as Senate 495 in 1980. It called for major cost reduction in seven areas of hospital operations estimated at $100 million statewide and would, the Trustees were told, "effectively guarantee that hospitals would operate at a loss." Opposition to it, led by MHA, was immediate and heavy. A massive protest by the hospitals, the first ever attempted on a statewide, coordinated basis, delivered the message. Senate 495 died and a replacement bill, which became Chapter 372, was passed two years later.

The new bill forced leaner staffing and, stressing as it did the need for improved productivity by remaining staff, accentuated the further growth of automation. In providing for reimbursement within fixed limits or "caps" on most procedures and admissions with dire penalties facing those who ignored them, it was a precursor of a 1986 Medicare regulation that limited reimbursement within diagnostically related groups of illnesses. It would create problems at many underfunded hospitals, but at Addison Gilbert the concensus was that it could be lived with. By reducing reimbursement it would require greater efficiency and careful management, and, as the eighties moved on, it would also accelerate a trend toward providing more services on an outpatient basis.

On the medical side, but also affecting hospital management, were Medicare-induced regulations covering practice and hospital utilization. Utilization Review (U.R.) was introduced as a means of shortening hospital stays, most notably those coming under Medicare reimbursement. It was deemed necessary in particular to cope with the long-standing AND problem, but unfortunately the U.R. process, designed to maintain pressure on cost increases, could not help solve the more basic problem of nursing-home availability.

Coupled with U.R. were the Professional Standards Review Organization (PSRO) regulations, which created related oversight boards. These were formed on a state-by-state basis, several in each state, for coverage of specific areas therein, and their function was to review each hospital's compliance with U.R. regulations as well as the necessity and appropriateness of its admissions.

Although the hospital and its Medical Staff adjusted satisfactorily for the most part, there were instances where neither the institution nor its patients and their families could understand decisions made. It was difficult and made for poor public relations to try to explain why an elderly person, unable to cope in a home environment and unable to find a nursing-home bed, could no longer stay at the hospital. These patients, kept simply because there was no other place for them to go, occupied beds needed by others, and, with third-party reimbursement for them reduced or eliminated, the hospital was forced to rely on whatever resources the patient had for payment or carry them as partial free care cases.

It was also difficult to understand the October 1979 review by the state U.R. board that disallowed reimbursement for 125 of the 1,300 patient days audited, said to be above the allowable quota, when 89 of those days were for three terminal cases. But the regulators had ruled that terminal care does not justify hospitalization, and that was that. The patients could not have been discharged with no place to go, and for the hospital and its Medical Staff it was a classic case of "damned if you do and damned if you don't" in which no one was satisfied, except possibly the regulators.

The problem's impact at AGH becomes obvious in view of the fact that of 38,097 patient days in 1979, AND cases accounted for 4,099. By March 1981 such patients occupied 30 percent of the available med-surg beds and had necessitated the reopening of Prentiss House. Adding insult to injury, in 1981 the state also reduced reimbursement for them to $70 per day, although the Rate Setting Commission approved a rate of $167 for semiprivate regular patients in October 1981. If maximum occupancy is taken as an ideal, then AND did its part; in 1983, with a psychiatric inpatient unit open and all other beds filled, the hospital logged a record 43,359 patient days.

Such was the world of regulation during the seventies and early eighties, and most assuredly beyond. Every decision would be influenced by these and many other such mandates, and Ted Scharfenstein and his management group could be assured of many hours of meetings and, beyond a doubt, some sleepless nights. The Planning Committee, created as a Board standing committee by new hospital bylaws in 1975, would become one of the key bodies, and five-year plans and consultants would be a regular part of hospital life.

The strong would survive, the weak would perish or merge with the strong; in either case, the days of freedom were finished. Whether regulation was effective in its primary goal of reducing health care costs must be left to future judgment, but it did arouse a consciousness of the need for greater efficiency and careful management.

Another outside influence affecting hospital management was the maturation of what might be called the ultimate in group practice, the Health Maintenance Organization (HMO) movement. The concept had its start in 1942 with industrialist Henry Kaiser's development of an idea for prepaid, preventive medical care conceived ten years earlier by Sidney Garfield, MD who joined Kaiser as cofounder of Kaiser-Permanente, originally a benefit program for Kaiser's California employees. It opened membership to the general public after World War II, and by the sixties it had become a model for the HMOs that followed.

The concept fitted nicely into the proposals for national health insurance then being explored at the federal level. Its proponents argued that if government wished to assure care for all, then the system should be based on health maintenance, the prevention of illness, via a prepaid, comprehensive plan. This had been the Kaiser concept, and it became the Nixon administration's proposal for privately operated health programs as opposed to a government-supported national insurance plan.

By the close of 1970 HEW had begun to promote the HMO movement. The next year some thirty had been organized, and further growth was being urged by several states. The concept was a milestone development — a program descended from the earlier ethnic charitable societies, once viewed as almost socialistically utopian, was being given conservative support. It was given credibility and formal acceptance in the Health Maintenance Organization Act of 1973, which required business to offer HMO membership as an option to its employees and fostered HMO formation with grants and loans. By 1979 there were 217, with 8 million members enrolled in the United States.

The Harvard Community Health Plan was established in the Greater Boston area in 1978. The AGH Trustees and Medical Staff were told to expect it to reach the North Shore, but it was a newer plan, Bay State Health Care, that in June 1979 approached the hospital and its physicians with a plan to solicit membership among Gloucester and Rockport employers. By November, with industrial interest apparently high, the hospital Planning Committee began a study to determine if indeed there was sufficient population to support an HMO on Cape Ann. Three months later its report offered "the general conclusion that Cape Ann is too small to support an HMO . . . a base population of between 100,000 and 250,000 people [being] necessary." Attracted by the idea nonetheless, it urged keeping the option open.

Later that year, although the two hospitals in Lynn were working on an area plan, the North Shore stood alone in not yet having an HMO in place, and the Medical Staff, or at least its younger members, was beginning to push for one. The Lynn plan, North Shore HMO, was by then raising funds among area hospitals to finance further study and apply for federal funding, a hope that dimmed in the face of cutbacks in the spring of 1981. Although North Shore HMO had five hospitals enrolled by June 1981, the AGH held back, relying on the Staff's opinion that it was "moving along too fast . . . [with] inadequate information for doctors to make an informed decision." This wait-and-see posture proved wise; in September North Shore HMO was denied federal support. Lacking the $1.5 million needed to start, it was judged unfeasible to continue.

The Boston-based Bay State Health Care returned to the scene in 1983, and in April the hospital contracted with it as a hospital provider and became eligible to accept patients already covered by Bay State. Although the Staff maintained a cautious attitude, with debate centering on "challenges [to] traditional medical care on Cape Ann," it also recognized the inevitable. Since Bay State was organized not as a true HMO but rather as an Independent Practice Association (IPA) that preserved existing physician-patient relationships, the Staff found it acceptable and joined the Trustees in voting for it over two other contenders, a Tufts University plan and one established by Blue Cross-Blue Shield. By 1985 Bay State was enlisting doctors for its preferred physician plan and enrolling further subscribers on Cape Ann. Although the Blues continued to cover many clients, the hospital itself adopted Bay State as alternative coverage for its own employee health plan. With that and with the physician's support, the new concept was soon firmly in place.

12

The Governing Body

WITH TUCKER VYE'S retirement, the man who had served with him as a Trustee during his entire twenty-five years and as the hospital's President for the last eighteen of them, longer than any of his predecessors in that post, also decided that it was time to step down. He announced his own resignation at the Annual Meeting of 1974, the twenty-second over which he had presided, four as Vice-President.

William S. Webber, Jr., Bill to all who knew him, was a man of many attributes. A native son whose ancestors first settled at Fresh Water Cove in 1725, he was a well-read man noted for his choice of the telling word, even though his formal education did not extend beyond Gloucester High School. He was for twenty-one years a member of the city Planning Board, was a long-time member of the Board of Cape Ann Savings Bank and a recognized municipal bond expert at the Boston offices of Advest, Inc., where he was affectionately called "the sage." And so he was, a man of considered judgment and firm convictions, an analytic thinker who could also lead, organize, prod and, above all, set an example of dedication for those with whom he worked.

His fellow Trustees made sure he would not be forgotten. An oil portrait of him was commissioned and completed in 1974 and today hangs with that of Dr. W. Warren Babson at the hospital. Of even greater significance, however, was the decision of the Trustees in 1978 that South Wing, Bill's first major expansion program, be renamed "Webber House." The dedication plaque unveiled at the Annual Meeting that year told the story in few words:

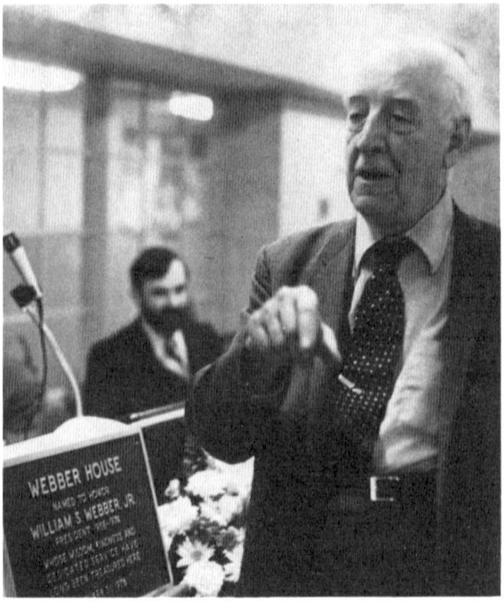

William S. Webber, Jr. at the 1978 Annual Meeting when South Wing was renamed Webber House in his honor.

"Named to honor William S. Webber, Jr. whose wisdom, kindness and dedicated service have long been treasured here."

The hospital governing board, which during this period would have two presidents, Harold Bell (1974—77) and Robert L. French (1977—84), would undergo change. Conscious of its growing responsibilities in the face of increasing strictures, it was essential that it enlist the best people available to serve, expecting informed participation at its meetings and those of its many committees.

Although the Chief of Medical Staff was *ex officio* a member of the Board, there had never been a Staff member elected Trustee.[1] So it was a historic first when the Corporation elected Dr. W. Warren Babson to the Board in 1975. Dr. Babson was followed by others of the Medical and Dental staffs after the traditional separateness of the governing body from the medical side was ended with new bylaws, approved in January 1975, which mandated at least two Medical/Dental Staff members on the Board of Trustees.

In an effort to keep the membership of the Corporation involved and of high calibre, the 1975 bylaws also established rotating six-year terms instead of almost automatic life tenure, and added revised criteria for selection. This reflected the judgment of hospital Vice-President and Bylaws Committee Chairman Bob French that selection of Corporators and Trustees should be based on a will to work as well as the possession of ability.

He carried this conviction with him to his later tenure as President, and one of his priorities in that office, which gained support from JCAH pressure for better-prepared Boards, was the thorough orientation of Trustees, old and new, as to their duties and responsibilities. All new Corporators and Trustees were expected to attend a series of luncheon meetings at which their acquaintance with the hospital and its people could be enhanced. French was instrumental also in producing a corporation manual during his first year, and in 1978 the Administrator was made responsible for producing and distributing to all Trustees and Medical Staff members a monthly report on pertinent hospital affairs.

More controversial was a proposal by President French in 1978 for a policy statement delineating responsibilities of Corporators and Trustees. In basic accord with nationwide trends assigning greater responsibilities and legal liability to hospital Trustees, the statement emphasized the need for ability and willingness to learn and contribute skills and service. As described at its introduction to the Executive Committee on May 16, 1978 it suggested periodic review of Board members and provision for replacing those failing to meet reasonable criteria of "performance, attendance and any other factors that may reflect interest."

In its earliest form the French proposal was an outline of his opinions as to criteria and needs of the hospital in a memorandum to the 1977 Nominating Committee, which was urged to judge performance and not hesitate to remove those not meeting standards. As presented to the full Board in July it had become a formal "Policy on Trustees and Corporators," which outlined Trustee responsibilities and qualifications in detail, set standards for a balanced membership and suggested steps to be followed in selecting new Trustees and Corporators. It also provided for nonrenewal of their terms if adherence to definite standards was deemed lacking.

The proposed policy was discussed "with a great deal of participation," a euphemistic description which masked an outspoken opposition focusing on procedures for renomination and performance review. The matter was referred to a joint meeting of the Executive Committee and the Nominating Committee, which would have borne the major share of responsibility for implementing the policy. The joint session resolved the most controversial issues, and a revised policy was accepted by the Board in October.

In retrospect the document, a detailed reinstatement of basic provisions of the bylaws, appears innocuous. Its intent was clearly to encourage more active and informed participation by the Trustees and Board committees with a membership selected from a broad range of skilled and dedicated people. In proposing it, President French, himself a hardworking and knowledgeable hospital volunteer, was expressing his belief that others should also, upon accepting election as either Corporator or Trustee, be ready to serve diligently while sharing any special skills they possessed. Through it, in principles that continue to hold true, he endeavored to give the hospital the strength he knew would be required by the changing times.

Bob French, the protagonist of change, was an informed, conscientious leader, possessing a vision of a strong, efficient hospital that blended well with that of the Administrator. The two worked closely together in bringing the institution through the trying seventies and early eighties. A man of strongly held beliefs and high ideals, a professional psychologist, he was sometimes impatient with others who perhaps thought more slowly or did not always agree with his ideas. He gave generously and wholeheartedly of himself, spending a great deal of time at the hospital and in committee work, rarely missing such meetings or those of the Board itself. He ranks high on the hospital's leadership rolls.

At the Corporation level more members were being given responsibility beyond attendance at the Annual Meeting, through assignment to the growing number of standing committees. Such service could also be used to discover those who might be Trustee material. Better programs for the annual meetings were also planned as a means of increasing interest and attendance.

In 1975 the practice of including an outside speaker on the program was inaugurated with David M. Kinzer, then President of MHA. This feature lasted through 1982 and brought leading figures from the health care field to enlighten the attendees and to receive a set of "Man at the Wheel" bookends in lieu of honorarium. Also begun in 1975 was the custom of inviting elected officials from Gloucester and Rockport as well as Cape Ann's members of the state Senate and Legislature and its Representative in Congress.

These moves were effective. A record eighty Corporators attended the 1976 session, and by 1983 the cafeteria, where buffet dinner was served, was being severely taxed for space with 91 of 170 members plus a large number of guests attending. It helped the ambience somewhat when the 1980 opening of a large meeting room in the newly renovated Nurses' Residence made it possible to hold a more comfortable business meeting there following the dinner.

NOTES

[1]Isaac Adams, MD, Trustee from 1892 to 1903 and the only physician elected prior to 1975, was not a hospital Medical Staff member.

13

On the Medical Side

The State of the Art

THIS PERIOD, most notably in its later stages, was one of continuing technological growth and change. The hospital's endeavors to adapt to modern techniques would not only improve patient care but help to attract outstanding specialists, the men and women necessary to assure the community that fine care was indeed available here at home.

Each year brought further advances in diagnostic and treatment capabilities. In 1974, for example, the hospital's surgery was enhanced by the acquisition of fibre-optical urological equipment, paving the way for a staff urologist. In that same year equipment necessary for joint replacement and advanced cataract surgery was added. By 1982, although only a year earlier the Medical Staff had deemed it a new procedure too sophisticated for smaller hospitals, the Ophthalmology Department was performing ocular implants.

Diagnostic advances resulted from the acquisition of the Auxiliary's nuclear scan and from the establishment of the Robert F. Brown Neuro-science Laboratory, utilizing an electroencephalograph given by the Cape Ann Medical Center. A state-of-the-art fetal heart monitor was acquired as a gift of the Isabel Babson Memorial Library Foundation, which continued its support of the Obstetrical Department. A B-mode ultrasound and a gamma camera for the Radiology Department in 1976 were followed three years later

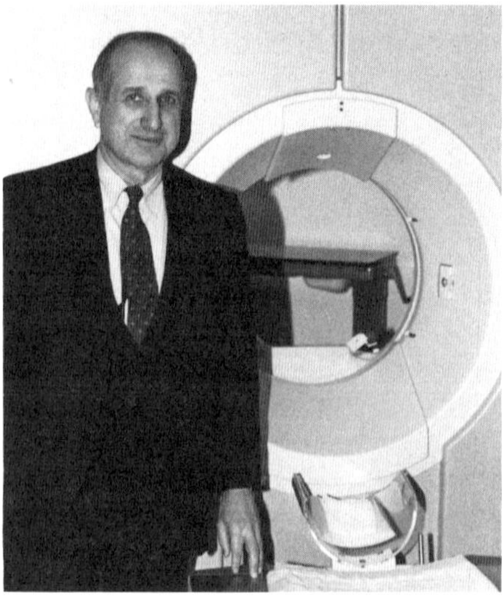

Bernard F. Gordon played a major role as plans for upgrading the Radiology Department progressed. His contributions were many and during the mid-1980s he helped make possible the acquisition of the hospital's C.T. Scanner.

by even more sophisticated ultrasound equipment and in 1981 by an advanced gamma camera. A partnership arrangement with Beverly and Hunt hospitals in 1980 made cardiac ultrasound available locally for the first time, and during 1983 the AGH acquired its own equipment, a General Electric Phased Array Sector System offering high-definition examination of heart structure and function.

Much of this and other state-of-the-art equipment became part of a new radiology unit housed in the Steele Wing's previously unfinished "shell" area, part of a major renovation project, the "Program for the Eighties." Five years later a computerized axial tomographic scanner, called the CAT scan, was added.

The new unit was made possible by the gifts and encouragement of Trustee Bernard M. Gordon of Magnolia. Mr. Gordon, the inventor/entrepreneur developer of much of the equipment involved, was founder and chief executive officer of Analogic Corporation, a supplier of components to the electronics industry. He made his first gift to the hospital in 1979, when he conveyed stock in his company with the suggestion that it be held to appreciate, sage investment advice indeed, as its growing value soon proved.

His interest whetted by his analysis of the hospital's growing capability, Bernard Gordon not only continued to offer major financial assistance, often in company stock, but added counsel and guidance as the Radiology Department was revamped during the expansion program. And thus it was, when the new department was dedicated, that his fellow Trustees found it

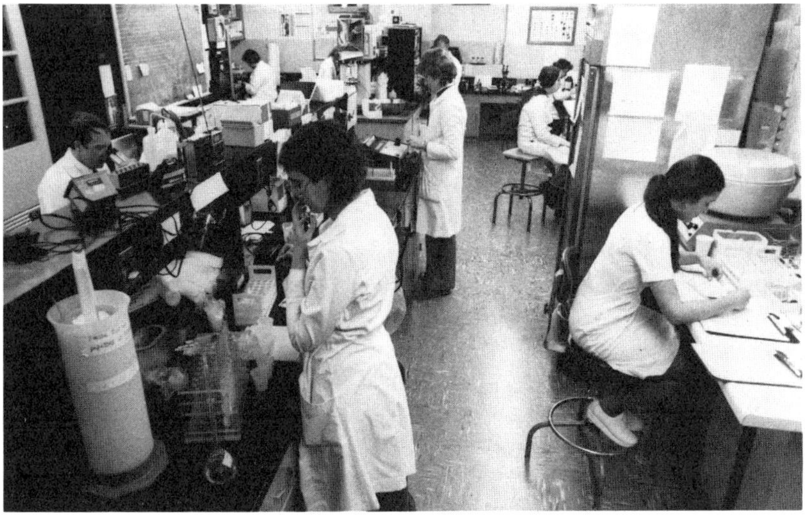

Prior to the 1980s expansion, the laboratory was still crowded and shared space with X-ray which in this view is behind the rear wall and around the corner to the left.

fitting to designate it in honor of his wife: "The Sophia Gordon Radiology Suite, given to assure community access to advanced diagnostic techniques."

The laboratory, since the earliest days physically adjacent to the X-ray area, was similarly growing as an important diagnostic unit. Still in what had become cramped and inefficient space between Prentiss and the West Wing, it did the best it could until the "Program for the Eighties" enabled it to expand into space vacated by radiology. As part of that program it was almost totally rebuilt — new work spaces, better layout, improved lighting — and for the first time, when the project was completed in early 1983, it could finally be considered truly physically adequate.

Meanwhile it had managed, within those space limitations, to maintain a sound equipment posture. With a full-time pathologist there was no need for reliance on Salem Hospital and its lab. Ongoing new equipment acquisitions soon minimized that traditional dependence, although Salem remained willing and able to assist as needed. In 1975 a DuPont ACA chemistry auto-analyzer made it possible to perform thirty-two different tests, singly or in batches, as needed twenty-four hours a day. Later came a multichannel gamma counter to permit a wide variety of radio-immunoassays including thyroid function, and in 1980 the well-equipped department was able to boast an Ortho-ELT-8 analyzer for a wide range of blood work, with results available in minutes.

In 1982 the lab was judged ready for accreditation by the College of American Pathologists and, after survey, was granted such status for a two-year period, recognition that has been regularly maintained since. Similar approval was given its blood bank by the American Association of Blood Banks. And it had become a busy place, performing 112,648 tests in 1983 in a trend that has continued since, with more than 160,000 tests annually now the norm.

Early 1982 found the hospital in negotiations with Cape Ann Medical Center, following the latter's proposal that studies be conducted to determine the feasibility of combining its lab and radiology functions with those at the hospital. As proposed in the required DON statement, the CAMC lab would continue to operate there but would be staffed and supervised by AGH personnel. This would permit most specimens, previously tested for the center by commercial Boston laboratories, to be analyzed inhouse. The CAMC radiology work would continue under Dr. Anne O'Donnell, but with interpretation done by the hospital's Department of Radiology. The proposal was seen as a mutual benefit offering lower operating costs for all.

Although approved by the DON authorities, the petition was delayed by the state Rate Setting Commission and then withdrawn in May 1983 pending a major change then under discussion concerning the hospital's corporate structure. The AGH lab meanwhile was authorized to provide serv-

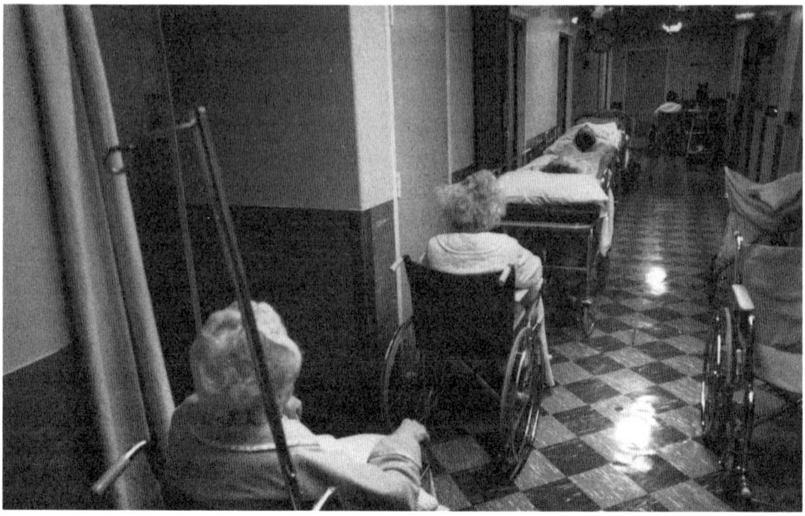

Crowded conditions in radiology characterized by this view of a narrow corridor, where wheelchair and bed patients faced long waits, were one of the many problems requiring attention.

ice to CAMC on an interim basis, and in 1984, with the hospital's reorganization in place, the two labs formally merged. Third-party reimbursement regulations made a similar merger of radiological facilities impractical.

Surgery was also changing. Many aspects of that specialty, once requiring lengthy hospital confinement, were being handled almost on an outpatient basis as one-day surgery became increasingly popular. First discussed here in 1975, prior to which only dental and certain gynecological procedures had been done on that basis, it was at first dismissed as not cost effective, since the same amount of operating-room expense would not be fully reimbursed. This changed with recognition by third-party payors that one-day surgery could be reimbursed at a more reasonable level and still save them money through length-of-stay reductions. By 1979, therefore, the concept could become part of the planning for the renovation program. Day surgery became fully operational during 1982, a long step from "the good old days" and indeed even from the forties, when Dr. Babson shocked the hospital community by getting his patients on their feet within a day or two of their operations.

Cardiac function and testing came into its own in 1977, when a long-time donor funded equipment for installation of a stress-testing program on the second floor of Prentiss House. Prior to this time, basic stress-testing, a matter of measuring pulse during variable pacing rates on a treadmill, had been done at the Gloucester YMCA. The installation at the hospital had medical supervision with constant monitoring and electrocardiogram printouts. It soon gained popularity under its directors, Dr. Douglas C. Fiero and nurse Virginia Webber, not only as a diagnostic or early warning tool but also among those planning a program of strenuous exercise or simply seeking assurance that all was well.

Two years later Dr. Fiero and Mrs. Webber established a cardiac rehabilitation program for post-coronary-attack patients. This also proved popular as a means of educating cardiac patients in proper diet, stress reduction, avoidance of risk factors and the possible need for psychiatric counseling. In ten two-hour weekly meetings, professionals from several departments, among them physical therapists, pharmacists, dieticians and social workers, work with each group, endeavoring, as Mrs. Webber describes it, "to allow them to live more comfortably with their heart." Its growth by 1983 made it necessary to consider adding a full-time director.

Advanced technical capabilities also raised questions of moral philosophy as desperately or terminally ill patients could now be sustained mechanically to a degree not previously possible. A 1977 Masschusetts Supreme Judicial Court decision requiring approval by that court before life-support could be withdrawn from incompetent patients led to broad discussion of the issue throughout the Commonwealth and at the medical staff level at each hospital. Such discussions here resulted in the July 1978 adoption of a "Do Not Resuscitate" policy, which concurred with the strict requirement that agreement by patient and family be well and carefully documented in the patient's medical record.

Savings lives of course remained the paramount concern, and by 1980 training in Advanced Life Support was made mandatory for Emergency Room staff and others whose duties required such certification. This combination of techniques, designed to forestall deterioration of vital functions during severe trauma, was also a matter of considerable discussion and medical concern during its introduction. It soon became standard practice, a positive benefit for cardiac and other trauma cases.

The Medical Departments

Among the medical departments the Emergency Room is probably the best known to the general public. Almost everyone eventually comes in contact with it as a patient or as the family or friend of a patient. From a public relations standpoint, therefore, its operation is just as sensitive as that of the inpatient work, more so perhaps since it must deal with a wide range of unexpected cases often requiring immediate care and with people often overwrought by whatever situation brought them through its doors.

Twenty-four-hour coverage by appropriate physicians is essential and, as has been described, this was one of the chores faced with something less than enthusiasm by the Medical Staff. Higher stipends in 1975 kept weekend coverage by Boston interns and residents intact with the always troublesome weekday summer coverage supplied by regular Staff volunteers at a fixed hourly reimbursement, an idea that worked better in the planning than in the execution. Basic to the problem was a lack of effective direction and coordination, and later in 1975 this was addressed by appointing a physician-manager who would be reimbursed for the extra duty at $150 a month. This concept was accepted by most of the Staff, in the belief that physicians in local practice were best suited for E.R. service and that its control should be a Staff function. A few argued for a full-time salaried director with staffing by physicians not in private practice.

The pros and cons were debated, often heatedly and at length, until March 1979 when, after an obviously outspoken discussion, the Staff voted "to endorse the creation of the position of Director of Emergency Services having total administrative responsibilities for medical activities centered in the Emergency Room on a part-time or full-time basis." Two months later Dr.

Michael Kelleher, in private practice at Cape Ann Medical Center, was appointed to the position on what a still divided Staff recommended be a six-month trial.

The six months became two years, until mid-1981 when Dr. Kelleher tendered his resignation in favor of his practice, but with the Staff now in agreement that the concept was sound and, as the Administrator told the Trustees, had resulted "in improved Emergency Room practice," he was persuaded to stay on. A year later he was formally appointed Director with a hospital-employed staff of E.R. physicians under his supervision.

Significant changes followed Dr. Kelleher's appointment. Long, frustrating waits for treatment became the exception and, if a wait was necessitated by a higher-priority problem, explanations were forthcoming. Specialist examination and treatment where indicated were more readily available. A Trauma Team composed of nurses and technicians from various departments, geared to respond on word that a severe injury case was en route, was also organized in 1981.

Care did not cease when the patient left after treatment. Each was given a set of after-care instructions detailing procedures to be followed at home. Provisions were made for monitoring and evaluating E.R. procedures and care with the patient brought into the process via a questionnaire which offered the opportunity to make comment and critique the service.

A good Emergency Room must also be ready for large-scale accidents, and since these are not everyday occurrences, it practices by holding occasional disaster drills. The Bradford Building fire on November 12, 1957, had proved the point. Two tenants died at the scene, and five firefighters, three tenants and an onlooker were all brought to the hospital injured or unconscious from smoke inhalation. A prearranged plan brought in seven physicians and several off-duty nurses and orderlies.

The crude but obviously workable plan then in effect was bolstered shortly thereafter by a JCAH requirement for a more structured approach. The resulting Disaster Committee, Drs. Lundberg and Ross plus Administrator Vye, working with the Police and Fire Departments, began a process that continues to the present day. By July 1961 the first formal Disaster Plan combining the hospital and local Civil Defense Unit was in place. Practice drills became part of the program two years later. Although a far cry from the realistic drills that were to follow, these at least gave the doctors and other staffers practice in responding to the telephone network calls for mock assistance.

More effective mobilization was possible in the expanded facilities after 1972, and subsequent drills that added police and fire participation proved their value in two real-life incidents. The capsize of the thirty-eight-foot *Aquarius* out of Portsmouth, New Hampshire, caught in a sudden snow squall off Annisquam on December 21, 1975, left one dead, two missing and three survivors at the hospital. The subsequent mobilization not only tested the disaster plan but showed the need to include the Public Relations Department to cope with eager newspaper and television reporters. A more serious incident occurred in January 1977 when the coastal tanker *Chester Poling* broke in two and sank off Dog Bar Breakwater. Again the planning paid off, with the P.R. people better prepared for what turned out to be far wider and more aggressive media coverage.

These two incidents demonstrated that drills must go beyond mere mobilization of staff. Realism including all outside units was seen to be essential. The first of these drills, a simulated tourist bus crash, was held May 15, 1979 complete with stage makeup wounds, designated injuries of many types, ambulances, police and triage stations on the scene and at the hospital. An educational success, it led to further refinement of the process, which again proved it could cope with such make-believe disasters as an explosion at Gorton's, a sightseeing boat collision in the harbor which brought the Coast Guard in as a participant, a plane crash on Dogtown Common and, in 1983, an ammonia leak at the Quincy Market & Cold Storage plant.

The city's ambulance service, a vital factor in accident or sudden illness, also changed in the early 1980s. Free service by city vehicles had been under question for several years, and it was thus no surprise when the issue came to a head in 1981. A tax limitation referendum, Proposition 2½, constrained municipal expenditures, and the Fire Department's well-trained and highly experienced Rescue Squad was among the services cut back except for emergencies. The hospital Trustees gave support to a proposal to charge a fee for ambulance use, offering to handle the billing for the city if that would help keep the service functioning.

The matter became moot in 1983 with formation of Beauport Ambulance, Inc., a locally owned firm. Beauport was able to offer EMT-trained ambulance staffs and would handle all nonemergency calls for a fee and act as backup for the Rescue Squad, which continued in use for emergencies and accidents. A brief liaison between the hospital and a larger off-Cape service proved unnecessary a year later as Beauport demonstrated its ability to handle the work.

Two other medical departments, Physical Therapy and Respiratory Therapy, each in being prior to 1970, came into their own during this period. Physiotherapy, to use an older terminology, had its first exposure here in 1929 following an ACS suggestion of its potential value. Dr. Harper E.

Whitaker, the Staff Roentgenologist and one of its early supporters, described its potential at a Staff meeting that September: "It may be used . . . in certain conditions not amenable to treatment by other measures . . . gastroptosis, arthritis, fractures [using] diathermy apparatus and the ultraviolet lamp." The Staff, however, had little interest in the subject, deterred perhaps by the ACS letter, which had also described the difficulty of finding qualified personnel.

Some ten years passed before the subject came up again, by which time nonmedical practitioners had demonstrated skills in therapy and massage and were anxious to add hospital-based work to their schedules. Requests for hospital affiliation by the local practitioners were received unenthusiastically by the Staff, and it was not until 1949, when three therapists were working on Cape Ann, that it began to acknowledge the possibilities. In December of that year it somewhat hesitantly granted all three the privilege of treating patients at the hospital under the supervision of the attending physician.

This arrangement continued until 1959 when Dr. Sydney S. Parker, trained in orthopedics and one of the few Medical Staff members with more than passing acquaintance with physical therapy, argued that "physical medicine is not well undertaken locally [and physicians need] education in it." He persuaded his colleagues to consider the establishment of what he called a physiotherapeutic department, and in March 1962, with space available in the old Maternity Wing after the 1956–61 expansion program, the Staff approved a Department of Physical Medicine and Rehabilitation with Dr. Parker as its director.

Rental of equipment and the appointment of Gertrude Cronin, a navy-trained therapist, followed. The fledgling department caught on almost at once and by October was performing 250 treatments each month at $5 each. During its first year it attracted 1,372 patients including five sent from Boston hospitals, among them many suffering from arthritis and the aftereffects of stroke, described by Dr. Parker as "the forgotten people left to vegetate at home." By 1963 the department had introduced a group therapy concept in which patients gained confidence by watching and talking to others; two years later the well-equipped unit was measuring and fitting "braces, supports and other appliances."

The Physical Therapy Department was firmly established by 1973, when Mordecai E. Berkowitz, MD, an orthopedic surgeon, joined the Medical Staff. Mrs. Cronin had a full-time assistant and an array of equipment — some of elemental simplicity, others modern versions of Dr. Whitaker's diathermy and ultraviolet light, and still others such as ultrasound therapy approaching sophistication. Despite this, Dr. Berkowitz, with more recent training and a wide experience, suggested that the department was not as current with modern practice as it could be.

It was a delicate situation. Dr. Parker and Mrs. Cronin, the department's founders, were still in charge but cooperated with the Staff's newly appointed ad hoc Physical Therapy Advisory Committee under Dr. Berkowitz. Dr. Parker, ready for retirement by then, took Honorary Staff status and moved to Florida in 1977. Mrs. Cronin stayed until 1979 when the Staff was advised that she had elected to take early retirement and was being replaced by a new Chief Therapist. She and Dr. Parker left a department that together they had brought from infancy to one which, during her last full year, had treated 6,693 patients. She was well deserving of the praise bestowed on her by the Staff as it officially acknowledged her departure.

The busy department needed more space and better equipment. Its needs became part of the planning for the expansion program then under way, and in that the hospital enlisted the counsel of Professor Norma Fisher of the University of Florida Physical Therapy Department. Professor Fisher, a native of Gloucester, was the niece of F. Burton Fisher, also Gloucester born, then living in Florida and nostalgic concerning his lifelong family ties to the area and its hospital.

The new Physical Therapy Department opened in spacious Steele Wing quarters in 1982. State-of-the-art equipment made it possible to add programs in sports medicine, pre- and postmaternity exercise regimens, industrial accident prevention and occupational therapy. By 1983 it employed a staff of five, which that year recorded 24,274 treatments.

Respiratory therapy (or inhalation therapy, as it was first designated) followed physical therapy on the local scene. Its earliest form, a simply oxygen tent used chiefly for coronary patients, had been in use for several years, but the first real step taken here toward establishment of the technique was in 1963, when the administrator was authorized "to purchase a positive pressure breathing apparatus" to be under the supervision of the anesthesiologist, Dr. Lloyd David.

By 1969, with recognition of the therapeutic value of the device, utilization had increased to the point where the Board found it necessary to "establish the position of Inhalation Therapist."

A year later the department staff numbered four and the Medical Staff was suggesting the need for a full-time physician to supervise the operation. By 1972 its eleven-person staff, still under Dr. David, was assisting post-surgery patients, the eldery and those with chronic lung problems, coronary patients and others. Its pulmonary function laboratory was analyzing arterial blood gases, and it was ready for more supervision than the busy Dr. David was able to supply.

Dr. Reza Dorrie, an internist with pulmonary experience, was appointed the first Chairman of the Medical Staff's Pulmonary Therapy Committee in 1972 and was the logical choice to become Director, a post he would be fully qualified to fill after a year of further training at Massachusetts General Hospital. He took over upon his return from that year in mid-1975 and was assigned office space on Prentiss II and given an enlarged pulmonary lab that could accommodate further diagnostic and treatment equipment. Six underutilized beds in the Steele I Intensive Care Unit were converted to respiratory treatment and care, and the hospital was then able to give its many chronic obstructive pulmonary patients — those suffering from emphysema, asthma and bronchitis — state-of-the-art diagnosis, treatment and care. It would shortly add a home-care capability with easily portable rental equipment, and by the end of the period it could point with justifiable satisfaction to its arrival at full maturity, with almost 36,000 treatments performed in 1983 alone.

By 1978 the Mental Health Center had well demonstrated the need for psychiatric care, but as a day-care facility only it could not adequately meet the needs of the more acutely ill. That need could, however, be served by an inpatient psychiatric unit, and the Medical Staff and Planning Committee opened exploratory discussion of the possibilities that summer. Despite concern over the financial feasibility of such a unit, other factors — community needs, inability to place patients elsewhere and the availability of space under a regional bed reduction program — favored the project. Under the urging of Dr. Cutter, by then Chief of Psychiatry, it gained Staff approval on August 10, 1978.[1]

It thus became part of the expansion planning and opened as a twelve-bed unit on the second floor of Webber House in 1981. Designed for relatively short stays, it was also among the first to admit non-voluntary patients. With its staff working closely with that of the Mental Health Center, it was able to assure complete psychiatric care within the community for all but the most severe cases.

The new unit suffered a severe blow in May 1982 when its Medical Director, Bruce A. Sayles, MD, was killed in an automobile accident. Dr. Cutter, retaining his post as Director of Outpatient Psychiatry, replaced Dr. Sayles, who was memorialized by his Medical Staff colleagues with the establishment of the annual Bruce Sayles Lecture, sponsored by the Continuing Medical Education program.

Two other services, maternity and pediatrics, had been going in the opposite direction as, with diminished utilization, they found themselves under constant pressure for regionalization by the North Shore Health Planning Council and state authorities. The maternity unit's struggle typifies the problem.

With 750 (a figure later increased to 1,500), births annually taken as the minimum to justify maintaining an obstetrical floor, the AGH, with 300 to 400 was an obvious candidate. There was no way to boost utilization by relying on the birth rate, however, and on a floor that must be kept free of infection and contagion, a solution was admittedly difficult. Partial solution was arrived at when, in May 1976, the Staff approved "clean" gynecological cases, those free of contagion, for admission to the Babson floor. Such cases fitted nicely with staff skills there, and their inclusion helped keep the unit viable. But the best justification for maintaining the service, which most effectively convinced the authorities, was to be found in Cape Ann's relative isolation and distance from other hospitals. This, plus the community's natural desire to have its children native Cape Anners, made it possible to keep the unit.

Development of an excellent prenatal program also helped. This had its genesis in 1970 when the hospital joined with the Isabel Babson Memorial Library in sponsoring an experimental four-session series under the direction of Ann Whiting, RN. A well-attended success, it was repeated three times that first year and became a regular feature, training both parents in all aspects of pre- and postnatal care. By 1980, still under Mrs. Whiting, the course had expanded to an eight-session format given four times or more a year.

Family-centered maternity training and care brought both parents and later even siblings into the birth event. By 1972 fathers who had participated in the course could attend the birth through labor and delivery. Fathers could also help care for the baby if the mother chose the "rooming-in" option, whereby the newborn stayed with her during the day rather than in the isolated nursery. Rooming-in also gave both parents an earlier opportunity to get acquainted with their child and learn more about its care under nursing guidance.

A homey birthing room was opened in 1983 to permit uncomplicated births to take place away from the institutional delivery room. Isabel Babson would have been pleased to see the old art of midwifery being revived as more mothers opted for the experience of natural childbirth with a nurse-midwife, a member of the obstetrical group practice, available to manage the procedure. By 1983 childbirth could, under some circumstances, be a twenty-four-hour procedure, with the mother up and on her way home after a single night at the hospital.

At the other end of the life cycle is geriatrics and its accompanying AND problem, which continued to plague the hospital. Senex House was born as a partial solution to those problems. Initial planning called for a four-bed unit on Steele II to be opened in early summer 1983. Expected to improve the quality of life for its patients while they waited in the hospital for nursing-home beds, it could also prepare them for transfer to the more active nursing-home type of care. The unit grew even as it was being planned and opened that June with twelve beds, a full-time nurse/director and a staff of eight. Available to it were occupational and physical therapists, a dietician, the Social Service staff, and a home-care worker to assist in development of self-care capabilities. Families were encouraged to participate in what was a significant departure from traditional hospital care.

Senex House, the hospital's short-term answer to the need for elder-care, was proving popular with patients and their families by 1983. It was a first small step toward the eventual development of a hospital-oriented, full-scale extended care facility, a badly needed additional local nursing home, which was looming ever larger in the minds of the hospital planners.

Hospital social service as a specific function came into its own during the 1970s. A liaison between a hospital and its patients, it had its origins in Medicare, utilization review and the accompanying need for someone to expedite nursing-home placements. Such a person joined the AGH staff in 1966 as Patient Coordinator and coped with increasing elderly patient loads and the persistent AND problem for the next ten years. By that time the demands had become such that a qualified professional social worker was needed.

Gertrude S. Bartlett, then on the staff of Cape Ann Children and Family Center, was appointed to direct the new Social Services Department in 1976. Her immediate task, discharge planning for patients requiring continuing home or nursing-home care, required close coordination with physicians, nurses, the visiting nurse agency and all the professional departments at the hospital. It was a sensitive position, in which she was expected not only to prepare patients for a change from hospital care but also to provide emotional support to them and their families.

Outside agencies were also becoming factors in care of the aging. Among these was Senior Home Care Service, a private nonprofit group with a program of health maintenance in cooperation with the visiting nurses. Its adult day care program, established in 1983, further addressed the increasing need for care of an aging population, and its hot midday meals delivered to the homebound or available at its Main Street headquarters complemented the hospital-based Meals on Wheels program of daily noontime delivery of meals to shut-ins.

Direct home health care was given by the expanding Gloucester District

Nursing Association. In 1973 it and the hospital established a cooperative training program for home-worker health aides. The district nurses also assigned a coordinator to work with the hospital staff in postdischarge planning and placement of nursing-home-eligible patients. By 1976 the GDNA had become Cape Ann Community Nursing Associates, flourishing under a working relationship with the hospital and Dr. Fiero, who served as medical liaison. Today, following a 1979 merger into the Visiting Nurse Association of the North Shore, the agency is even stronger, a key member of the Cape Ann health care team.

Some Problems of Privilege

Among the areas where Trustees and Staff work together is the granting of hospital privileges, a jealously guarded prerogative that can sometimes lead to problems. The Staff examines each applicant and makes a recommendation to the Board, which then conducts its own study and makes the final appointment. Usually the two bodies have no difficulty, but every so often there is a depature from the norm, sometimes involving an applicant who does not appear to meet Staff standards or, more rarely, a nonmedical specialist seeking hospital privileges.

The 1974 application for podiatry privileges is an example of the latter. Podiatrists are not MD degree holders, so when Dr. Francis Powers of Gloucester requested Medical Staff membership permitting him to admit and treat his patients at the hospital the response was sympathetic but cautious. The general feeling was that "it is unwise to admit someone to an overlapping practice [such as surgery] who is not as well qualified [medically]," and the application became the subject of intense debate. The issue was further complicated the next year by a similar inquiry by two more podiatrists and by the Staff's discovery that no other hospital closer than Boston granted such privileges.

By March 1976, after a year of discussion concerning limits of treatments and the long-standing bylaw restriction of privileges to MDs and dentists, the Staff was leaning affirmatively toward the appointment of one of the three applicants, Dr. William Edgerton, whose credentials were excellent. Encouragement was also offered Dr. Powers and Dr. Sylvester Smith, and amendment of the bylaws to permit limited appointments was under consideration. A special committee of the Staff held several meetings with the applicants in an effort to reach agreement, but two years passed without resolution of the issue.

The old bylaws did permit affiliation of podiatrists as Allied Health Personnel (AHP), a category that offered no admitting privileges but which allowed treatment at the hospital under medical supervision. Dr. Edgerton, however, chafed under this restriction, believing that his training and experience deserved better, even to the point of performing surgery under general anesthesia. It was an unresolvable impasse further complicated by American College of Surgery rules that made it impossible for a relatively small Medical Staff to monitor advanced podiatric practice. Although Dr. Edgerton's AHP status lapsed, he continued a practice at Cape Ann Medical Center. Drs. Powers and Smith also continued their Gloucester practices.

AHP affiliation surfaced again in 1983 in granting Medical Staff status to licensed PhD level psychologists. Needed to perform testing and counseling in a new psychiatric inpatient unit, they were granted limited privileges to work under supervision by the unit's psychiatrists, all fully qualified MDs.

A privilege issue of a more common type was that which followed the September 1977 application of Dr. Ottfried von Waldenberg, a graduate of a Canadian medical school. His family practice in Rockport had attracted a considerable following, and he needed privileges to allow him to admit his patients who might require hospital care. His first meeting with Medical Staff members raised questions, most of which concerned his training and qualifications.

Data submitted subsequently were found to be incomplete to the point that his application could not be reconciled with bylaw requirements. Worse, his references did not respond to requests for further information and there were flaws in his credentials. Despite these information gaps the Staff Council voted in April 1978 to pass the matter along to the full Staff, which further evaded the issue by voting to forward the application "without recommendation or endorsement" to the Board of Trustees. On advice of its Personnel Committee, the predecessor of today's Professional Affairs Committee, the Board returned the matter to the Staff Council for continued research and documentation.

The facts, when they came out, were devastating. Von Waldenberg had been convicted and reprimanded in Newfoundland for submitting inappropriate charges to the Canadian Medical Care Plan and for false statements on his application to practice there. The Maine Board of Registration had refused to license him for falsifying his application. Von Waldenberg's request for privileges to the AGH was judged faulty in its failure to disclose these matters. Meanwhile he had continued and expanded his Rockport practice with his patients apparently liking him but puzzled at his inability to have them admitted to the hospital. Staff members who admitted and treated his patients in the hospital were further concerned as to the apparent quality or appropriateness of his treatment method. But until all the facts were in and his application for Staff membership processed, public comment or judgment as to his competence was impossible.

His request for further review in January 1979 was withdrawn to await a finding by the Massachusetts Board of Registration and Discipline, which some months later issued a somewhat ambivalent report. A series of meetings during the summer of 1980 with a special Staff committee were called "cordial" but were inconclusive, with no compromise possible in view of his history and his inability to reconcile what he described as "the difference between Canadian and U.S. practice."

The long period of discussion and study ended in 1983 when Dr. von Waldenberg decided to close his Rockport practice. Although not all the questions had been resolved, the Staff had done its best to accommodate him and his patients within the scope of its rules and its concern for the practice of good medicine. It is to the credit of all involved that the issue was one of standards and a refusal to compromise a commitment to them.

Another aspect of medical privileges, that of delineation or definition of their limits for each doctor, is directly connected to the trend toward specialization. This first received major attention here when a new Staff rule required each member to define his or her own limits of practice by stating a primary specialty and listing which of the many subdivisions within that specialty were included in that practice. Under pressure by the JCAH and sensing that concurrence might be a defense in case of litigation, all Staff members were soon in compliance. Strict delineation of privilege became an aid in making and renewing Staff appointments, and all applicants must now submit such definition before approval. They also became elements in a maturing peer review process.

Peer Review

Medical peer review has existed informally since the beginnings of medical practice as doctors critiqued the performance of their colleagues, sometimes privately and on occasion more publicly. We have seen examples of it here previously, but it took a long step forward at AGH when, in 1950, the Staff noticed that a high percentage of excised organs and other surgically removed tissue did not show significant pathological changes from the norm. Staff concern at this discovery led that same year to the establishment of a Tissue Committee. A unique concept at the time, with only one other known to have been formed (in New Jersey), it was a pioneering step toward formal medical quality review. The committee's charge was to review all surgical specimens (removed tissue and organs) that showed no abnormalities, and, if the case record revealed no mitigating conditions, to discuss the case with the physician involved.

Dr. Lawrence Ross, its first Chairman, would fill the post for the next twenty years. The Staff seems to have accepted the concept easily, perhaps, as Dr. Babson once observed, because they saw it as being directed chiefly at the surgeons. Indeed, one immediate result was a reduction in the number of older men who, without a regular surgical practice and often with little retraining since medical school, were allowed to perform in the operating room.

The committee's value became apparent with its first full year report in 1952. During its first year, covering six months of 1950, of 281 cases studied, ninety-four (33.4 percent) showed no pathology (abnormality), and of these, thirty-seven (13.2 percent of the whole) were described as not clinically justified. By 1952, of 517 cases studied, seventy-three (14.1 percent) indicated no pathology, with a mere twenty-eight judged unnecessary. The committee was further encouraged shortly thereafter by a JCAH survey that gave the still unique concept high praise and adopted it as a model for others to follow.

Ten years later fewer than 2 percent of 699 cases showed no pathology with only one of these called not justified, a record described by Pathologist Nickerson to be "as good as any of our country's best operated hospitals." Improvement continued, and in 1975, when the committee was absorbed into the work of the new full-time pathologist, a final report showed a single unjustified case among 2,474 surgical procedures studied. This record has been maintained under Dr. Cornetta and demonstrates excellence by any standard.

The first Peer Review Committee for oversight of the entire Staff was appointed in May 1971, with Dr. Hamer Lacey as Chairman. During the next year it established a program to review a series of specific illnesses as an educational tool and as a "measure [of] the quality of care given at this hospital and compared with other hospitals." By 1973 it was regularly reviewing the work of all physicians prior to annual reappointment, and by 1976, when it became the Medical Care Evaluation Committee under Dr. David Sauer, it was examining applicants' credentials, monitoring attendance at committee and clinical meetings, and in general probing and analyzing the overall quality of care.

The new committee, basing its procedure on techniques devised and recommended by the JCAH, was expected to report six times a year to the Medical Staff and Trustees. Each report was to cover a different medical field and to be based on the study of several cases within that field. Variances from established norms could be pointed out and in many cases become the subject of future Staff education programs. The Trustees as well as the Staff recognized its value as a safeguard in the face of an increasingly litigious climate as the 1970s closed.

Concern over the trend toward litigation led to further JCAH recommendations for more stringent quality assurance standards. In 1981 the Medical Evaluation Committee was replaced by a joint Quality Assurance Committee to be chaired by a Trustee and employing a full-time coordinator. The Board, aware of its own responsibility and liability, had also established its own Professional Affairs Committee for examination of applicants for Medical Staff membership and of Staff members' qualifications prior to annual renewal of privileges. The two committees were charged with "vigorous review of physician privileges, practice, performance and continuing abilities."

Continuing Medical Education

The commitment to medical excellence was also reflected in a recognition of the need for continuing education. Like peer review, ongoing learning dates back to the earliest days as physicians discussed their cases in doctors' lounges or in the corridors of the hospital. A more formal sharing of experience through monthly discussion of all deaths in the hospital was begun here under Dr. Thomas Conant, who chaired the Medical Board until 1915. Though well intended, these discussions suffered from a lack of what Dr. Mooring called depth and substance and, until autopsies were more routinely performed, were indeed often inconclusive. Periodic discussions continued spasmodically until 1947 when the Staff, urged by Dr. Babson, decided that more could be gained from a study of interesting or unusual cases where the patient had recovered, eliminating discussion of all but nonroutine deaths. This concept, encouraged by the JCAH, continued and, with the addition of outside speakers and films, improved into the 1960s.

Medical society meetings offered another opportunity for the sharing of information and experience, sometimes in the form of "papers" but more often in one-on-one conversation. Drs. Babson and Ronald Hallett, for example, were instrumental in 1935 in promoting clinical reports as an agenda item when it became, once each year, this hospital's turn to host a meeting, usually featuring a lobster dinner, of the Essex South District Medical Society. Such report programs caught on and were frequently presented here and elsewhere until the sixties, when specialization and the need to devote more time to discussion of developing socioeconomic trends – Medicare, malpractice and the like – made them no longer feasible.

The conscientious doctor, realizing that things were changing and that what he didn't know was not going to help his patients, also made an effort to keep up with advances through independent study – reading medical journals, attending specialty or general medical meetings and taking seminar courses at one or another of the nation's medical schools.

The 1960s brought a general realization that medicine was advancing so fast that a more formal approach to continuing education was essential. The first Postgraduate Medical Institute (PGMI) of the Massachusetts Medical Society was established in 1965 to supply speakers and work materials to hospital medical staffs. An initial session was held at AGH that October with others scheduled monthly thereafter, funded through an annual $25 assessment on each Staff member. Attendance was optional, however, and the seminars may not always have reached some who needed them most.

This problem was partially corrected by a 1972 vote by MMS requiring fifty hours annually of formal continuing medical education in order to remain a Fellow of the Society. Further impetus was provided by a state Board of Registration requirement for fifty hours of approved credit study for annual relicensing. The big step forward came in 1974 when the MMS formed its Committee on Continuing Medical Education to guide individual medical staffs and to replace the old PGMI format.

The AGH Staff was quick to take advantage of the opportunity to improve its own program. With enthusiastic Trustee approval of "an expanded continuing education program" and with Dr. Babson's appointment as Director of Medical Education, the local program was in place by December. In March 1975 it became one of the first five Massachusetts hospital programs to be accredited with "approved status" for one year. As the Staff proudly informed the Trustees, "the body of surveyors were quite impressed with what we have done."

The hospital's Continuing Medical Education (CME) program was firmly in place the next year, offering two sessions monthly with local and outside speakers. Its program credits were acceptable toward mandatory government educational standards, and it was recognized with a two-year accreditation. It was further honored that year in being selected one of three cosponsors of a major symposium offered by MMS to promote wider establishment of similar programs. In 1978, when there were forty-three CME programs in the state, it became one of the very few granted the maximum four-year accreditation.

Dr. Douglas Fiero replaced Dr. Babson as director in 1978, and it was again awarded full accreditation in 1982. An excellent ongoing program had found wide acceptance as one that, together with regular credit participation in out-of-town seminars, could offer assurance that the people of the community were being cared for by men and women who themselves cared enough to be the very best.

The Medical Library

A good educational program requires a good library. In its earliest form here the Medical Library, a small, miscellaneous collection of books at the start, was hampered by lack of space, and most doctors probably relied on whatever texts were available to them in their own offices. The first mention of the subject, in 1900, notes that "several valuable books were added to the medical room by purchase from the fund donated by Dr. E. S. Eveleth . . . Gray's Anatomy, colored plates $6.40; Atlas of Operative Surgery $3.50; Stinson's Fractures and Dislocations (2 vols.) $6.00; American Textbook of Surgery $8.00."

Beyond that, except for occasional mention of periodicals available, there is no record of activity until 1942, when the first Library Committee was appointed. It can be assumed that there was a fairly active library at that time, as the committee chairman was directed to "interview the Superintendent regarding missing books from the staff room," but a first-time assessment of $3 per member voted February 12, 1942 suggests that its growth had been slow and its control somewhat haphazard. Better facilities were available at Salem Hospital, which shared its library under its Hospital Community Plan of 1945 and continued to do so after the breakdown of that Rockefeller Foundation venture. But also, by 1949 the AGH Library Committee could report the purchase of magazine and book racks and the start of a planned book purchase plan, which made the use of the distant Salem library less essential.

Annual assessments of $5 by 1956 hardly allowed more than minimal acquisition, however, and in any case space in the Doctor's Room, relocated in 1934 to quarters now occupied by Administration, was limited. Despite these limitations, the 1957 appointment of Dr. John Gale as Library Committee chairman proved to be a major turning point. Encouraged by a $548 Friendship Fund grant designated for the library by the family of Murdock MacInnis, he increased the assessment to $10 and proceeded to update the collection to the point where a year later the *Annual Report* was able to describe "a marked modernization of our medical library . . . so we have up-to-date reference books and journals in every field of medicine."

Construction of a new Doctors' Lounge and Library as part of the Babson Wing program in 1961, plus a $1,000 fund established by the MacInnis family, gave major impetus to library development. By 1964 its size required cataloguing, with assistance by Gloucester's Sawyer Library staff, and four years later it was designated one of eighteen New England hospital libraries to participate in a Core Library concept developed by Harvard Medical School and the PGMI. The appointment of a librarian/medical staff secretary in 1969 provided control for the expanded facility which improved further with a National Institute of Health grant of $3,300 in 1971 to install a Nursing Core library and enlarge the earlier PGMI core.

Other gifts followed, among them one by the Isabel Babson Memorial Library for books on obstetrics, and by 1977, when he resigned as chairman after twenty years of almost continuous service (he had been replaced by Dr. Robert Kline for a brief period between 1967 and 1974), Dr. Gale could look with satisfaction at a fine medical library. Open to nurses and technicians as well as physicians, it was serving well as a source of information for all who wished to avail themselves of it.

Medically the seventies and early eighties had been a time of increasing diligence in maintaining standards, for conscientious self-examination and reeducation and, to the satisfaction of all involved, for relative harmony among Trustees, Administration and Medical Staff. The well-trained and respected Administrator regularly attended the monthly meetings of the Medical Staff and its Staff Council. The Joint Advisory Committee, a combination of Staff and Trustees, met regularly to discuss and recommend in the many areas of shared concern. And, a small but significant indication, the Medical Staff Annual Dinner gave way to joint affairs, well attended by Board and Staff members socially on a common ground. As the period closed, the Staff continued to seek improved communication with Administration and the Board of Trustees. It was a better relationship, but not yet perfect.

NOTES

[1]Dr. Cutter was replaced as Chief of Psychiatry by Danuta Stachiewicz, MD in 1983.

14

Hospital Management and Personnel

THE SCHARFENSTEIN management style was quite different from that of his predecessor. Tucker Vye can be seen as more of a "loner," only infrequently meeting with his administrative staff and seldom seeking input from it. He tended to allow each department to perform on its own while holding himself ready to intercede if performance did not meet his standards. Although he began to meet more frequently with his top divisional managers after 1971, before then it was chiefly at JCAH time that he conferred with them or with department supervisors. His method was one of delegation, but it faced the risk that coordination would be lost. It was a method that worked well in a less complicated day but no longer sufficed under a growing list of new rules and outside influences.

Ted Scharfenstein, on the other hand, while also a delegater, tended to keep a firm hand on the tiller. He established weekly meetings of his divisional managers, the Administrative Council,[1] and also met each month with all department heads. In establishing this program of regular meetings he hoped to improve interdepartmental communications and coordination of effort wherein each component of the chain of command had familiarity with the operation as a whole and could better understand how his or her department's function fitted in. Each divisional head was further expected to meet regularly with subordinate department heads within the division, and these in turn held at least monthly meetings with the members of their departments.

Was it an effective method? By the standards of the seventies and eighties it met the demand for an informed management, and, insofar as possible, it helped avoid surprises. It was a more open management method, which would appear a factor in the general improvement during this ten-year period which, to everyone's concern, did not open comfortably.

Management

Fiscal 1973 had closed with the largest operating deficit in the hospital's history. The $5 million budget for the year to come set another record high. Creditors' demands and rising prices had forced further borrowing from outside and from endowment, and, since hospitals remained under price controls after the rest of the business community was freed of them, it was impossible to adjust rates. An entire nursing floor had been closed due to persistently low census figures, which created further income problems, although it made some staff reduction possible. The year 1974 was also a time of economic recession, made more uncomfortable by energy shortages instigated by a newly confident Arab-led oil consortium. It was, taken as a whole, not the best of times for the new Administrator.

High among his priorities was correction of the precarious financial situation. In May he announced a more aggressive collection procedure calling for submission of delinquent accounts to a collection agency after ninety days. Room rates, freed of federal controls on April 30, could be brought more in line with costs, and at its May meeting the Executive Committee recommended an increase of approximately 10 percent. A further $4 increase that autumn brought all private rooms above the $100 per day rate for the first time. By then, too, the census was back to normal, but with only slight relief for the cash pinch.

The holdover state Medicaid backlog demanded constant pressure on the Department of Public Welfare, and such efforts reduced it to $158,000 by July, after the state resorted to a bond issue partially enabling it to meet its multimillion-dollar obligation to hospitals, physicians and pharmacies. This problem was to continue through the balance of the seventies.

Opportunities for possible economies were constantly sought. A new inventory-control system, initiated by Tucker Vye, plus cautious buying showed results by October. So too did an energy-saving effort through more efficient boiler operation and control of heat loss. The use of disposables, common since the sixties, was curtailed, especially in anesthesia and respiratory therapy. A new food distribution system authorized in late 1974 was expected to reduce staff requirements and amortize its costs within the first year, and new delivery carts the next year not only improved the quality of patients' meals but saved another $20,000 a year.

The "every little bit counts" theory was effective. Although preaudit predictions of an end to red ink proved somewhat optimistic, 1974 closed with an operating loss about a third of that the previous year, and after "other income" was added in showed a small net surplus for the first time since 1960. Scharfenstein described the year in his first annual report: "[It] was a difficult one at best [but] much has been accomplished and much remains to be done."

During that first year he had gained the respect and confidence of the Trustees and Medical Staff and was then able to concentrate more on long-range plans. A $6 million budget and a rate increase were made necessary by the continuing national inflation, but by then the Trustees could face the need for higher room rates with greater equanimity. A $5.00 increase, carefully documented for the new Massachusetts Rate Setting Commission, was approved in November, and these were to become almost automatic each year from then on as costs of goods and services escalated. The AGH budget ballooned along with everything else and by 1983 had reached almost $17 million with a private room costing $190 a day, too high in the minds of many, but necessary and even then lower than all but one other hospital in the immediate area.

It helped that utilization remained high throughout 1975. Although made less attractive by continuing collection problems and slow pay by the heavily involved third parties, the 40,275 patient days that year were a new high. This trend carried into 1976 when the Trustees could feel satisfaction, until they realized that many of these patients were part of the troublesome AND problem, on another record of 42,723 patient days and an 81 percent average occupancy rate. Such high utilization perhaps kept the financial situation from being worse but could not offset inflation and slow pay for services. Fiscal 1976 closed with a record $486,616 operating deficit.

Continuing inflation, the need to maintain a competitive level of wages, a cut in Medicare reimbursement, the higher cost of borrowed funds plus an unpredictably fluctuating census all combined to intensify the cash flow problem during 1977. With accounts receivable at $2,300,000 by October, more than half of which was from third-party payors, it became extremely difficult to meet suppliers' bills and the payroll. Staff was reduced, two nursing floors were closed, inventories were reduced to starvation levels, and even coffee service for the seemingly endless series of meetings was eliminated.

Fiscal 1977 came to its September 30 close with a shocking operating deficit of just over $1 million, on a total budget of $8 million. That highly unwelcome record was bad enough, but a hastily called special meeting of the

Executive Committee on October 6 was to cap even that climax.

The session opened with a statement by Treasurer Harvey H. Bundy that he had learned only the day before that federal and state withholding and Social Security taxes totaling some $500,000 had not been paid since early May. His shocking disclosure, which had been discovered during a routine conference with Controller Lewis S. Chase, indicated that the failure to pay was a decision made without consulting anyone by Mr. Chase, a member of the staff since his appointment as Accountant and Office Manager in 1959. Bundy further revealed that an Internal Revenue Service agent had already scheduled a visit for the next day, the purpose of which had not been given but doubtless involved an investigation into the tax nonpayment.

The agent's visit on October 7 was made easier by the fact that hospital authorities could communicate their awareness of the problem, concede its existence and state their determination to correct it. The agent advised that under the circumstances no criminal charges were indicated but that minimum penalties and interest, totaling 13 percent of the overdue amount from October first until payment in full, would be imposed. He made arrangements for weekly visits to assure that priority was given to back and current payments and placed a lien on all hospital assets pending full payment.

Lew Chase was permitted to resign on early retirement, and the hospital's public accountant was appointed Acting Controller. Collection of receivables was further strengthened. Staff layoffs were scheduled and pay increases postponed in an effort to generate cash. A dejected Administrator confirmed his ultimate responsibility as chief executive officer, although he had had no indication of his subordinate's failure to make required tax payments until it was revealed by Treasurer Bundy.

It is easy to lay blame for the fiasco on Controller Chase, but as Scharfenstein and former President Bill Webber agreed: "We are all partially at fault." There was, as Scharfenstein further conceded, "a breakdown of the reporting system to both the Administrator and the Board of Trustees [in which] decisions were made by individuals and not communicated to those in authority." For that Lew Chase can be faulted, but what he did was free of any taint of ulterior motive; he was simply doing what he thought would enable the institution to pay its bills, meet its payroll and, above all, remain solvent. His intent was good, but his method was wrong.

It is ironic – and perhaps excuses Lew Chase to some degree – to note that during this time the hospital was party to two suits against the state to recover funds owed on AND and Medicaid payments. The first of these had been entered by the hospital in late 1977 to collect $542,000 owed on back AND charges and the other as a class action suit by the MHA entered in May 1979 in an effort to speed up payment of back Medicaid billings. The state settled the MHA suit in 1980 after a new budget had been approved by the Legislature, and $280,000 was finally won in 1981 on the AND suit. Had it not been for the lack of these funds and other cash flow items, the Lew Chase affair might not have occurred.

By mid-December 1977 $105,000 had been paid the IRS under an arrangement which kept the hospital operating on a very strictly supervised cash basis.[2] Receivables had been reduced, a new post of Patients Accounts Manager was to be filled by year end, and an additional collateral loan pledging endowment funds was authorized. And of greatest significance, a young man named Brian F. Dealy was appointed Controller to take office early the next year.

Dealy was a product of the modern school of hospital financial management with a firm grasp of the need for internal control and accountability. In the mainstream of the computer age, he soon discovered flaws in AGH procedures and organized steps to correct them. Above all, he agreed with the Administrator that never again could the financial structure of the hospital be permitted to operate without a firm and knowledgeable director.

The long-standing accounts receivable problem was first to come under scrutiny. A continual review procedure with better follow-up of insurance and third parties and a new credit and collection policy with provisions for financial counseling of patients were in place by late that spring. Tighter personnel policies, especially covering vacation and time off, were installed, and better planning for wage and salary management was under study. A change of audit firm and more diligent Board surveillance brought sterner financial review throughout the year rather than merely at the close of the fiscal year. Unlike his predecessor, Dealy also knew how to deal with third-party payors and especially with the Medicare-Medicaid program. It helped further that, conceding the problems, Medicare was more promptly reimbursing documented AND cases.

The new financial management approach was effective. The collateralized $200,000 line of credit at Cape Ann Bank & Trust was canceled as no longer required in September 1978, when it was also noted that the AGH was believed well able to meet the terms of a statewide voluntary cost-reduction program negotiated between MHA and the Commonwealth. This conclusion was doubtless made easier by the fact that the hospital was by then skilled at making cuts and that costs had already been reduced to a bare minimum.

The year also showed an all-time high of 5,242 patients admitted, a figure not, however, reflected in total patient days because of a trend toward shorter stays. Of more importance, due in no small measure to better financial management, the year closed with an operating deficit of "only" $215,000 on an $8.5 million budget, a loss offset by a record high $353,000 from the always helpful "other income."

A report to the Trustees in May 1979 revealed what was described as "a strong cash position," permitting discounting of suppliers' invoices for the first time in several years. The positive financial condition continued to improve with careful monitoring of accounts receivable and the impact of the Board's departure from its traditional "break-even" philosophy and the establishment of a new policy that would henceforth budget an excess of operating income over operating expense. At year's end Treasurer Bundy could report that "it gives me the greatest of pleasure to present our financial results for 1979," with warm credit to the new Controller and his reconstituted Business Office staff. It had indeed been a good year, closing in the black for the first time in a decade with an operating surplus of $405,000.

The next year was even better, with $976,000 of back payments received from third parties and what the Administrator described as "benefits equivalent to $2.6 million . . . from settlements and improved management." Good management from then on could assure that despite regulatory strictures and further reimbursement reductions the hospital would continue to operate in black ink. Spurred by the requirements of a construction bond issued in 1981, which mandated a 1.5 to 1 ratio of revenue over expense, it did so each year through 1983 and for several years thereafter. Although Brian Dealy resigned in mid-1983 to take a similar post at St. Elizabeth's Hospital in Boston, his legacy of strict financial control remained.

Hospital Staff

A hospital's staff employees are its most important asset, and also its most costly in terms of its operating budget, with payroll at most not-for-profits accounting for between 60 and 65 percent of expense each year. Because they are vital to it, a hospital's employees must if possible be recompensed on a scale commensurate with their skills and at a reasonable parity with commercial enterprise and other hospitals. Ted Scharfenstein's prior experience had taught him this, and his philosophy called for pay increases at regular intervals based on an orderly plan with due regard for skill and performance.

With the worst of the financial problems behind him he could concentrate more effort on payroll and other "people matters." An MHA-sponsored "job description and equity compensation survey [which] will identify the differences in jobs and salaries within this and other area hospitals" was described to the Trustees in August 1978. The AGH share of this statewide survey was $3,000, and, taking it as a first step toward an improved personnel policy, the Trustees approved participation.

From it came a completely new salary program and an immediate adjustment in those job classifications judged too low in comparison with nearby hospitals. From it also came a program for establishing wage bases within the newly identified job classifications with periodic adjustments on a "step" basis ranging between 5 and 8 percent each year. This type of planning worked well in assuring predictable payroll levels and a sense of fair play to those involved. Because a "step" basis eventually tops out, the program phased out five years later, to be replaced in 1982 with a new classification schedule and a return to annual across-the-board adjustments.

The pension program of 1965 required amendment following enactment of the Employees Retirement Income Security Act (ERISA) in 1976. Broader coverage and greater benefits put in place that year actually went beyond ERISA requirements and kept the AGH plan in line with similar plans at neighboring hospitals. Employee discounts on hospital services and hospital payment of 70 percent of health insurance premiums were maintained, with dental coverage added in 1981. That same year a life insurance program for all employees was installed, with premiums within specified coverage limits paid entirely by the hospital.

The concern for employee health was further addressed in a policy originally proposed in June 1975 by the Medical Staff's Infection Committee. From that concept, assisted by pressure from the JCAH, came the Employee Health Plan (1978), which required Emergency Room examination in case of any injury or illness on the job and clearance, with health counseling if indicated by the Employee Health Nurse before return to work following an illness or accident leave.

Good employee relations go beyond pay and other material benefits. Recognizing this, in early 1975 the Administrator described to the Board his ideas for a service pin program similar to that of the Auxiliary. That November he presided over the first Employee Service Awards Evening at which 120 employees with service covering five to thirty years received pins engraved with the hospital logo and the number of years employed. Three, Martta Blanchet, nurse Ellen Coull, and Leona Mitchell, each with thirty years or more, also received engraved pewter bowls. Attended by family members and several Trustees, it was a popular innovation that became an annual event, complete with newspaper coverage.

The hospital family also came together in recreational activities. Christmas parties for all employees had been introduced in 1966. Held in the cafeteria with a tree and other decorations, they included a somewhat disguised employee Santa Claus invariably shown in a *Times* photo with a comely young lady on his knee. Further entertainment by a Nursing School choral group under Claire Chaffee's motherly eye was also a feature until 1977.

Christmas had been a rather special time at the hospital long before 1966. Brightening the season for patients brought outside groups in to decorate the corridors, with much activity by local garden clubs and the Auxiliary. The annual visit of the Gloucester Fire Department's carollers complete with treats distributed by their own Santa dates back many years, as do visits by church and club groups with everyone trying to make Christmas hospitalization as easy as possible.

An employee Activities Committee was formed in the mid-1970s to plan off-campus events. A clambake at Stage Fort Park in 1974 initiated a series of such affairs, which included dinner dances, shopping trips, bus tours, a softball team and an occasional float in Gloucester's annual Fourth of July Horribles Parade. News of employee vacation trips, marriages, babies and other accomplishments was covered after 1975 in a periodic bulletin coordinated by the committee and the hospital Public Relations Department. Retirement parties were encouraged, some as teas at the hospital, others as dinner parties at Cape Ann's several function rooms. Gifts and certificates of appreciation became the order of the day at these affairs, all of which offered respite from the daily routine and brought the family – Trustees, Medical Staff and employees – together.

The Nursing Staff

The nurses continued to be the dominant force among the employees. A growing sense of profession had become more evident as they increased their skills and were, when qualified, authorized to perform tasks once confined to physicians. This, together with chronic shortages and the consequent competition for their service, gave them considerable clout.

The need to maintain and improve skills was of high priority, and this had to be more than simple on-the-job learning by watching and doing. Organized inservice training had its start at AGH in a small program developed by Dr. Lloyd David about 1963 which, according to one of the nurses who recalls it, "would meet perhaps once a month if we could arrange it, and with his busy schedule we might have it two afternoons or at night." Among its teaching tools was the hospital's first Rescusci-Annie,[3] bought by Dr. David for his classes.

The benefits of this early course led in 1967 to a suggestion by Dr. John Gale for "a continuing teaching course for nurses" to augment the optional program, which by then included voluntary attendance at monthly Medical Staff clinical conferences. The Gale program was firmly established by 1969 and included off-campus course work in addition to that done in house, with attendance at out-of-town seminars encouraged and expenses partially underwritten by the hospital. The expanding program gradually acquired its own library of textbooks and films and gained further credibility with the 1971 appointment of the first Inservice Coordinator. In 1976 it was expanded beyond the nursing service to include orientation for new employees at any level, plus managerial training for department heads and other supervisors.

As the program grew, further financial support became essential. This was gained with help from a trust established many years earlier by Amos Story of Gloucester, who left a sum of money to be used in teaching "plain cooking and sewing, free to girls and young women who are residents of Gloucester." Changing times led to lack of demand, and the accumulation of unexpended funds had prompted its trustee to suggest in 1934 that such teaching could be done at the hospital's School of Nursing, a change of purpose in which the Probate Court concurred. When the school closed in 1978 the court approved a further change of purpose whereby all the trust income could be used to support the Inservice Program. The funds thus generated assured the hospital an outstanding program well supported by the Medical Staff and fulfilling its goal of more highly skilled employees at all levels.

During 1981, when inservice training was placed under a revamped Staff Development Department, the Medical Staff formalized what it called a "professional interface" with the nurses, which included seminars on professional topics, a patient care conference system and a generally better liaison between the two groups. The program was significantly enhanced in 1982 when the AGH was selected as one of three in Massachusetts to offer weekly evening courses at the hospital under the auspices of the Boston University School of Nursing. The program, in which B.U. faculty and others participated, granted credits toward the coveted Bachelor of Science (Nursing) degree and were open to nurses from other area hospitals. They were popular and ceased in 1987 only because B.U. eliminated its School of Nursing.

Hiring and keeping nurses remained a problem, exacerbated by the closing of many hospital nursing schools. Relatively low pay and the lure of easier and more lucrative career choices also reduced interest in the profession. Competition for nurses became more aggressive as hospitals of all sizes endeavored to maintain adequate staffs, with many forced to close entire floors during acute shortages such as that in 1979, which forced closing of the AGH subacute-care unit for several months.

Hospitals everywhere engaged in active recruitment with innovative steps beyond media advertising, much of which touted the attractions of a hospital's community along with opportunities for advancement and other enticements. The AGH held "Coffee and Dessert Nights" during 1979, the worst year. These were aimed at attracting nonworking RNs to return or at least to join the nursing pool, from which they could be called for part-time work as needed. The idea was effective, and the "Nights" were repeated during the next two years.

Unpredictable variations in census made the task of maintaining an adequate staff even more difficult. Although periods of low utilization and the tenuous financial situation through 1977 made it easier to operate shorthanded some of the time, the occasional extra heavy patient loads were severely taxing. At times, with the hospital filled to capacity, overtime work, double shifts and lost vacations replaced normal operating policy.

It was probably inevitable that this situation, coupled with what some nurses considered too low pay and lack of appreciation, led to an interest in unionization. Although in 1974 the National Labor Relations Board had brought all hospital employees under its jurisdiction, such interest lay chiefly with the nurses. A more natural target as an easily definable group, they also had the clout to make themselves heard. The Massachusetts Nursing Association, eager to enroll them and represent them with a united voice, soon began to make its presence felt.

In early 1980 a group of AGH nurses, already under pressure from the aggressively recruiting Teamsters Union, approached MNA for advice. Although lacking full support among their colleagues, they described gains made by the already unionized LPNs and cited low pay and what they viewed as unfair promotion practices in justifying their position. The sympathetic MNA, claiming to represent 13,000 nurses within the state, was eager to enter the arena. The NLRB agreed to hold an election in which a choice, yes or no as to affiliation, could be expressed, but only if a majority of the nursing staff joined in requesting it, a requirement they met in April 1980.

There the matter rested while the makeup of the bargaining unit was argued, MNA wanting only nurses in any unit it controlled and management holding to its belief that if a union must be established, it should cover a broader spectrum of employees. The issue dragged on amidst growing unrest, and, facing what they saw as a threatening situation, the Trustees sought guidance beyond that offered by the Massachusetts Hospital Association. They retained a professional counseling firm, Modern Management Methods, Inc., a no-nonsense, hard-hitting group specializing in labor-management relations. Enlistment of "Three Ms" was seen by the restless nurses as "union busting" and was surely responsible for growing antagonism, with charges and countercharges from both sides. Complicating matters even further, the nurses themselves were hardly unanimous, as attested by private statements and letters to the newspaper against the union.

The long stalemate over the composition of the bargaining unit continued through the summer and fall while the NLRB considered the matter. It finally broke in January 1981 with a decision for a nurses-only unit, and the long-awaited election was scheduled for February 6. Both sides increased efforts to convince what was perceived as a large undecided faction. When the day came and the ballots were counted, it was almost anticlimactic — the AGH nurses had voted down union affiliation by a vote of 79 to 33.

It had been an unhappy year, and both sides were equally relieved to see it over as they joined once more with a renewed sense of purpose and a desire for constructive harmony to replace the long period of recrimination and unrest. From the experience came the opportunity for the nurses to air their concerns, and from it also came the realization that what the RNs really wanted was status as health care professionals. That perception brought several changes, among them the move toward altered Medical Staff-nurse relationships. Communications between the two groups were further improved with the establishment of a joint Nursing Liaison Committee. Changes in policies dealing with job responsibilities, salaries, benefits and working conditions also proved beneficial. On the supervisory level, a system installed in 1975 that had given control to Clinical Supervisors was replaced by a return to the traditional floor-based control.

Among the LPNs, negotiations with the Licensed Practical Nurses Association had gone reasonably well through 1979, with wage levels the major issue. A change in that ten-year affiliation, however, came in 1980 when the Service Employees International Union (SEIU), a branch of the CIO/AFL, entered the scene. This group had for some time been successfully organizing hospital employees, and the independent LPNA, seen by many of its members as somewhat complacent, was an obvious target for a more aggressive approach promising more effective bargaining.

The local LPNs were among its targets, as the Trustees learned after a successful reaffiliation election in June gave bargaining rights to the SEIU. Contract negotiations that fall were rigorous and were held, in a break with past practice, at an off-campus location. It appeared obvious from the start that the SEIU hoped to gain stature by winning a large pay increase, while the nurses were more interested in terms that would give them professional recognition.

Negotiations that first year were protracted and often acrimonious and, after a hospital offer was turned down, moved toward threats of a strike. A tentative agreement staving off that action collapsed over the issue of professionalism, and, despite intervention by the Federal Mediation Service and further negotiations, the union issued a strike notice effective January 20, 1981. To the LPNs' credit and contrary to what their union representatives were saying, they stated publicly that they did not want to see the hospital closed, giving tacit approval of its plans to keep it staffed and operating.

Agreement was reached before the deadline. The settlement gave the LPNs the same increase in pay received by all other employees three months earlier and won them concessions on professional duties, greater access to inservice training and a stronger voice in nursing policy discussions. Other provisions of the new contract remained essentially as before, and, most important, it and the RNs' antiunion vote the next month restored peace.

Despite fears of difficult negotiations at the annual contract reopening the next fall, things remained calm, with federal mediators again present. Agreement was quickly reached with no change beyond ratification of the general wage increase already granted the other employees. The 1982 contract followed a similar pattern, although closing it took six bargaining sessions and renewed federal intervention. Negotiations were by then free of rancor and open antagonism, and subsequent contracts have been settled in relative calm.

NOTES

[1]The Administrative Council included the Controller (after 1977 called Director of Fiscal Services, becoming Director of Finance after 1982), the Director of General Services and Purchasing (after 1976 Director of Administrative Services), the Director of Professional Services (after 1976 Planning was added to this title), the Director of Nursing Services, the Director of Development and Public Relations, and, until 1977, the Medical Records Administrator.

[2]The federal lien was removed in July 1978 with the final payment to IRS. A balance of $30,000 still owed the state was paid shortly thereafter to close an affair that had been a serious embarrassment for all involved.

[3]A name describing the manikin used in demonstrating and teaching cardiopulmonary resuscitation.

15

Other Aspects of Hospital Life

Fund Raising and Bequests

GIFT SUPPORT, so long a tradition at the Addison Gilbert, continued to be a significant factor in the hospital's own health. Robert L. French, then Vice-President, had replaced Carroll Steele in 1975 as Chairman of the Development Committee, newly formed and separated from the Finance Committee in a bylaws change that year. The Annual Giving Program remained the keystone of the philanthropic effort, but under French would come additional and more sophisticated elements.

Perhaps the most important of these was introduction of an active bequest and deferred-giving program in 1976. This had its formal beginning that summer when a Wills Clinic was offered on a trial basis with Terry D. Mayo, a nationally known estate planning consultant, as lecturer. The success of the initial program led to two further sessions that fall during which the still enthusiastic summer audience explored the subject in more depth. It was the start of an educational program in which a three-session format was repeated annually, sometimes twice a year to meet what was correctly described as popular demand.

It was also for hospitals a pioneering approach to a subject that had long been treated deferentially. Just as the AGH had been an early proponent of formalized annual giving, so it was in estate planning, and in 1978 it was asked to share its experience with others by presenting a panel discussion

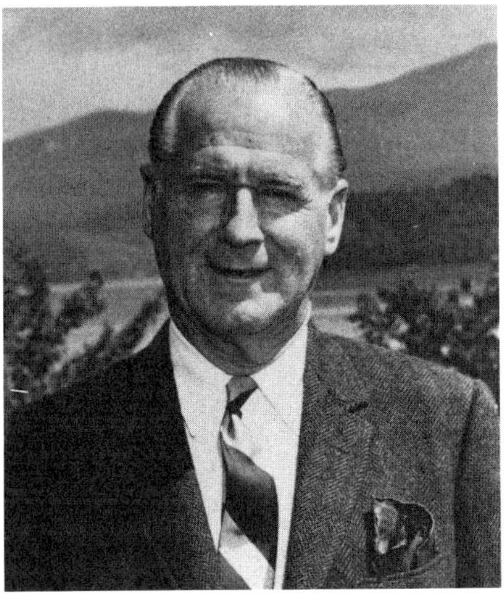

F. Burton Fisher's generous bequest at his death in 1980 made the Fisher Ambulatory Care Center a reality as a part of the expansion program of the 1980s.

at the annual convention of the National Association for Hospital Development. Many hospital fund raisers from across the nation later adopted similar programs.

The new program was a long step forward from the simple reminders that had been on the back cover of every annual report until 1974. Its success as a method can only be proven with time, but if interested and attentive audiences can be taken as a guide, then the estate-planning seminar approach was effective. It, like other forms of deferred giving, has been likened to an acorn – the one who plants it is not likely to sit under the oak tree's shade, but eventually someone benefits from its growth.

Additions to endowment in the form of bequests were significant during the period, although it was too early for them to have been influenced by the new program. Between 1974 and 1983 there were forty-one bequests totaling $1,063,036 plus two major unitrusts, one established by Carroll Steele and the other by his brother Quentin, with future benefits to accrue to the hospital. A single bequest by F. Burton Fisher of $750,000 in 1981, the largest the hospital had yet received, was an outstanding factor in that total.

Burton Fisher, "Bud" to his friends, was a Gloucester native who, though not resident here since his boyhood, never forgot his heritage. His grandfather was Sylvanus Smith, one of the original Trustees of the hospital and its Treasurer until 1904, when his son Horace succeeded him. In a long correspondence with hospital authorities during which his bequest planning developed, Mr. Fisher often recalled his family ties.

He had first contacted Tucker Vye in 1963 to broach the subject of a $100,000 bequest designated for construction of a facility adjacent to the hospital to assist those living alone in bridging the gap between hospital discharge and the eventual return home, an idea derived from his own bachelorhood and his hotel management background. As the years passed, during which government regulations became more restrictive and study of the original purpose made it appear infeasible, he continued to discuss ideas and enlarge his plans for future beneficence.

The hospital's need for new ambulatory care capabilities, plans for which were being developed by 1978 and included physical therapy, led to a mutually acceptable designation of purpose. The planned bequest, which Mr. Fisher later advised might go as high as $750,000, would be used for ambulatory care, and he warmly accepted the proposal that a new center should bear his family's name. And so it was that at his death in 1980 $400,000 was designated for the Fisher Ambulatory Care Center, then under way as part of the Program for the Eighties, with the balance put to the F. Burton Fisher Fund for the purchase of equipment for the new center.

It is perhaps possible to envision Sylvanus Smith's pride in his grandson's gift. And, although Mr. Fisher never mentioned it and, indeed, may never have been aware of the unfortunate affair involving his Uncle Horace, his beneficence can perhaps be seen also as a final, if unintended, act in that episode half a century earlier.

Two gifts of real estate made in early 1978 illustrate further the growing sophistication of the development program. J. Humphrey Wilkinson, a longtime summer resident of Rockport, made an unrestricted gift of his Eden Road residence in memory of Dr. C. Bruce Brown, who had died the previous year. With approval of the donor, the property was sold that summer for $146,000 and thus became one of the largest outright gifts recorded to that time. Another summer resident, Natalie F. Friend, offered a five-acre plot of undeveloped land adjoining the hospital property. The Trustees agreed to the conservation restriction she placed on the rock-strewn uplands bordering Route 128, and, although it gained no material benefit from it due to the restriction, the hospital was thus enabled to join the escalating movement toward creation of a "green belt" along Route 128 and in other parts of Cape Ann.

The AGH was also beneficiary of a unique form of gift support via the "Wishing Well," located outside the Pewter Shop on Rockport's Bearskin Neck. This annual presentation of a sizable coin collection had begun in 1962, and going to Rockport to pick up the weighty coffee cans full of pennies, nickels, dimes and quarters became something of a post-Labor Day event for the Development Office staff, which also had to count and carry them to the bank. The Wishing Well gifts, designated by the originator, for pediatrics had totaled $10,000 by 1974, and by 1983 a further $10,000 had been collected from what a *Times* story described as "that little hole in the ground over in Rockport."

The combination of so many efforts was without doubt a major factor in restoring the hospital to financial viability. A total of just over $5 million from all sources – annual and capital fund gifts plus bequests – over this ten-year span would put this small community hospital on a par with the largest. On a per bed basis it outdid many of them and set a standard for others of its size and type to strive for.

The enthusiastically perseverent French, never hesitant to ask support for a cause he knew was worthy, gained wider recognition of his unique talent in 1983. In voting him its annual award for Distinguished Service to Philanthropy that year, the New England Association for Hospital Development took note of the high standards set by the Addison Gilbert under his leadership. Never one to rest on his laurels, Mr. French reassumed the chairmanship of the Development Committee in 1986, after ten years as hospital President and Board Chairman.

The endowment portion of these funds, together with those from past years, had as always to be invested. The policy under which the Investment Committee made its decisions still held to the tradition of emphasizing preservation, with moderate growth, of capital, while providing necessary income. With just over $1 million entrusted to it, the committee, chaired since 1970 by former President Frederick (Fritz) Bundy, had sole decision-making power, using Cape Ann Bank & Trust and David Babson as advisors. By January 1980, when Mr. Bundy relinquished the chairmanship to his nephew, Harvey H. Bundy, the funds totaled $1,793,000.

Meanwhile in 1976 the law governing funds management was changed. Among other features it permitted trustees of charitable institutions to delegate investment responsibility to outside counsel and pay for such service, in effect relinquishing considerable power to professional managers. The revised law also gave trustees more flexibility in expending or accumulating income and capital and was, moreover, permissive only, leaving the decision for any change in method to individual boards of trustees.

Some members of the AGH Board had felt for some time that investment performance could be improved. In March 1982, when it was also facing the stringent financial requirements of a pending bond issue, they voiced that belief in voting to direct that "the Investment and Finance Committees report on investment objectives and the best means of accomplishing [them]." A joint meeting of the two committees conceded that the structure as established was slow and cumbersome in requiring approval by all Investment Committee members prior to portfolio decisions and suggested that perhaps power should be given to outside management, with monitoring by the committee. They also suggested "that in consideration of the long term relationship [of] the Hospital and the Bank, that [Cape Ann Bank & Trust] be selected for a one year period" as fund manager.

A problem with that proposal lay in the fact that Harvey Bundy was also a top executive of the bank. Recognizing the potential for conflict of interest, he stated his intention to resign as committee chairman when the bank became investment manager. He also stated his opinion that until the change was made his financial expertise would be of value in setting new policies and objectives. The Board, President French in particular, was unwilling to simply appoint the bank as manager in view of what was perceived as its less than satisfactory investment advice in the past. The bank could, however, be among those to be considered for the post.

Bundy defended the past performance by pointing out that, as a mature fund which under a long-accepted policy had emphasized long-term bonds rather than growth equities, the bank was to some degree locked into the situation. When compared with other, younger portfolios such a policy could appear less than successful, but even so, over a period of years, it had substantially tracked commonly accepted indexes. He argued that a balanced fund using "prudent man" guidelines in place for many years would never compare with a pure common stock portfolio. He could also point out that, during his brief time in office, the funds, admittedly with major assistance from bequests, capital funds awaiting expenditure and the hospital's then current operating surplus position, had grown to about $6 million. From his point of view he had done a good job, and, having pride in his capabilities, he took exception to what he viewed as undeserved criticism of himself and the bank. He resigned as committee chairman forthwith, and since he had already (in January 1982) been appointed to the honorary position of Life Trustee, the service of a dedicated hospital volunteer came to a close.

The situation appeared quite different from the Board's point of view, however. For years the hospital had been bank oriented, and many Trustees felt that the size of the portfolio required independence from such control. It was time, as Bob French describes it, to abandon "the pretense that a few local bankers could pick stocks in their spare time." The Cape Ann Bank though among the candidates was not to become investment manager for the AGH.

That appointment went to the Boston firm of Standish Ayer & Wood for management of the hospital's endowment. Similar management responsibility for the smaller pension plan funds had already been awarded to Gardner & Preston Moss., Inc., also of Boston. The Investment Committee retained the authority to set policy and give broad oversight to the portfolios, with day-to-day investment decisions left to professional management.[1]

The Hospital's Art Collection

Although not part of the hospital's formal giving programs, gifts of art over the years have resulted in a fine collection of work by Cape Ann artists. Such gifts had been made since the earliest days, but until the Thompson/Vye reporting system of the 1940s little was recorded, and the origin of many items is uncertain. Lack of records also supports the belief of many that some of the earliest pieces were damaged and discarded. We do know that Trustee Robert F. Brown attempted in 1972 to trace some of the more valuable pieces, with only partial success; the work he did was also the first attempt to appraise their value.

A few of the earliest acquisitions can be documented, however. There is mention in Board records of what seem to have been the first received, two paintings titled *Morning* and *Night* given by Mrs. Eleanor W. Rowe in 1898. Except for an oil portrait of President Charles H. Pew given in 1907 by his widow, there is no further mention of the subject until 1930. Even an unsigned museum quality portrait of Addison Gilbert has no documentation, although it is generally believed to have been part of his estate and is perhaps one of those he left to Sawyer Free Library or to City National Bank.

In 1930 John A. Cook and Charles Winter each gave a painting in support of the Prentiss House program. Cook made further gifts of his watercolors in 1932 and 1933, when Oscar Anderson also shared his work with the hospital. Other paintings during those earlier days were undoubtedly given to pay for a hospital stay, but again this is an assumption that lacks documentation. Several paintings were also given during the late fifties to assist the South Wing campaign, among them works by Anthony Thieme, Don Stone and Stanley Woodward.

The Depression era WPA program was another source of work by local artists. This public works program offered support to many unemployed citizens among whom, at this time when scarce money went for necessities and not for art, were many artists. Supported by government grants, they were encouraged to continue their work, which the program later distributed to appropriate institutions. The AGH received many by Cape Ann artists in this way. Prominent among those whose paintings still hang here are Bertha Baxter, Maude Berneker and Bertha Peyton.

It was only after Ted Scharfenstein became Administrator, however, that the work of Cape Ann artists was actively sought as a means of enhancing the decor of the hospital. It was he who, with a newcomer's appreciation of one of the area's unique assets, conceived the idea of a hospital gallery where artists could display their work, and from its opening in April 1977 the AGH Gallery was never without an exhibit, always for one month and most often consisting of "one-man shows." The hospital also gained as many exhibitors, after showing there, gave it a specimen of their work for its collection. This first gallery, somewhat cramped in the corridor off the Washington Street lobby, was replaced in 1983 by the Pat Maynard Memorial Gallery in the Fisher Lobby. Mrs. Maynard, a talented artist and ardent Auxiliary member, was thus honored by her artist husband following her death in 1984. Joe Maynard, himself to die the following year, was a Boston advertising executive and a dedicated AGH Trustee.

Other artists were encouraged to share their work with the hospital by Dr. C. Bruce Brown of Rockport. Dr. Brown, a self-described "Sunday painter" of considerable skill, had a working acquaintance with many members of the Cape Ann art colony, and some of the better paintings in the AGH collection were acquired during the seventies as a result of his gentle persuasion.

The entire collection contained more than 200 items by 1983 and included works by many of the best-known artists, past and present, who have called Cape Ann their home. Only once has a piece been sold: *Adrian*, an oil marine by MacFarlane, was relinquished in 1971 for $15,000, with which to purchase equipment essential to complete the Steele Wing Intensive Care Unit.

By far the most valuable item in the collection is *The Old Fort and Ten Pound Island*, a large oil by Fitz Hugh Lane. As is the case with others of the early acquisitions, the donor of this painting is unknown, although legend attributes it either to the estate of an unidentified benefactor or to the Prentiss family to be hung in Prentiss House. It did hang in the corridor there for many years, until Tucker Vye had it rehung in the Nurses' Residence for its protection. It was removed to the Cape Ann Historical Association in 1964 for display and security and has hung there on loan, part of the Association's own extensive Lane collection, since then.

Any asset as valuable as this painting is bound to raise questions as to the propriety of holding it, and, after interest was expressed by art dealers in 1979, it became the subject of intense debate by the Trustees. A committee, appointed "to consider possible disposition of the painting and to de-

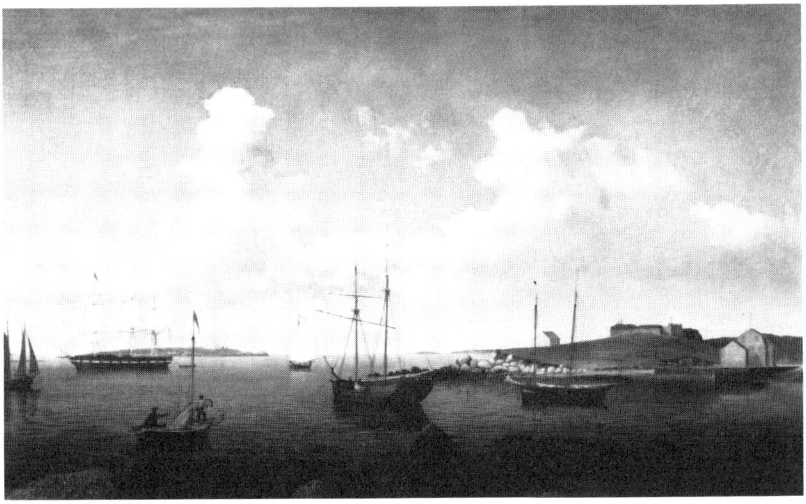

Among the best known and certainly the most valuable asset in the hospital's large collection of Cape Ann art is Fitz Hugh Lane's "The Old Fort and Ten Pound Island," known within AGH circles as "The Lane." It hangs on loan at the Cape Ann Historical Association.

velop a policy for unrestricted gifts of this nature," recommended "that at some point [the painting] be sold . . . proceeds [to be] used for capital expenditures." The report, presented to the Board on April 24, 1979, was discussed with considerable emotion and heat, one faction describing the painting as a Gloucester heritage to be retained while others more pragmatically suggested eventual sale.

Recognizing that the Board had considerable responsibility for control and management of "the Lane," which in January 1982 was appraised at $300,000, President French sought legal advice. Counsel's report made two major points: 1) that, lacking evidence to the contrary, the hospital was the outright owner and 2) that retention of the work, though not within the health care purposes of the hospital nor an income producing asset, was justified "as long as the Trustees believe in good faith that it is in the best interests of the Hospital to do so." It supported the compromise view later expressed by Mr. French that the painting be held "until the hospital stands in dire need of the funds that selling it would realize."

Advice in late 1983 of a pending offer that would net $400,000 to $450,000 revived the 1979 arguments, which subsided when the tentative offer failed to materialize. There the matter rested. The hospital still owns the Lane, and although sale may become necessary in the future, it meanwhile remains publicly displayed for the enjoyment of the community and art connoisseurs.

And in point of fact, even at its estimated current value it represents only a very small portion of the hospital's total assets.

Marketing and Public Relations

Competition among health care providers became much more intense during the 1970s and 1980s. The HMOs vied to increase their share of the market; walk-in clinics and "surgicenters" drew patients away from the physician's office and hospital emergency rooms, and hospitals themselves were attempting to expand their traditional service areas. Public relations took on a new aspect, marketing: the offering of specific services, wider territorial mailing lists and, once unthinkable, hospitals advertising their services in the newspaper or on television.

A good example of such aggressiveness appeared close at hand as Beverly Hospital began attempts to broaden its area coverage. Its 1979 acquisition of the closed Cable Memorial Hospital in Ipswich allowed it to open an emergency center there, with referrals and admissions naturally to go to Beverly. It also ran large display advertisements proclaiming its expertise in many Essex County newspapers, including that in Gloucester. Its Birth Center, a separate facility on its hospital campus, was promoted in this way and even on roadside billboards.

Some hospitals, Addison Gilbert among them, responded by expanding community programs already in place, with its Community Health Education Program a case in point. Although the maternity service here had long sponsored prenatal clinics, other aspects of preventive medicine through public education had not yet become generally known. The first tentative effort at AGH had been made in April 1974, when three nonhospital groups sponsored a health fair with participation by the hospital and other agencies, an event that was encouragingly well attended. By 1977, further encouraged by the success of an on-going hypertension clinic sponsored by the NSHPC, area hospitals were beginning to establish their own programs, among them the Heart Saver Program established here in 1977.

The Auxiliary formed a Committee for Health Education that year to study the possibilities, and the hospital, using a questionnaire, sought to ascertain public opinion as to the need and to garner ideas for program content. With strong support by the Medical Staff, the first seminar in the fledgling program was scheduled for October 1979. A panel discussion led by Drs. Fiero, Jedrey and Wedmore explored aspects of hypertension. That program was followed the next month by one on first aid by Dr. Gunn, and such discussions soon became a regular part of hospital activity, open to the public at no charge.

The idea caught on, with programs covering such topics as sports medicine, perspectives on aging, life-saving for pool owners, cardio-pulmonary resuscitation, poison prevention and treatment, Alzheimer's Disease, and several psychiatrist-led sessions. The first Health Works, a one-day free public clinic to screen and explore a variety of health problems, was held April 30, 1981. It was the first of several held statewide, proposed and sponsored by Boston TV Channel 5, WHDH radio, Shawmut Bank of Boston and the American Red Cross. This well-attended affair became an annual event, with one of its most popular features, a blood-pressure check, adopted in 1983 by the hospital as a no-charge weekly walk-in clinic.

A medical information service supplying taped commentary by telephone on more than 200 assorted health topics was established in 1981. This program, despite its good intentions and attendant publicity, never lived up to the hopes the hospital had for it, but it remains in place for those wishing to avail themselves of it. Newsletters and other printed material which put information directly in the public's hands were also widely used after 1981.

The establishment of satellite medical offices was seen as a means of gaining patients from Cape Ann's fringe areas, in particular Essex, Magnolia and Manchester. The first was opened in 1979 in Essex, after that town lost its only resident physician. The town offered to provide office space to any doctor or group wishing to open a practice, and, after negotiations with the hospital and members of the Medical Staff, it opened that spring. Shortly thereafter the Administrator was able to tell the Board that "the Essex office [provides] medical services to many individuals who [have] not seen a physician for a long time." The office was soon generating a good patient flow with admissions, if needed, coming to the AGH.

The *Annual Report*, since the earliest days a somewhat stodgy pocket-size booklet with limited distribution, underwent major changes under the new marketing program. It broke with tradition in its 1974 edition with a change of size, content and format. More important, it was distributed via the hospital's mailing list to some 6,000 residents of the area. Over the next ten years this annual exposition of hospital activities was further improved with professionally prepared copy and photographs.

A survey conducted for the hospital in the fall of 1981 stimulated further efforts toward achieving its recognition as a high-quality community asset. By suggesting the need for even more public exposure the survey was a factor in the improvement of all hospital publications. It also encouraged the use of the newly opened cable television network, paid newspaper insertions, a medical directory and a "Medical Emergency Handbook," and a further change in the hospital logo.

Other efforts to involve the community were initiated during this lively period. One evolved from discussions with the NSHPC concerning the Council's requirement for community involvement in planning for changes covered by the state Determination of Need program. As proposed during the first year of the active, hands-on French presidency, there would be a Community Advisory Panel which, in addition to meeting NSHPC requirements, could suggest health care needs and act as a sounding board for plans to meet those needs. As described by the Planning Council, the panel should represent the adult population proportionately as to age, sex, income and national origin, a mix that presumably could speak for those it represented. Suggestions for candidates were solicited from varied sources – city and town officials, residents, social needs agencies and industry.

Six meetings of the panel were held between July 1978 and February 1980 before it ceased to function. Although minutes were kept for only the first three of these, there seems to have been enthusiasm for the concept and considerable discussion of suggestions generated by the panel as well as the hospital. A questionnaire seeking ideas at the first session elicited many worthwhile possibilities, many of which later came to fruition. It was during these meetings that the Program for the Eighties received its first public airing as the panel learned of and endorsed the planning for it.

The Community Advisory Panel was, in retrospect, better in the concept than in the fulfillment. Able only to comment and recommend without power to act, it could not actively follow through and convert its proposals to reality. Irregularly scheduled meetings that later too often lacked content destroyed continuity and whatever sense of purpose it may originally have had. Such a function was perhaps not sufficient for its more knowledgable members whose early enthusiasm was overcome by frustration. To its credit, many of its suggestions were sound and led to changes, some of which might not have otherwise been made.

On a more intimate basis, opinion was also sought from those well-suited to offer it, the patients. A 1975 proposal for "a patient suggestion system" became a short questionnaire to be mailed after discharge to all house patients during one month each quarter, a system that sampled about a third of the patients each year. This relatively simple device, used for several years until replaced after 1983 by a patient's ombudsman program, brought favorable response as well as criticism and provided the basis for a number of improvements. A similar survey method later garnered comment as to Emergency Room service.

The Auxiliary and the Alumnae Association

The most involved affiliated group continued to be the Women's Auxiliary, but it also was changing. Although the activities and devotion to service that had always characterized it remained, outside influences relentlessly took their toll. Rarely able even in the best of times to muster a membership exceeding five-hundred, it watched its numbers diminish as the young women on whom it depended for new life and for volunteers increasingly turned to paying employment. Combined with home and family responsibilities, this made it difficult for them to assume other activities.

Despite losses, the women of the Auxiliary stuck to their sense of mission. Older members worked the Coffee and Gift shops, and these two profitable ventures continued to fund the never-ending series of hospital projects the group took on. The younger women chiefly performed the "Ways and Means" function, those events for which the Auxiliary had long been famous. Old standbys were carried on with occasional new ideas – fashion shows in 1976, 1978, 1979 and 1981; round-the-Cape "Booze Cruises" in 1982 and 1983; tours of the Newport, Rhode Island mansions in 1981 and 1982; golf and tennis tournaments and other one-time events – and these, although becoming more difficult to organize and staff, continued to add to the funds raised.

Direct service to the hospital continued and was reinforced. The sewing group, temporarily shut down a few years earlier in the first flush of the new Medicare rules, had been revived, and this service, the most senior of any Auxiliary function, continued to supply simple cloth items. In 1982, with the Fisher Lobby about to go into service, there was need for staffing at its information desk and for guides and escorts to augment the outpatient assistance group already functioning. The junior program was enhanced in 1979 when the Auxiliary awarded its first annual $500 scholarship to the graduating "Junior of the Year," and after 1982 junior members could also earn class credit at high school for hospital work performed after a period of training.

Efforts to increase the attendance and interest of younger working women led to a change in the monthly meeting format in 1977, when a noon luncheon preceding a short program replaced the traditional midafternoon tea with program. The recognition of volunteers was further emphasized in 1978 by replacing the annual recognition tea as a feature of one of the monthly meetings with a hospital-sponsored program recognizing all volunteers. And, in a milestone shift of emphasis, a new constitution adopted in 1979 changed the name to "The Addison Gilbert Hospital Auxiliary" and made men eligible for membership. This move, anticipated some eighty years earlier when an 1898 proposal to admit men was soundly defeated, was well meant but ineffective, as the men apparently had not found discrimination a problem.

By 1980 it was becoming increasingly difficult to find volunteers to staff the Coffee and Gift Shops and the various service functions. Some consideration was given to employment of a paid Director of Volunteers by the Auxiliary, but the women decided to continue on their own and save the money for their projects. Three years later, however, with volunteers needed in the new ancillary service area as well as in the two shops, the hospital itself employed its first Volunteer Coordinator to work independently of the Auxiliary. And with that the pendulum began to swing back as newspaper items and word-of-mouth recruiting brought both men and women to give a few hours of time each week.

These concerned people were no less dedicated than the Auxiliary women, but they were not members, and although the two groups worked well together, the fact that they were under separate control made coordinating their efforts difficult. It was not to happen for several more years, but change to come was presaged at a Planning Committee meeting in May 1983 when the opinion was expressed that "the Auxiliary and volunteers have gone as far as they can with their present structure."

In redefining the role of volunteers it was becoming inevitable that the Auxiliary and the nonaffiliated volunteer group must eventually merge. Whether this would mean the end of an organization which, like the Board of Trustees and the Medical Staff, is one of the hospital's roots to its past was open to conjecture. Were that to happen, however, one thing seemed certain – the hospital would be the poorer without the love and dedication of the women of the Auxiliary.[2]

Along with its larger, more affluent sister organization, the Nurses' Alumnae Association was also feeling the pangs of maturity. Except for the occasional addition of honorary members and a 1956 decision to open membership to registered nurses on the hospital staff, it had had no new members since the old school graduated its last class in 1949, and that membership was aging. It maintained its traditional supportive loyalty, with gifts to every building program (a room in Steele Wing bears its name in silent tribute) and regular, smaller gifts for equipment as needed. Its members had held a highly successful fiftieth reunion in 1964 and an equally good sixtieth ten years later, but by 1984, instead of planning for a seventieth, talk was instead of a predictable though unwelcome future.

In November 1984 the dwindling group held its last formal meeting, at which the members elected a final slate of officers in hope of continuing.

But they could only reminisce as President Edith Lord did eloquently in March 1987 in her final communication announcing the group's termination, summing up three-quarters of a century of service:

We can all look back with fond memories of the many years we had together . . . our meetings, social events, fund raising and our reunions. We can be proud that our nurses have gone on to hold key positions in hospitals, military service, industry and school and college health services. We can also be proud that we supported our hospital financially and by donating many articles of equipment when we were active and financially able.

And even in the demise of their association the alumnae made a final gesture toward the institution of which they had so long been a part. A nostalgic vote turned over their now small remaining treasury to the hospital as a last gift — or, in this case, perhaps, bequest. The Nurses' Alumnae Association will always have a unique place in the hospital family, and the modern AGH can do no less than say: "Thank you for all you've meant to *your* hospital."

NOTES

[1]At the close of fiscal year 1988 the endowment portfolio, still managed by Standish Ayer & Wood, totaled $14,637,702.

[2]The change anticipated in 1983 came on May 18, 1988 with the adoption of bylaws for a new organization, The Addison Gilbert Auxiliary Service, which replaced the ninety-year-old Auxiliary and combined it with the previously nonaffiliated volunteers. The new group, under hospital control, soon demonstrated its own value and dedication to its mission of service.

16

Bricks and Mortar

WITH THE NEW front entrance of 1972 stimulating thoughts of further improvement of the Washington Street side, the Trustees had to consider its landscaping. In 1975 it accepted the offer of the three local garden clubs to take on planning and execution of some of that work, to include building a small patio just south of the entrance. Two damaged spruce trees, all that remained of these given in 1919 by the Nurses' Alumnae Association (the others having been lost to hurricanes in 1954), were removed to expand the parking lot. Removal and replacement of some of the poorer shrubs and trees closer to the street, plus a program for annual flower planting around the circular driveway, completed the project. The front was further enhanced by the later addition of "Tony's Flagpole," given by his family in memory of Tony Freitas, a retired police boat skipper and an early member of the hospital security force.

Inspired by the work outside the building and needing more space for their popular Coffee and Gift shops, in 1975 the Auxiliary proposed changes to the upper lobby. Plans were prepared by Gloucester architect Donald F. Monell and $100,000 was pledged to fund their proposal. The switchboard/reception desk was shifted to a more practical location nearer the entrance, with an enlarged Gift Shop to occupy the space thus vacated. The Coffee Shop could then expand into the space released by moving the Gift Shop, almost doubling its capacity. Another part of the project entailed opening up and restoring the old original fireplace, paneled over years before, as a feature of a renovated waiting area comfortably furnished in a homelike setting.

One thing always seems to lead to another. The revamped lobby made the administrative area and its corridor look shabby. When removations were completed there in 1976, the Nursing Service offices had been relocated to West Wing (the old Maternity Wing), and Medical Records moved from West Wing to the eighty-year-old North Wing's second floor. The Administrator's office left the old operating rooms for larger and more attractively accessible quarters across the corridor. The North II floor was refitted as additional office space, and the decrepit old elevator serving all four floors there was completely rebuilt.

Renovation of the Pediatrics Unit followed in 1977 as the result of recommendations by JCAH. This $41,000 project, which revamped the entire South I floor and gave pedi a modern nurses' station, was partially funded by a $22,000 gift. Another renovation, which culminated in reopening the nineteen Prentiss House private rooms, was made possible by a major gift from Margaret Farrell Lynch, whose family had taken a benevolent interest in the wing since its beginning. Used for some time as offices and as quarters for the cardiac and respiratory services, it was restored to its original purpose in 1981 to replace beds taken over by the Psychiatric Unit. The renovations added private bathrooms, new air-conditioning and furnishings, complete redecoration and a life-support system for each room – and, in a prime example of the crew's ability, the work was done almost completely by the hospital maintenance department. Although the second floor was again closed under a state-required bed-reduction program a few years later, the first floor remains in use by patients preferring its small though attractive private rooms.

The closing of the nursing school in 1978 left the old residence available for other purposes. The Board had decided in September 1977 "to evaluate the building for purposes and use," and retained Don Monell to study it. A few months later, after a report that included the finding that the building was "sufficiently sound for meaningful renovations," plans were in place pending the graduation of the school's final class in 1978.

The second and third floors were converted for use by the Mental Health Center outpatient unit. Once again the Auxiliary came to the rescue, with a pledge of $100,000 in February 1980 for conversion of the first floor to conference and office space. When that project was completed a year later there were available a large conference room, seating more than a hundred, and two smaller meeting rooms, one on the first floor and the other in the basement in a former classroom. Office space was provided for the later

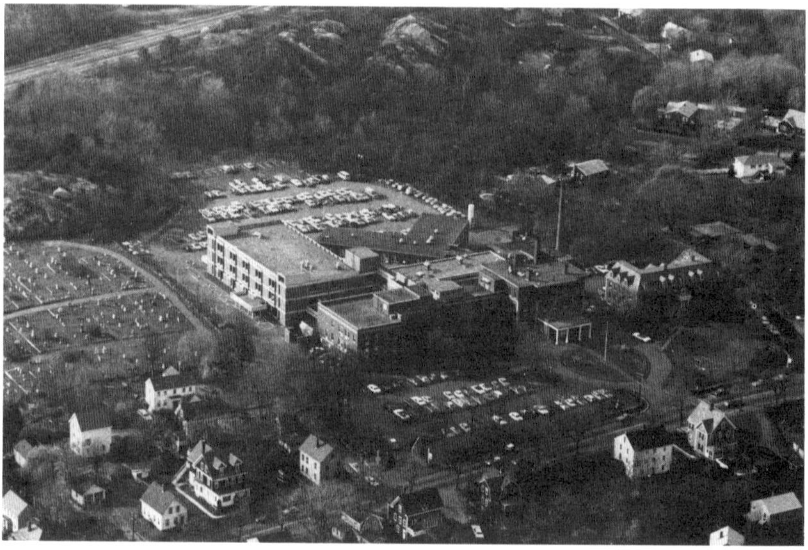

The AGH of 1980 was a far larger institution than envisioned by its founder. Three years later the storeroom between the Steele and Babson Wings was converted to the Fisher Lobby, and further change was even then on the drawing boards.

move of the Development Department to the new center, and the Auxiliary gained an office and a small kitchen for its use. The Longan Room was redecorated but left essentially as Patrick Longan had last seen it. And a few years later the final touch was added when the leaky old tunnel to the hospital was waterproofed and its stained cement walls and ceiling covered and painted in keeping with the decor of the new center.

No longer would it variously be called the Nurses' Residence or the School of Nursing Building. In 1981 it became the Conference Center, and in January 1985 it was redesignated The Robert L. French Center "in honor and recognition of a friend and to express our affectionate appreciation for his leadership." It seems appropriate to assume that Fred and Mabel Barker would have approved this sentiment and the purposes for which their old building remains in daily use.

On a more mundane note, the disposal of rubbish created a problem in 1976 when the then new federal Environmental Protection Agency cited the hospital because of the discharge from an incinerator installed in 1958 and from the boiler stack. This issue had previously arisen in 1971 following complaints to the state Board of Health, which censured the hospital and ordered smoke sensors installed.

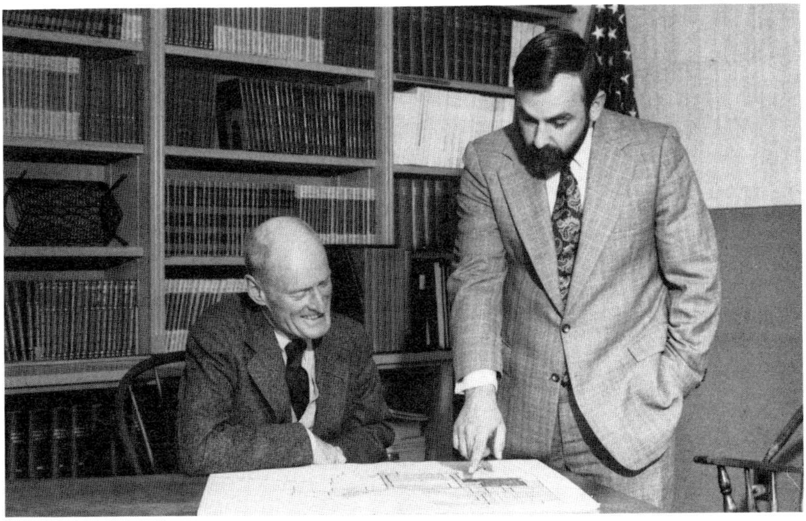

President Robert L. French and Administrator T.R. Scharfenstein confer in the medical library during the planning stages of the "Program for the 'Eighties."

A new incinerator installed in 1977 to permit burning off all rubbish was further refined a year later with the addition of a heat recovery system, a $60,000 installation put in place by the busy maintenance department. Like so many other special projects it was funded by gifts, about half by the Gorton Group companies. It performed as promised and in 1980 was reported as saving 38,000 gallons of fuel oil annually while adding to the essential steam-generating capacity. In 1983 it received official recognition when the hospital was selected to represent Massachusetts at an International Energy Day, and that October the state's Secretary of Energy visited here to personally inspect the system.

The Program for the Eighties

These developments, significant though they were, were overshadowed by the ambitious "Program for the Eighties." The so-called shell area originally planned for radiology when Steele Wing was built had stood empty except as a place to store obsolete or unneeded furnishings since 1972. As the radiologists continued to struggle with inadequate space, pressure to do something with such a valuable vacancy was overwhelming. Other motivating influences, earlier foreseen in the first state-mandated "Five Year Plan" in 1977, included a trend toward changing concepts in health care — emphasis on preventive medicine and more outpatient or ambulatory treatment, for example — and a growing pressure for lower operating costs which would require the highest possible efficiency.

Formal long-range planning, eventually to be served by a Board standing committee and a professional director, was necessary to meet the increasing demands of the government planners themselves. The five-year plans that followed that of 1977 were regularly updated as the Trustees attempted to identify future plant, equipment and staffing requirements, all closely tied to the availability of capital funds and the overall budget process. It was a procedure in which the Medical Staff participated eagerly as, like the Trustees, it recognized the benefits well-executed advance planning could bring.

One of the first positive steps had been taken by the Staff, which in December 1974 proposed "a long range plan for future development of the X-ray Department [as] a prototype for future planning efforts with the Staff and Board of Trustees." The Board responded a few days later by authorizing architectural counsel to study and report as to the feasibility of improving both radiology space and the laboratory. The tenuous financial situation through 1977 made any solution impossible until that problem was corrected.

By mid-1978 further needs were becoming evident as the Board and Staff faced increased regional pressure to reduce beds and consolidate services, demands which seemed best met by identifying new uses for phased-out beds and upgrading older services. The Medical Staff, for example, after considerable discussion was the first to recommend creation of an inpatient psychiatric unit as part of the 1978 five-year plan and another piece in the developing program. A year later in a major presentation by the Staff and Administrator to the Trustees the final pieces of a massive reconfiguration of the hospital fell into place.[1]

The Determination of Need request covering the entire project presented and approved at that meeting contained 464 pages of narrative and supporting data, and had been months in preparation. After several public hearings, as required by the determination process, and protracted deliberations by state authorities, the DON procedure was finally completed in June 1980. With state approval the project could move to the next step — funding.

A public fund-raising campaign, already approved by the state's Commissioner of Public Health, was scheduled to open in July. Several months earlier the Trustees had selected John F. Rich Company of Philadelphia to direct this largest-ever effort, and, anticipating DON approval, a campaign brochure and audiovisual materials were ready.

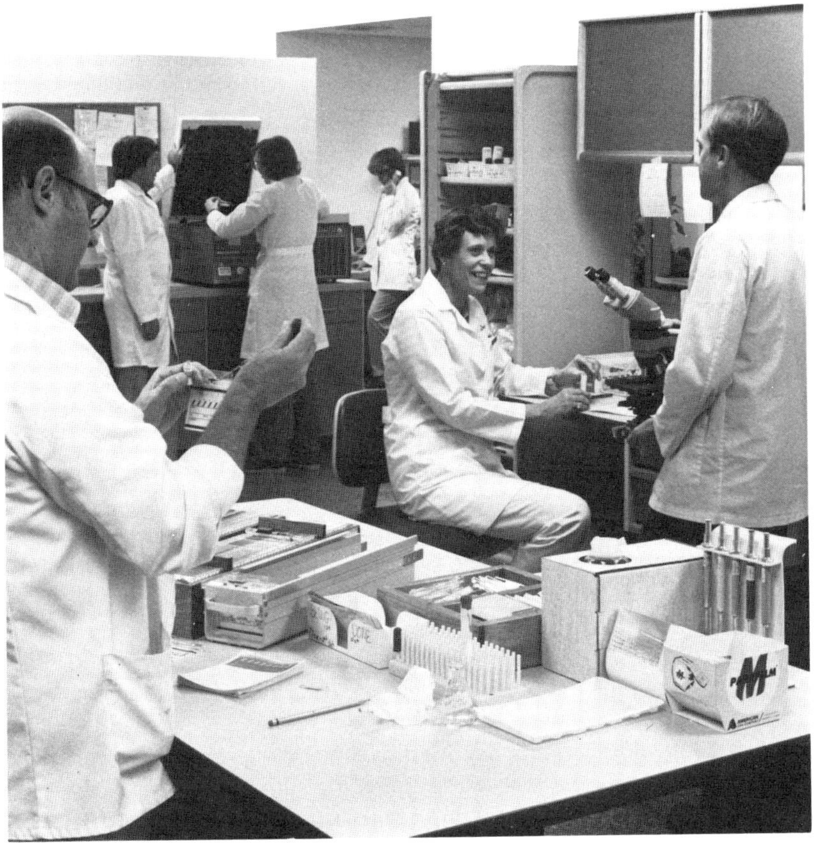

Laboratory space was expanded and laid out much more efficiently as a result of the "Program for the 'Eighties" completed in 1982.

The initial commitments to the $2.5 million program came from those most intimately involved. Despite some members' doubts as to its ability to achieve it, the Auxiliary accepted a challenging pledge of $250,000. The Trustees pledged the same, and, not to be outdone, the Medical/Dental Staffs suggested that they could also commit a quarter-million dollars. With 30 percent of the goal pledged, the campaign could "go public."

Ross N. Clouston, Chief Executive Officer at Gorton's, became General Chairman of an effort which, before it was over, enlisted 392 workers at various levels and covered the Cape and surrounding communities. By the end of July a further $750,000 had been pledged as the leading gift prospects made commitments. Massive publicity, many presentations of the descriptive slide show, hundreds of personal visits and a community-wide mail campaign followed, and by December President French, who had personally raised just over $1 million of the total, could confidently state that the goal had been met.

It had been more than met. A final report listed 1,396 gifts for a total of $2,594,599. The Trustees' gift totaled $361,380 including the gift by Bernard Gordon for use toward the Sophia Gordon Radiology Suite. The Medical and Dental staffs surpassed their goal at $253,450. The Auxiliary, in yet another demonstration of the power of a group of determined women, took

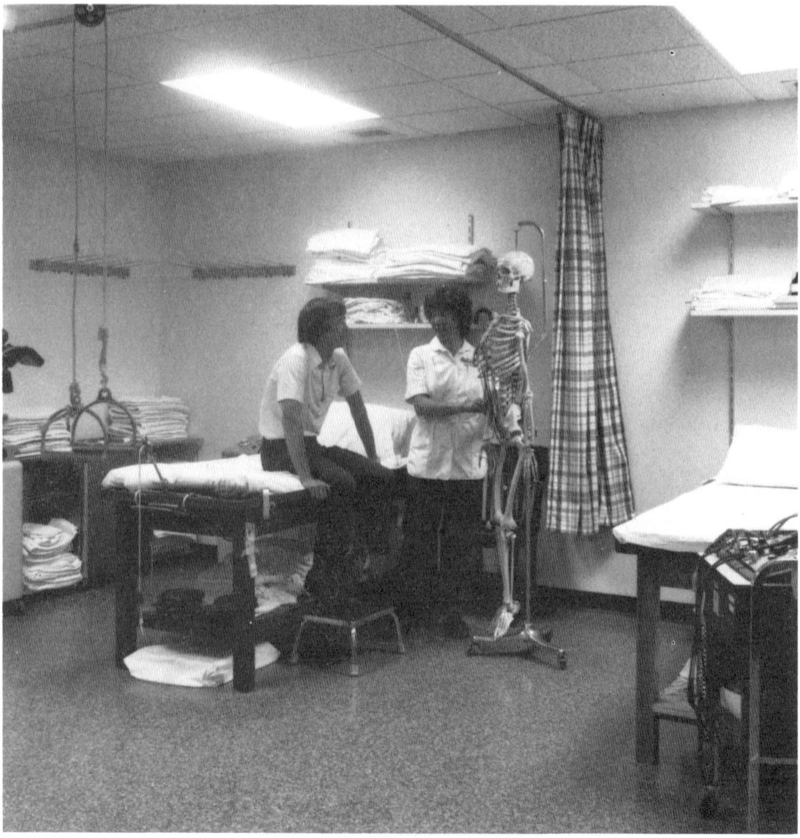

Completion of the program also resulted in relocation of physical therapy to larger and better-equipped space adjacent to the emergency room.

longer with its pledge and completed it in May 1987. The balance, including $1,200 from the aging Alumnae Association and $250,000 from the Gorton Group and its parent, General Mills, came with broad support from Cape Ann's industries and individuals. Fund-raising counsel's final report described it as "a classic campaign in every sense of the word," concluded in a brief six months and unusual in attracting so many large gifts.

The balance required for the project was obtained through a $6.5 million bond issue backed by the Massachusetts Health and Educational Facilities Authority (HEFA). Despite qualms as to the wisdom of assuming massive debt, but reassured by the success of the campaign and the favorable report of the hospital's auditors, the Board voted on July 21, 1981 to enter an agreement with HEFA for an issue to go on sale that October. At 12.5 percent interest and collateralized by the hospital plant and the campaign proceeds, the A-rated tax-free bonds sold quickly, and the funds with which to complete the project were assured.

Construction costs were firm at $3,849,936. All other expenses, including $1,348,000 for equipment and $705,941 to refinance the balance of the Steele Wing mortgage, totaled $6,548,941. The miscellaneous nature of the construction work did not lend itself to the standard general contractor procedure, and counseled by Bernard Gordon, for whom the firm had recently done a major building project, the Trustees appointed Minton Construction Corporation as construction manager. Minton had performed several large hospital and industrial jobs, and under the firm's experienced direction the work proceeded on schedule to its dedication on October 22, 1982.

An Open House that day celebrated the new main entrance and lobby at the rear of the hospital and, above all, the establishment of the ambulatory care center, which henceforth would bear Burton Fisher's name. The relocated Radiology Department, occupying most of the Steele Wing ground floor and almost totally reequipped, fulfilled the retired Dr. Wells' most extravagant dreams. Also shown that day were the enlarged Physical Therapy Unit, spacious new laboratory quarters, and the Psychiatric Unit, which occupied the entire second floor of Webber House.

The Pharmacy was moved to newly built space attached to Babson Wing. Next door within the same subproject was a Doctors' Lounge, which opened into the older Medical Library. Medical Records and the Cardiopulmonary Service had new quarters off the lobby to which had been moved the switchboard, reception desk and admitting service. Although never having a formal chaplaincy, the retrofitted hospital was further enhanced by the addition of a small chapel-meditation room adjacent to the Prentiss I nursing floor.

The Program for the Eighties marked a most significant move to meet changing health care concepts, which emphasize ambulatory care and preventive medicine. It was the denouement of many of the developments already described, and with it years of planning and contemplation of change were concluded. The old hospital was ready to enter a new era as it moved that day into the 1980s and beyond.

NOTES

[1]See Appendix D for excerpts from the record of this meeting, which was held August 28, 1979.

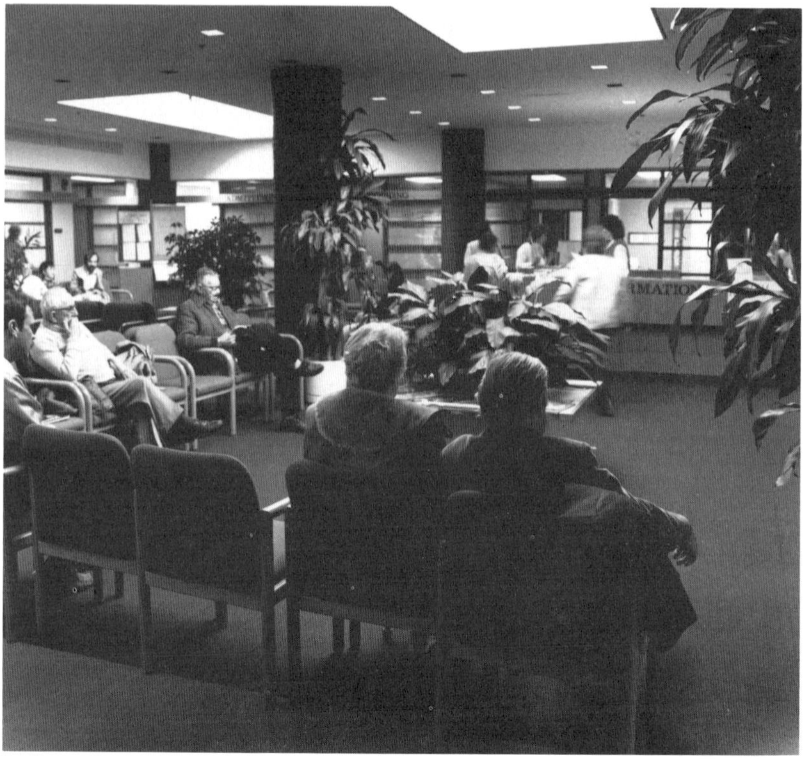

The Fisher Lobby was converted from the storeroom and was a key element in the "Program for the 'Eighties."

17

One Final Milestone

ALTHOUGH MEDICAL STAFF bylaws had been revised and amended frequently through the years, those of the hospital stood the test of time well. The revision of 1949 remained in place except for occasional minor amendment until 1975. Then, with impetus from JCAH recommendations that all hospitals should periodically review and revise their bylaws, President Harold Bell appointed Robert French chairman of an ad hoc Bylaws Revision Committee. Intent on making any changes fit the world that had emerged since 1949, the committee began by retaining legal counsel.

It recognized from the start the need for the Board to face new responsibilities and the existence of increasingly complicated factors – changing operations, new and ever-changing statutory limitations, legal liabilities – that made service as a Trustee more demanding and required high standards for membership. After a year of study the committee came back with recommendations that addressed these and other points with changes that set new criteria for selection of Corporators as well as Trustees. Also spelled out were revised responsibilities for Board standing committees and a control mechanism covering conflict of interest, liability and indemnification. As the committee pointed out when their revision was approved by the Board on October 21, 1975, they came into comformity with then current practice with less change than expected, which as Mr. French said was "a tribute to the old bylaws."

They were to be short-lived, however, as in 1983 machinery was put in motion that would alter the entire corporate structure of the hospital. A radically different concept of hospital governance and management, first seen during the late 1970s, was becoming popular as increased competition from many directions forced all hospitals to consider means of diversification. In order to understand the changes that were taking place, an insight into the nonprofit tradition is helpful.

Most community hospitals like AGH are "not-for-profit" entities and thus enjoy a tax-exempt status. Commercial business, including stockholder-owned or proprietary hospitals, are "for-profit" and taxable. While their not-for-profit status does not prevent them from operating at a reasonable surplus as long as that surplus remains as hospital funds, it does permit such hospitals to receive gifts which, in turn, are tax deductible to their donors. On the other hand, the nonprofit hospital cannot operate a for-profit enterprise as part of itself without jeopardizing its precious nontaxed status. Under the law such for-profit activities can, however, be carried on by a separate corporation, which holds title to the nonprofit hospital and the separate profit-making subsidiaries.

The possibilities for the latter are almost limitless, although for practical purposes they are usually confined to health-related enterprises. They presumably would make a taxable profit which, through the parent foundation, could be used to benefit their nonprofit sibling, but in any case they would add flexibility in responding to community needs. Each — the parent, the hospital and the other subsidiaries — has its own governing body as trustees or directors.

By 1983 the movement toward the concept had reached a point whereby the independent hospital that failed to seek the ability to diversify was in danger of losing its identity through merger or outright absorption by more prosperous and forward-looking institutions. It was in this climate that President French opened the milestone year of 1983 with appointment of an ad hoc Corporate Reorganization Committee. The new committee, of which he was Chairman, retained legal counsel and was ready to make its first report by April. That report described the major purpose of change as identifying "profitable endeavors which would support the charitable purposes of the institution [together with] a modification of the hospital structure . . . in which to pursue [that] mission."

On September 6, 1983 the committee brought to the Board a detailed report that revealed a totally revised corporate structure providing for a nonprofit parent with two subsidiaries, one the not-for-profit hospital, the other a proprietary for-profit holding company, which could itself establish and own any number of diversified subsidiaries. The name Addison Gilbert

Foundation was suggested for the parent with the for-profit subsidiary to be called Seacoast Health Systems, Inc. The eight page report suggested as objectives of the reorganization: creation of a more flexible structure suitable for future diversification; sheltering of endowment funds with increased focus on fund raising; increased marketing effectiveness; continuity of management; and, perhaps most important, the isolation of for-profit activities free of the restraints under which the hospital by itself was more and more being forced to operate.

The membership of the ninety-four-year-old hospital Corporation would transfer from the hospital to the proposed foundation, which, in addition to being parent to the subsidiaries, would manage the endowment funds and assume fund-raising responsibility. Its separate governing board would be responsible for strategic planning, approval of all subsidiaries' budgets, determinations of need, and control of borrowing and, if the need arose, would oversee any sale of assets and become custodian of the receipts therefrom. The hospital's Board would remain in charge of its operation, and boards of directors would govern the affairs of the for-profit subsidiaries. And in at nomenclatorial change the Administrator would henceforth be President, and each body of trustees would be led by a Chairman of the Board.

A formal report was prepared for a milestone meeting on October 25, 1983 at which the Trustees voted unanimously to accept the plan to become effective on November 3. The state issued the charter formally establishing the new entity on October 26, and a special meeting of the hospital Corporation was set for November 2, when the plan would be explained and the new bylaws voted on. The Corporators, agreeing with committee opinion that, more than a legal stratagem, this was indeed a plan capable of responding quickly and flexibly to changing needs, voted to accept the proposal. And with that vote the AGH became one of twenty other Massachusetts hospitals which, along with hundreds across the nation, were preparing for the future.

History was made that day, just as it had been on February 18, 1889. It was the end of an era, but not the end of a Cape Ann institution that had stood the test of time, its tribulations and its glory. It was simply a new beginning.

EPILOGUE

In 1983 the story of Addison Gilbert Hospital moved from history into the future. The events set in motion then are still unfolding and will continue to do so for many years to come and thus become a tale to be told later and by others. Meanwhile, as the saying goes, "Stay tuned."

The unfolding story will undoubtedly be told as it develops just as it has always been – in the newspaper and hospital publications – by the hospital's communications office. We are confident that even as its problems of the past were solved while Addison Gilbert's hospital developed into the fine institution of 1983, so too will be those which it and others like it face today and in the future.

APPENDICES

A

The Brown Farm Purchase

Brown agreed to settle the *fee determinable* question by putting his property in trust and empowering the trustee to sell it. In a letter from Henry Parmenter to George Marsh a few days after Parmenter received the June 27 agreement, however, it appeared that some doubts still remained. After expressing his frustration at the long delay, he raised the question of the trusteeship: "Whom can we agree upon? Brown suggests John Remby. It does not quite commend itself to me. What do you think of it? . . . He has asked whether I or Dustin would act as trustee, I believe, but I think it would look better to have someone not in our board. And I think the Judge will think so."

Two weeks later the hospital's Boston attorney, W. C. Russell, gave his opinion that Brown could give good title "but the authorities on this question are so doubtful that I should by no means advise you to accept [it]." He went on to suggest two possible avenues to pursue, the first being the trusteeship and the other, eventually taken, that Brown sue the corporation for nonperformance of the purchase and sale agreement which would allow the court to decide the question of heirs. On September 7, 1891 the committee gave its final report recommending the property as "a proper location" with a purchase price of $10,000.

A new purchase and sale agreement was then executed, a binder of $100 paid, and on October 6 Brown filed suit as plaintiff versus Addison Gilbert Hospital, defendant, in Essex County Superior Court. The suit was quickly heard; the defendant agreed with the stipulations, and the plaintiff testified that he "never has been married and has never had any children [and that he] is the only son of the testator's son Jonathan Brown" and thus there was no other issue nor were there any other heirs of his father, Jonathan. The Court issued its decree the following day ordering the hospital to perform on its agreement and pay, upon execution of "a proper deed and conveyance," the balance of $9,900 plus plaintiff's court costs.

Further delays continued to hold up closing, however. Although a third purchase and sale agreement was executed in accordance with the Court's order, it was not until four years later, on January 1, 1896, that payment was made and the deed filed and passed. There is no indication of a cause for this hiatus although it is probable that a search for any heirs may have been required.

B

Regulations of the Addison Gilbert Hospital

A Medical Board, of three members, appointed by the Trustees, shall provide for the medical service of the Hospital, according to such rules and regulations as shall be prescribed by them and approved by the Executive Committee.

The Medical Board shall meet at the Hospital the first Monday of each month, at eleven o'clock.

Special meetings may be held at the request of the chairman.

The medical service of the Hospital shall consist of Consulting Physicians, Visiting Staff and Assistant Physicians. These appointments shall be made by the Executive Committee on recommendation of the Medical Board.

At least two members of the Visiting Staff shall serve in the hospital at the same time, and to them, as far as may be practicable, the patients shall be assigned, alternately, as admitted.

Patients shall be visited daily, from 8 to 12 A.M., and at such other times as may be necessary.

A daily record of the history and treatment of each case shall be made by the attending physicians, in books provided by the Hospital, to be kept in the building, in custody of the Medical Board.

No complicated fractures shall be treated, or important operations be performed without consultation with, and the approval of the Medical Board.

The entire staff of the Hospital shall be invited to all important operations.

The Physicians of the Staff and all other physicians who may attend patients in the Hospital, shall attend gratuitously all recipients of the Hospital's charity, and all other patients not otherwise provided for.

Attending Physicians may call in counsel the members of the Staff and with the consent of these may call any other physician, provided it is done without expense to the Hospital.

Any changes in, or additions to these rules approved by the Executive Committee and Medical Board, shall be binding.

The Matron of the Hospital shall be an educated and skillful nurse, capable of taking charge of the Hospital and of instructing pupils in nursing. She shall have had a training in hospital work, at least equivalent to that furnished by Hospital Training Schools. She shall have the whole responsibility for the conduct of the Hospital, according to such rules as she may find necessary to prescribe, and as may be approved by the Executive Committee. She shall act as Superintendent of the Training School, and registrar of the directory for nurses; shall have power, with approval of the Executive Committee, to appoint and to discharge pupil nurses, assistant nurses and domestics. She shall not expend any money or contract any debt without the authority of the Executive Committee. She shall keep a record in detail of all moneys received and disbursed by her, which shall be open at all times to the inspection of any member of the Executive Committee and Trustees, and render monthly to the said Committee a full account of all her receipts and expenditures.

She shall keep an accurate account of bedding, table linen and other furnishings, take charge of all moneys or other property not in use, belonging to patients, and keep a record of the same and deliver it to patients upon their leaving the Hospital, taking receipts therefor. She shall, when a patient dies, furnish the Executive Committee with an inventory of all the effects of the deceased, and the Committee shall direct their disposal. As the Treasurer's agent collect for Hospital and nurses' service and perform any other duties that pertain to the office.

Patients will be admitted to the Hospital by the Matron with the approval of the Medical Board.

Persons having acute venereal or contagious diseases shall not be admitted, nor incurable cases be received except for reasons satisfactory to the Executive Committee.

Emergency cases may be admitted at all times.

In the wards, patients will be charged at the rate of ten dollars per week for board and nursing services. In private rooms the charge will be from fifteen to twenty-five dollars per week.

Abatements of the regular Hospital charge and admission to the free beds of the hospital may be granted by the Executive Committee.

The Board of Trustees shall be the Executive Committee.

These rules and regulations may be amended at the annual meeting of the Trustees, or at a special meeting called for that purpose.

Adopted June 25, 1897.

Attest,

JOHN K. DUSTIN, JR., *Clerk*

C

Physicians of Cape Ann Association of 1925-1926

Hospital Medical Staff 1925-1926

*Harold N. Baker, MD,
Assistant Physician
*Harry C. Burrell, MD,
Etherizer
*Hanford Carvell, MD,
Attending Physician
*Ezra E. Cleaves, MD,
Attending Physician
*Snow P. F. Cook, MD,
Oculist/Aurist
*John J. Egan, Sr., MD,
Attending Surgeon
*Edward B. Hallett, MD,
Attending Physician
*Ira B. Hull, MD,
Etherizer
*Scott W. Mooring, MD,
Attending Surgeon
*Charles M. Quimby, MD,
Etherizer
Philip Rowley, MD,
Attending Surgeon
Elwood E. Shields, MD,
Attending Physician
*Augustus M. Tupper, MD,
Consultant
*Harper E. Whitaker, MD,
Roentgenologist

Former Hospital Medical Staff in Cape Ann practice 1925

Parker Burnham, MD
(resigned 1919)
*Roy Garland, MD
(resigned 1924)
*Philip P. Moore, MD
(resigned 1919)
*Charles H. Morrow, MD
(resigned 1919)
*Percy C. Proctor, MD
(resigned 1919)

Other Physicians in Cape Ann practice 1925

Silas H. Ayer, MD
Mary Dakin, MD
William Hale, MD
*Avis M. Keith, MD
F. Albert Oakes, MD
Mary Parker, MD
*Howard L. Quimby, MD
*George Rust, MD
George Vogel, MD

*Indicates member Physicians of Cape Ann

D

Program for the 'Eighties

This excerpt from the record of the August 28, 1979 meeting of the Board of Trustees well expresses the needs which motivated the Program for the 'Eighties.

The Board then turned to consideration of the capital project and the Determination of Need request. President French introduced members of the Medical Staff who discussed needed improvements in their departments' facilities.

Dr. Steven Geary described problems in the Radiology Department. Built in 1958, the radiology facilities are characterized by poor lighting, unreliable equipment and high maintenance costs. The Joint Commission on Accreditation of Hospitals (JCAH) has cited the department for both inadequate space and equipment. Proposed expansion of the radiology facility will permit improvements in procedures currently performed, as well as addition of new procedures.

Dr. William Cornetta described the work of the Laboratory in performing 270,000 different tests each year. Its space is divided into small, unworkable compartments, resulting in inefficient conditions. Problems in both space and lighting have formed the basis for citations by the College of American Pathologists, the JCAH and the Massachusetts Department of Public Health. Changes proposed in the capital program will result in improved working conditions and greater efficiency.

Dr. Mordecai Berkowitz described the improvements planned for the Physical Therapy Department. The new facility will be four times as large as the old one, permitting longer patient visits and thus longer and more effective care. Access to the facility will be improved by relocating it near the entrance.

In summarizing other aspects of the expansion of ancillary services, Administrator Theodore Scharfenstein explained that centralization of ancillary services reflects the growing emphasis on outpatient rather than inpatient care. The physical proximity of ancillary departments resulting from the capital project will enhance their ability to function as related components of the Hospital.

Dr. Sebastian Aparo described addition of the day surgery unit as being primarily a conceptual rather than physical change. Growing emphasis on outpatient care, particularly by third-party payors, and the need to control costs require that the hospital provide this service.

Dr. Philip Cutter discussed the conversion of twelve medical/surgical beds to use as an inpatient Psychiatry facility. He noted that the lack of inpatient psychiatric care represents a significant gap both in the medical service provided by the Hospital and in the mental health service available on Cape Ann. Its inclusion in the capital project reflects a growing consensus that treatment in the community, when feasible, is superior to institutionalization at another location.

Mr. Scharfenstein concluded by describing the overall changes in bed complement, reducing the total from 144 to 124. The change results mainly from elimination of three- and four-bed rooms and an increase in the number of single rooms. The project will leave the hospital with only private and semi-private rooms, but with flexibility to respond to short-term census increases.

Roger Wilson of the John F. Rich Company presented in detail the conclusions of his firm's feasibility study of a capital gifts campaign. Summarizing a written report which was distributed to the Board, Mr. Wilson noted that the hospital was generally well-regarded in the community and that its particular strengths included the quality of its Medical and Nursing Staffs, its identification with the community, the relationship between Board, Staff and Administration, and its leadership. He observed that 96% of those individuals interviewed by his firm approved of a capital gifts campaign and 77% expressed a favorable opinion of the proposed changes in the Hospital's plant. Based on interviews as well as on independent investigation his firm views a goal of between $2,000,000 and $2,500,000 as reasonable and suggests for present planning purposes an amount of $2,250,000.

Craig Anderson of Ernst & Whinney described his firm's analysis of the hospital's financial structure. It was their conclusion that with a $2,000,000 equity contribution (from a capital gifts campaign), the hospital can afford a $5,800,000 building program and the debt necessary to complete it. The project will add $5.00 per patient day to cost, and will require increased revenue of $11.00 per patient day to offset these costs. Ernst & Whinney considers this to be a favorable basis upon which to proceed and projects that it will improve the hospital's financial picture even with additional debt.

There having been discussion following these presentations by members of the Medical Staff, Administratioin and consultants, on motion made and seconded,

IT WAS UNANIMOUSLY VOTED: To approve the Determination of Need Request.

E

Hospital Trustees 1889-1989

- Abbott, E. Raymond 1948-1982
  - Life Trustee 1974-1982
- Adams, Isaac, MD 1892-1903
- Anderson, Alfred M. Jr. 1943-1955
- Andrews, Richard L. 1968-1969, 1972-1986
  - Life Trustee 1984-1986
- Babson, Daniel T. 1909-1940
  - Vice President 1917-1926
- Babson, Elmer W., DVM 1917-1944
  - Vice President 1931-1944
- Babson, Nathaniel 1900-1927
  - Vice President 1914-1917
- Babson, W. Warren, MD 1975-1987
  - Life Trustee 1977-1987
- Banks, Neill K., Jr. 1969-
  - Vice President 1977-1981
- Barker, Fred A. 1903-1939
  - Vice President 1906-1914
  - President 1914-1923
- Bell, Harold 1960-
  - Vice President 1972-1974
  - President 1974-1977
  - Life Trustee 1977-
- Bermingham, John 1983-1984
- Bernstein, Melvin I. 1948-1954, 1958-1973
- Blackman, David F. 1987-
- Blatchford, Robert E., DDS 1977-1980
- Bolger, Thomas P. 1919-1943
- Bonney, Weston L. 1977-1980
- Bradley, Temple A. 1942-1978
  - Assistant Treasurer 1949-1950
  - Vice President 1950-1951
  - Life Trustee 1964-1978
- Brooks, Laurence F. 1956-1961
- Brown, C. Bruce, MD 1976-1977
- Brown, Jane P. 1973-1979
- Brown, Robert F. 1949-1973
  - Vice President 1966-1973
- Brown, William G., Jr. 1929-1949
- Bruni, Francis A. 1980-1986
- Bundy, Frederick McG. 1942-1981
  - Vice President 1944-1950
  - President 1950-1952
  - Life Trustee 1964-1981
- Bundy, Harvey H., Jr. 1961-
  - Treasurer 1974-1979
  - Life Trustee 1982-
- Burbank, Charles G. 1968-1979
- Cahill, John R., Jr. 1940-1975
  - Assistant Treasurer 1950-1956
  - Vice President 1956-1966
  - Life Trustee 1966-1975
- Cahill, Peter J. 1970-
- Cameron, George E., Jr. 1963-
  - Life Trustee 1983-
- Carroll, Eben C., Jr. 1960-1963
- Carroll, Thomas J. 1930-1947
- Chane, Leo S. 1964-1979
- Clark, C. Richard 1967-1977
  - Life Trustee 1976-1977
- Clouston, Ross N. 1980-1986
- Corliss, John 1889-1897
  - Vice President 1889-1897
- Cornetta, William J., III, MD 1988-
- Costello, John T. 1957 only
- Cunningham, John 1909-1933
- Cunningham, John D., III 1981-
  - Vice Chairman 1985-1986
- Cunningham, Sylvester 1889-1909
  - Vice President 1897-1906
  - President 1906-1909
- Curcuru, Benjamin L. 1948-1978
  - Life Trustee 1969-1978
- Curtis, James W., Jr. 1971-
  - Vice President 1974-1979
  - Life Trustee 1987-
- Davis, Arthur C. 1929-1964
  - Vice President 1935-1942
  - Life Trustee 1949-1964
- Dean, William J. 1956-1974
- Dexter, Harold C. 1960-1978
- Dexter, Stephen F. 1989-
- Dustin, John K., Jr. 1889-1909
  - President 1889-1897
  - Clerk-Secretary 1897-1901
- Faulk, N. Alston 1964-
  - Life Trustee 1976-
- Feldman, Michael L. 1968-1969
- Fiero, Douglas C., MD 1984-
- Fisher, Charles E. 1906-1929
- Fisk, Ann L. 1978-1985
  - Vice President 1981-1983
- Foster, F. Lee 1983 only

French, Robert L. 1970-
    Treasurer 1971-1974
    Vice President 1974-1977
    President 1977-1983
    Chairman 1984 only
    Life Trustee 1988-
Frost, Joseph H. 1980-
Goldman, Sidney 1974-
Gordon, Bernard W. 1980-
    Life Trustee 1987-
Griffin, J. Hollis 1929-1971
    Life Trustee 1949-1971
Greely, Gerald D. 1973-1982
Guittarr, Alexander J., Jr. 1969-1979
Gunn, Kari S. 1988-1989
Hagstrom, Edward A. 1956-1959
Hall, Arthur J. 1943-1955
Hall, Chaney N. 1935-1947
Hammond, John Hays 1909-1917
    President 1909-1913
Hanson, Conrad R. 1923-1948
    Clerk 1923-1939
Hart, Lawrence J. 1946-1971
    Life Trustee 1969-1971
Heberle, Charles T., Jr. 1948-
    Treasurer 1968-1971
    Life Trustee 1975-
Horvitz, Joel R. 1979-
    Treasurer 1980-1983
    Vice Chairman 1987-
Howard, John T. 1980-
    Life Trustee 1984-
Hubbard, William H. 1943-1944
Jodrey, H. Lawrence 1963-1972
Jones, Donald R. 1954-1956
Jones, Henry A. 1983-
Kart, Robert J., DVM 1987-
Keating, Nancy M. 1985-
Kerr, Benedict A. 1948-1969
Lattof, Thomas M. 1979-
Littlefield, Paul D. 1986-1989
Loeffler, Frank R. 1945-1963
Lowrie, Charles W. 1962-
    Vice President 1968-1972
    Life Trustee 1983-
Lundberg, Robert N., MD 1978-
    Life Trustee 1988-
MacInnis, Murdock N. 1954-1956
MacInnis, William J. 1948-1974
    Life Trustee 1974
MacLean, George E. 1957 only
MacLeod, Edward J. 1964-1966
Maddocks, Harold 1934-1963
    President 1942-1947
    Life Trustee 1949-1963
Marsh, David L. 1984-
Marsh, George J. 1889-1896
    Clerk-Treasurer 1889-1896
Maynard, Joseph A. 1981-1985
McEwen, Lawrence C. 1954-1980
    Assistant Treasurer 1956-1976
    Life Trustee 1974-1980
Merrill, George Frye 1922-1925
Monroe, Elizabeth G. 1987-
Moore, William 1948-1967
    Vice President 1956-1967
Moore, William F. 1911-1919
Moores, Carl 1975-1978
Morse, Carol 1986-
Morton, Arnold L. 1954-1970
Murch, Arthur S., Jr. 1943-
    Vice President 1948-1949
    Secretary 1968-1979
    Life Trustee 1974-
Norton, Frederick H. 1966-1986
    Life Trustee 1976-1986
O'Connell, Francis A. 1976-1980
O'Connor, William F. 1984-
Oliver, Frank V. 1943-1954
O'Neill, Gilbert W. 1945-1946
Otis, W. Harold 1929-1973
    Life Trustee 1954-1973
Parmenter, Henry A. 1889-1891
Parsons, Roy L. 1946-1954
Parsons, William Emerson 1926-1931
    Treasurer 1926-1931
Patch, Isaac 1914-1964
    Life Trustee 1949-1964
Pearce, Charles F. 1943-1954
Pearce, Frank C. 1909-1934
    Vice President 1932-1934
Peterson, Lawrence N. 1954-1978
    Life Trustee 1974-1978
Pew, Charles H. 1897-1906
    President 1897-1906
Phillips, Ezra L. 1909-1938
    Treasurer 1925-1926
Phillips, N. Carleton 1923-1952
    President 1926-1942
    Life Trustee 1949-1952
Radcliffe, John A. 1928-1944
    Vice President 1944
Ramsden, Janice J. 1981-1988
    Secretary 1985-1988

Reed, William G. 1949-1961
Richardson, David L., Jr. 1984-
  Secretary 1988-
Robinson, William H., Jr. 1940-1960
Rogers, Allan 1889-1913
Ross, Lawrence, MD 1976-
  Life Trustee 1986-
Rule, Mary 1983-
Shackelford, Fred A. 1906-1956
  Clerk 1909-1923
  President 1923-1926
  Vice President 1926-1931
  Treasurer 1932-1939
  Life Trustee 1949-1956
Shute, Kilby W. 1906-1930
  Clerk of the Corporation 1901-1909
Simonds, Lincoln S. 1909-1956
  Life Trustee 1949-1956
Simpson, Barbara M. 1975-1979
Simpson, Robert 1959-1967
Smith, Benjamin A. 1906-1923
Smith, George A. 1906-1907
Smith, Horace A. 1909-1925
  Treasurer 1904-1925
Smith, Sylvanus 1897-1909
  Treasurer 1897-1904
Somes, John E. 1889-1900
Stanley, John L. 1906-1908
Steele, Carroll K. 1943-1975
  President 1947-1950
  Life Trustee 1964-1975
Steele, Richard C. 1920-1923
Stelluto, Janis D. 1974-1982
Stevens, George 1981-
Stickney, Arthur E. 1985-
Sudbay, Donald E. 1978-
Sullivan, Frank B. 1940-1965
  Vice President 1949-1952
  President 1952-1956
  Life Trustee 1960-1965
Swanson, Ernest B. 1943-1949
Tarr, Frederick H. 1925-1944
Tarr, Frederick H., Jr. 1945-1956
Thompson, Robert F. 1937-1967
  Clerk 1939-1949
  Treasurer 1939-1967
  Secretary 1949-1967
  Life Trustee 1960-1967
Tornberg, Ingvar E. 1976-1978
Waring, Lloyd B. 1974-
  Life Trustee 1980-
Webber, John S. 1974-1979
Webber, William S., Jr. 1948-1984
  Vice President 1952-1956
  President 1956-1974
  Life Trustee 1968-1984
Weiner, Barry Y. 1982-
  Secretary 1982-1985
  Chairman 1985-
Weiner, Gordon M. 1969-1980
Weiner, Susan S. 1988-
Weld, Philip S. 1964-1973
Wilson, Alan 1979-1987
  Secretary 1979-1981
  Vice President 1982-1984
  Vice Chairman 1984-1987

F

Hospital Trustee Presidents, 1889-1989

John K. Dustin 1889-1897
Charles H. Pew 1897-1906
Sylvester Cunningham 1906-1909
John Hays Hammond 1910-1913
Fred A. Barker 1913-1923
Fred A. Shackelford 1923-1926
N. Carleton Phillips 1926-1942
Harold S. Maddocks 1942-1947
Carroll K. Steele 1947-1950
Frederick McG. Bundy 1950-1952
Frank B. Sullivan 1952-1956
William S. Webber, Jr. 1956-1974
Harold Bell 1974-1977
Robert L. French 1977-1985
Barry Y. Weiner (Chm.) 1985-

Appendices

G

Foundation Trustees, 1983-1989

Brooks, Laurence F. 1983-
  Secretary 1983-
Clouston, Ross N. 1983-1984
Cohen, Martin E. 1983-
Davis, Chandler N. 1986
  Chairman, Seacoast Health Systems
Foster, F. Lee 1983-
  Vice Chairman 1985 only
  Chairman 1986-1988
French, Robert L. 1983-
  Chairman 1983-1986
Gordon, Bernard W. 1983-1986
Horvitz, Joel R. 1983-
  Treasurer 1983-
Howard, John T. 1983-1989
Keating, Nancy M. 1986-
Littlefield, Paul D. 1989-
Lundberg, Robert N., MD 1983-
  Vice Chairman 1986-1988
  Chairman 1988-
Maynard, Joseph A. 1983-1985
  Vice Chairman 1983-1985
O'Connor, William F. 1985-
Ramsden, Jancie J. 1988-
Silva, Richard R. 1988-
Weiner, Barry Y. 1985-
  Vice Chairman 1988-
Wychgram, Clifford 1983-1987

H

Hospital Medical and Dental Staffs, 1897-1989

Aaronson, Michael J., MD 1983-
Ackerman, Edward S., MD 1985-
Adams, J. Randolph, MD 1977-1983
Adels, Barry R., MD 1973-1975
Ahern, Charles F., DDS 1969-
Ahlin, Jeffrey H., DDS 1977-1985
Ames, Melvin, MD 1933-1934
Amiralian, Donald T., MD 1986-
Anastasia, Gaspar W., MD 1989-
Andrews, Earle R., DMD 1957-1988
Andrews, Gary L., DDS 1964-1965
Anscombe, Roderick J., MD (C) 1987-
Ansello, Alan L., DMD 1986-
Aparo, Sebastian J., MD 1966-
Apshaga, Bronie J.P., MD 1958 only
Arena, Joseph F., MD 1968-1978
Arnason, Barry G., MD 1972-1976
Arsenian, Michael, MD 1989-
Babson, W. Warren, MD 1932-1987
Bailey, George Guy, MD (C) 1954-1979
Baker, Harold N., MD 1926-1976
Baker, J. Wain, DMD 1957-
Balasekeran, Saroja, MD 1980-1981
Bargoot, F. John, Jr., MD (C) 1976-1983
Barkin, Neil J., MD 1977-1979
Barnard, Bryant, MD 1972-
Barrett, Steven A., MD 1977-1979
Bauer, Anne C., MD 1987-1989
Becker, Daniel I., MD 1972 only
Belliveau, Robert E., MD 1985-
Benoit, Richard P., MD 1971-
Berkowitz, Mordecai E., MD 1972-
Biron, Pierre, MD 1972-1973
Bland, Edward F., MD (C) 1959-1978
Blatchford, Robert E., DDS 1964-1981
Bloombergh, John H., MD 1947-
Boswell, Reid T., MD 1988-
Bramble, A. Dwight, MD 1983-1986
Brand, Jeffrey B., MD 1987-
Bray, Walter A., MD 1935-1936
Breed, Frederic B., MD 1946-1950
  1956-
Brenner, Mark J., MD (C) 1986-1989
Brett, A. Leo, MD (C) 1937-1967
Brewer, Robert D., MD 1949-1952
Brewster, Thomas G., MD 1976-1983
Broder, Benno M., DMD 1957-1969
Brown, C. Bruce, MD 1948-1977
Brown, Richard E., DMD 1960-
Brownstein, Carlton S., MD (C) 1975-1989
Bryan-Brown, Peter, MD 1969-1971
Bubley, Glenn J., MD 1982-1983
Burnett, Francis L., MD 1928-1945
Burnham, Allen S., DMD 1919-1930
Burnham, Parker, MD 1908-1919
Burrell, Harry C., MD 1926-1967
Byrne, John J., MD (C) 1960-1980
Caldwell, Kenneth C., MD 1977-1978

Callahan, William J., DMD 1957-1973
Carey, Robert W., MD (C) 1972-
Carvell, Hanford, MD 1915-1942
Caudill, Estill L., MD 1973-
Chamberlin, Donald T., MD (C) 1948-1951
Cherry, H. Elisabeth, MD 1972-1979
Choate, Cynthia P., MD 1983-
Clapp, John C., MD (C) 1977-1979
Clark, Chester E., MD (C) 1976-
Cleary, Francis X., MD (C) 1985-
Cleaves, Ezra E., MD 1924-1950
Cohen, Bernard S., DMD 1957-
Cohen, David J., MD 1937-
Collins, James F., MD 1940-1945
Collins, Paul J., MD 1966-1967
Conant, Thomas, MD 1897-1919
Cook, Snow P. F., MD 1897-1934
Cooper, Herbert L., MD 1965-1978
Cornetta, William J., III, MD 1974-
Cornwell, David R., DDS 1979-1985
Courant, Reginald, DMD 1957-1981
Coy, Willard A., DMD 1957-1971
Crabtree, E. Granville, MD (C) 1931-1948
Culhane, Richard H., MD 1970-1972
Cunningham, Ralph E., DMD 1957-1959
Curtis, Ever, MD 1948-1979
Cutter, Philip D., MD 1970-
David, Lloyd G., MD 1961-1983
Davies, John A. V., MD (C) 1948-1973
Denis, Leonard J., MD 1986-1987
Dexter, Milton A., MD 1935-1937
Dienes, Robert S., MD 1987-
Dillon, Raymond A., MD 1949-
Dorrie, Reza, MD 1970-
Dorsey, William R., MD 1980-
Doyle, George M., MD 1935-
Driesman, Mitchell H., MD 1979-1981
Duff, John F., MD 1962-1978
Edwards, Michael G., MD 1987-
Egan, John J., MD 1897-1944
Egan, John J., Jr., MD 1932-1980
Ernlund, Carl H., MD (C) 1931-1949
Eveleth, Edward S., MD 1897-1916
Feener, Lester C., MD 1927-1929
Feingold, Murray, MD (C) 1964-
Feldman, Merrill I., MD 1968-1975
Fetting, John H., MD 1978-1980
Feiro, Douglas C., MD 1972-
Finegan, Daniel J., MD 1912-1919
Fingert, Howard J., MD 1987-
Finkelstein, Lawrence J., MD (C) 1976-1986
Fisher, B. Philip, MD 1979-
Fitzgerald, James, MD 1972-1975
Fitzpatrick, Amy B., MD 1984-1985
Flanagan, Walter A., MD 1971-1978
Floru, Marietta, MD 1989-
Fortunato, Robert 1984-
Frigoletto, Frederic D., Jr., MD (C) 1976-1987
Fritz, Robert T., MD 1977-
Gale, John S., MD 1953-
Garland, Albert S., MD 1897-1921
Garland, Joseph, MD (C) 1897-1902
Garland, Joseph, II, MD (C) 1931-1947
Garland, J. Everett, MD 1897-1907
Garland, Roy, MD 1908-1924
Geary, Steven R., MD 1975-
Gemmellaro, Salvatore P., MD 1979-1983
Gewin, Edward Evans, MD 1951-1953
Giorgio, Louis A., MD 1989-
Gleason, David C., MD 1969-1983
Glovsky, C. Joel, DMD 1961-
Goldberg, Bruce A., MD 1983-
Goldberg, Edward L., MD 1971-1973
Goodale, Robert L., MD (C) 1949-1983
Gorsline, John W., MD 1985-
Gotlieb, Norman E., MD 1987 only
Greene, Earl F., MD 1930-1972
Gross, Peter D., MD 1975-1976
Guanci, James J., MD 1986-
Guillemont, John G., MD 1972-1974
1985-
Gulati, S. Patrick, MD 1989-
Guldemond, Theodore A., DO 1984-
Gunderson, Paul L., MD 1972-1975
Gunn, Alexander N., II, MD 1972-1989
Haines, Samuel, MD (C) 1960-1978
Hallett, Edward B., MD 1897-1939
Hallett, Ronald P., MD 1930-1984
Halprin, Arthur H., MD 1979-1980
Hannon, William E., MD 1980-1983
Hartfelder, Ronald C., MD 1988-
Harvey, Norman A., MD 1949-1950
Hayden, Edwin Parker, MD (C) 1938-1975
Hazen, Lois Fesler, MD 1951-1958
1964-1969
Hellman, Paul V., MD 1978-1981
Hickey, John J., DDS 1972-
Himel, Harvey, MD 1984-1985
Hodgson, John S., MD (C) 1937-1942
Holteen, W. Paul, MD 1961-1972
Hooper, N. Abbott, DMD 1957-
Horowitz, Leonard G., DMD 1979-
Hubbard, Edward D., MD 1912-1923
Huffnagle, Frederic T., MD 1969-1973
Hull, Ira B., MD 1926-1946
Irving, William R., MD 1930-1968
Jackson, Richard R., MD 1987-
Jacobs, Edward E., Jr., MD 1973-1974
Jedrey, Robert L., MD 1963-

Johnson, Lewis F., MD 1954-1958
Jones, Chester M., MD (C) 1931-1939
Jones, Daniel F., MD (C) 1919-1937
Joplin, Robert J., MD (C) 1950-1954
Kace, Alan J., DMD 1971-
Kaplan, Henry, DMD 1979-
Kaplan, Melvin S., MD 1973-1974
Kaufman, S. Donald, MD (C) 1981-1983
1986-
Kaufmann, Jill R., MD 1989-
Kaulbach, Maximilian G., MD (C)
1976-1979
1985-
Keane, Geoffrey P., MD 1949-1980
Kelleher, Michael H., MD 1979-1986
Kenyon, Paul B., Jr., DMD 1961-
Kincaid, Catherine G., MD 1979-1981
Kline, Robert M., MD 1966-1974
1981-1982
1986-
Knowles, James H., MD 1897-1919
Knowles, Robert K. B., MD 1906-1914
Koch-Weser, Peter T., MD 1976-1983
Koh, David, MD (C) 1984-
Kolb, David A., MD 1985-
Kopelson, Gene, MD (C) 1982-1983
Kossayda, Norman P., MD 1980-1985
Kramer, Lewis L., MD 1979-
Krukonis, Edward E., MD 1972-1975
1985-
Kubik, Charles S., MD (C) 1947-1977
Kwon, Chal K., MD 1989-
Lacey, Hamer, MD 1956-
Lakritz, Kenneth B., MD (C) 1986-
Lazarus, Hans, DMD 1957-1964
Lebwohl, David J., MD (C) 1977-
Ledbetter, John S., MD 1985-
Leiter, Andrew B., MD 1981-1983
Leland, George A., Jr., MD (C) 1931-1942
Lemmer, Lodewyk A. S., MD 1987 only
Lempert, Mark B., MD 1987-
Levin, Morton A., DDS 1971-
Levine, Julius, MD 1973-1975
Lodge, Edmund A., MD 1944-1972
Logan, Frank P. T., MD 1901-1919
Lord, Frederick P., MD (C) 1918-1941
Lovejoy, Frederick H., Jr., MD (C) 1983 only
LoVerme, Stephen R., Jr., MD (C) 1979-
Lundberg, Robert N., MD 1951-
Lydiard, R. Bruce, MD 1979-1981
MacDonald, Alexander S., MD 1981-1983
MacDonald, John B., MD 1959-
Maletz, Leo, MD (C) 1954-1975
Mann, Neil N., MD 1969-
Mark, Konrad A., MD 1986-
Matthews, Terence J., MD 1972-1973
McCarthy, Humphrey L., MD 1928-1930
McGee, Michael, MD 1989-
McKee, Kathleen E., MD 1962-1963
McManus, Richard A., MD 1960-
McNamee, H. Brian, MD 1974-1975
McPeak, Clarence N., MD 1936-1940
Meachen, J. W., MD (C) 1930-1936
Mehta, Pradip M., MD 1989-
Melamed, Jeffrey S., MD 1984-
Menges, Ernest, MD 1938-1939
Mercurio, John P., DMD 1960-
Mesaros, Marie, MD 1977-1980
Meyer, Gregory C., MD 1976-1979
Meyers, Robert D., MD 1971-1974
Miceli, Frances A., DDS 1971-
Miceli, John, DMD 1977-
Miceli, Robert C., MD 1981-1983
Michaelson, Ira B., MD 1981-1983
Michelson, Jost J., MD (C) 1947-1989
Mihm, Martin C., MD (C) 1975-
Miller, Brian F., DO 1987-
Miller, Wallace C., MD 1940-1942
Mooney, Philip, MD 1897-1914
Moore, Philip P., MD 1901-1919
Mooring, Scott W., MD 1905-1962
Morrow, Charles H., MD 1897-1919
Morse, Abbie S., MD 1897-1914
Morse, Frank P., MD (C) 1953-1980
Morse, Frank P., III, MD 1973-1981
Morse, George, MD 1897-1904
Moser, Hugo W., MD (C) 1961-1974
Moulton, Robert T., MD (C) 1953-1963
Mulvey, William A., MD 1947-1950
Munro, Donald, MD (C) 1942-1973
Murray, George G. B., MD 1976-1981
Nelson, Kevin R., MD 1983 only
New, Peter S., MD 1967-
Newell, John L., MD (C) 1946-1975
Nicholas, William R., MD 1974-1981
Nickerson, Donald A., MD 1945-1973
Niehoff, Joan N., MD 1986-1987
Oaks, James Howard, DMD 1960-1977
O'Connell, Timothy A., MD 1987 only
Odeneal, Thomas H., MD 1936-1944
Oder, Frederic E., MD (C) 1972-
O'Donnell, Anne R., MD 1978-
O'Donnell, Walter E., MD 1960-
O'Keeffe, Augustine P., MD 1976-
Osborn, Lawrence W., MD 1972-1982
Ott, Brian R., MD 1985-
Palmer, Robert S., MD (C) 1959-1976
Paly, Sidney N., MD 1965-1982
Paradise, Carolyn M., MD 1981-1986

Parker, Sydney S., MD 1951-1981
Pearce, Thomas S., MD 1986-
Peinert, Richard A., MD 1985-
Pett, Morris H., MD 1948-1976
Philbrick, Roscoe H., MD 1930-1939
Pinegar, Richard L., MD 1987-
Piro, Anthony J., MD (C) 1981-
Pohas, George J., MD 1938-
Poland, Warren M., MD 1939-1983
Pomeroy, Irving H., Jr., DMD 1931-1953
Poor, Hooshang D., MD 1986-1987
Powers, Walter J., DMD 1957-1976
Powers, Walter J., Jr., DMD 1960-1978
Prather, George C., MD (C) 1948-1965
Prescott, Charles S., MD 1957 only
Preston, Robert C., DDS 1977-
Prien, Edwin L., MD (C) 1942-1980
Pritchard, Rowland W., MD 1972-1974
Procter, Percy C., MD 1897-1919
Proppe, Karl H., MD 1977-1980
Prusty, Somnath, MD 1984-
Quimby, Charles M., MD 1926-1938
Quimby, Sumner F., MD 1897-1914
Rabe, Edward F., Jr., MD (C) 1986-
Rane, Philip S., MD 1969-
Reeves, John R., MD 1984-1987
Regier, Darrell A., MD 1972-1975
Reveno, Peter M., MD 1971-1983
Richardson, Brenda E., MD 1979-
Ritter, Sherwin H., MD 1967-1985
Roberts, John C., MD 1959-1962
Rosansky, Allan B., MD 1972-1985
Rosenberg, Bruce M., MD 1969-
Ross, Lawrence, MD 1945-
Rotner, Howard E., MD (C) 1971-
Rowley, Philip W., MD 1919-1926
Rowley, William, MD 1897-1922
Rust, George S., MD 1930-1971
St. Onge, Richard A., MD 1972-1973
Saks, Joel W., MD 1970-1973
Sandfield, Russell, DDS 1973-
Santos, John C., MD (C) 1975-
Satwicz, Paul R., MD 1987-
Sauer, David W., MD 1973-
Savage, Louis D., MD 1957-1983
Savett, Laurence A., MD 1967-1969
Sayles, Bruce M., MD 1981-1982
Schwartz, Alvan R., MD 1976-
Schwartz, Stanley, M., DMD 1983-
Scudder, Charles L., MD (C) 1909-1948
Shah, Arpena M., MD 1975-1976
Shahani, Maya, MD 1983-1987
Shale, John H., MD 1976-1979
Shelkrot, Joel W., MD (C) 1986-
Shields, Elwood E., MD 1915-1926
Shinn, Philip A., MD 1919-1921
Slager, Michael, MD 1986-1987
Slater, Kenneth C., MD 1979-1987
Smith, Thomas P., MD 1973-
Snell, Kenneth B., MD 1963-
Spatz, Edward L., MD 1968-1982
Spector, Michael A., MD 1987-
Splaine, Edward F., MD 1985-
Squires, Thomas S., DMD 1965-
Stachiewicz, Danuta, MD 1975-
Steeve, Philip E., MD 1976-
Stelluto, Michael R., MD 1965-1986
Stetson, Richard P., MD (C) 1947-1961
Stuppy, William P., MD 1979-1980
1985 only
Sudarshan, Alexander P., MD 1987-1989
Sudarshan, Yvonne A., MD 1987-1989
Summergrad, Paul, MD 1982-1985
Swartz, Jacob H., MD (C) 1937-1973
Swiggett, Robert L., MD 1985-1989
Taylor, George H., DMD 1919-1989
Teeling, Brendan J., MD 1973-1982
Torrey, Arthur S., MD 1912-1924
Treibeck, Theodore, MD 1986-
Tupper, Augustus M., MD (C) 1924-1930
Underkofler, Richard S., MD 1986-
Upchurch, Ralph H., MD 1981-1983
van Sonnenberg, Eric, MD 1979-1981
Vance, L. Alexander, MD 1949-1963
Wachman, Amnon, MD 1969-1973
Weber, Eric T., MD (C) 1979-
Wedmore, Sydney M., MD 1974-
Weidemann, Michael T., MD 1979-1980
Welch, Charles A., MD 1973-1976
Wells, Edward P., MD 1957-
Wertz, Michael P., MD 1987-1989
Wheeler, Roy R., MD (C) 1940-1949
Wheeler, Roy R., Jr., MD 1961-1965
Whitaker, Harper E., MD 1915-1933
White, Robert E., MD 1975-1977
Wile, Kenneth J., MD 1971-
Williams, Austin T., DMD 1961-1977
Williams, Marny L., DDS 1974-
Williamson, Paul K., MD (C) 1984-
Wilson, Stanley A., MD 1942-1955
Wolfe, John C., MD 1974-
Wolfe, Stephen A., MD 1972-1973
Wonson, Carroll W., DMD 1957-1981
Wysocki, John P., MD 1975-1987

(C) indicates a member of the Consulting Staff.

I

Hospital Medical Staff Chiefs, 1897-1989

J. Everett Garland, MD, Chairman of Medical Board	1897-1907
Thomas Conant, MD, Chairman of Medical Board	1907-1915
Snow F. P. Cook, MD, Chairman of Medical Board	1915-1922
Edward B. Hallett, MD, Chairman of Medical Board	1922-1929
John J. Egan, Sr., MD, President of Medical Staff	1929-1934
Ira B. Hull, MD, President of Medical Staff	1934-1942
Thomas H. Odeneal, MD, President of Medical Staff	1942-1944
Harold N. Baker, MD, President of Medical Staff	1944-1945
John J. Egan, Jr., MD, President of Medical Staff	1945-1946
Harold N. Baker, MD, Chief of Medical Staff	1946-1950
John J. Egan, Jr., MD, Chief of Medical Staff	1950-1955
Lawrence Ross, MD, Chief of Medical Staff	1955-1961
Robert N. Lundberg, MD, Chief of Medical Staff	1961-1966
C. Bruce Brown, MD, Chief of Medical Staff	1966-1969
W. Warren Babson, MD, Chief of Medical Staff	1969-1971
Hamer Lacey, MD, Chief of Medical Staff	1971-1975
Edward P. Wells, MD, Chief of Medical Staff	1975-1977
Walter E. O'Donnell, MD, Chief of Medical Staff	1977-1979
John S. Gale, MD, Chief of Medical Staff	1979-1981
Sebastian J. Aparo, MD, Chief of Medical Staff	1981-1983
Bruce M. Rosenberg, MD, Chief of Medical Staff	1983-1985
Alexander N. Gunn, II, MD, Chief of Medical Staff	1985-1987
Douglas C. Fiero, MD, Chief of Medical Staff	1987-

J

Hospital Auxiliary Presidents, 1898-1988

Nella J. French	1898-1899
Maria H. Bray	1900-1915
Carrie A. Newell	1916-1920
Hannah V. P. Merchant	1921-1922
Una E. Parsons	1922-1927
Suzanne Carter	1928-1929
Una E. Parsons	1929-1930
Eleanor B. Doremus	1930-1932
Theresa Maddocks	1933-1936
Elizabeth L. Alling	1937-1942
M. Esther Blatchford	1943-1946
Mary A. Hall	1947-1950
Alice H. Bradley	1951-1952
Pauline Chekares	1952-1953
Margaret W. Arnold	1954-1955
Beatrice H. Albert	1956-1957
Dorothy Marshall	1958-1960
Marjorie O. Ross	1960-1962
Kathleen M. Steele	1962-1964
Clara M. Keefe	1964-1966
Eleanor Harris	1966-1967
Marion A. Boudreau	1967-1969
Gwendolyn L. David	1969-1971
Janis D. Stelluto	1971-1973
Renee A. Sarofeen	1973-1975
Betty Anne Good	1975-1977
Norma P. Tarr	1977-1980
Carolyn M. Swett	1980-1982
Kari S. Gunn	1982-1984
Carol Morse	1984-1986
Susan S. Weiner	1986-1988

K

Glossary of Acronyms and Terms

ACR — American College of Radiologists

ACS — American College of Surgeons

AGH — Addison Gilbert Hospital

AHA — American Hospital Association

AHP — Allied Health Personnel

AMA — American Medical Association

AND — administratively necessary days (Medicare patients held at the hospital beyond allowable stay due to inability to place in nursing home)

Auxiliary — The Women's Auxiliary to the Addison Gilbert Hospital

Blues — Blue Cross-Blue Shield

CAMC — Cape Ann Medical Center

CCU — Coronary Care Unit

CME — Continuing Medical Education

CPR — Cardiopulmonary Resuscitation

DON — determination of need (a state function required to determine validity of a hospital capital program)

DPM — a degreed podiatrist

EMT — Emergency Medical Technician

ENT — Ear, nose and throat specialty

ER — Emergency Room

GCAHS — Greater Cape Ann Human Services, Inc.

GDNA — Gloucester District Nursing Association (now called VNA or Visiting Nurse Association)

GMA — Gloucester Medical Association

HEW — United States Department of Health, Education and Welfare

HMO — Health Maintenance Organization

HSA — Health Systems Agency

I, II, III — used to designate floors beyond ground level within a hospital wing

JCAH — Joint Commission on Accreditation of Hospitals

LPN — Licensed Practical Nurse

med-surg — medical-surgical (usually refers to a floor unit or beds for the care of acute, but nonintensive, care cases)

MHA — Massachusetts Hospital Association

MLPNA — Massachusetts Licensed Practical Nurse Association

MMS — Massachusetts Medical Society

MNA — Massachusetts Nurses Association

MSPCC — Massachusetts Society for Prevention of Cruelty to Children

NLRB — National Labor Relations Board

NSHPC — North Shore Health Planning Council

OBS — obstetrics or obstetrical

OPD — Outpatient Department

OR — Operating room

PGMI — Postgraduate Medical Institute

PSRO — Professional Standards Review Organization

RN — Registered Nurse

RSC — Rate Setting Commission (a state body for oversight of hospital charges)

SEIU — Service Employees International Union

T & A — tonsils and adenoids

TBC — tuberculosis

Times — *The Gloucester Daily Times*

UR — utilization review (a Medicare requirement to monitor length of patient stays in the hospital)

WPA — Works Progress Administration (a Depression era public works program)

Appendices

Illustrations and Credits

Appendices

Index

A page number followed by a numeral in parentheses indicates more than one reference to that subject.

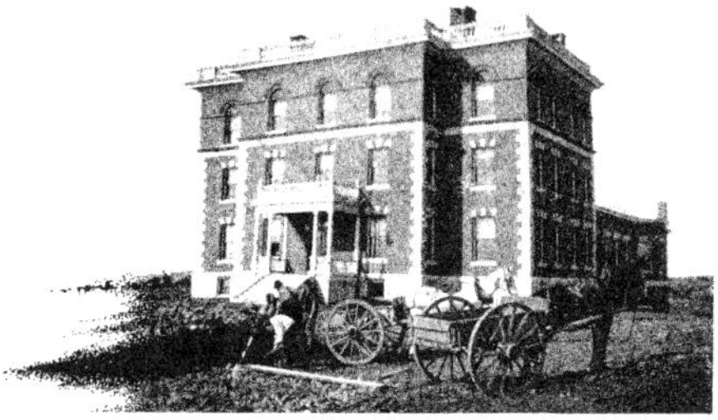

Designed by A. L. Morris,
the text of this volume was composed in Paladium
and printed by Knowlton & McLeary
in Farmington, Maine on Mohawk Text.
Endleaves and jacket were printed
on Curtis Tweedweave Text
and the binding, in Holliston Mills Roxite,
was executed by New Hampshire Bindery
in Concord, New Hampshire.

o admit as patients

uch inhabitants of th

emergency such others

as may need medical

reatment and to provi

and treatment to the i

expend for such purpo

they shall see fit, the

of the principal of the

receive from any othe

may be contributed fo